Dr.F's Fightology

Takuya Futaesaku

&

Fightology World Team

ISBN: 9781983042355

DEDICATION

This book is dedicated to
PRINCE & JOHN BLACKWELL

"For all of us, life is death without adventure, and adventure only
comes to those who are willing to be daring and take chances."
Prince 1958-4ever

ACKNOWLEDGMENTS

I would love to thank my family. Hiroko, Sheila, Nate, Mam, Dad,
and Toru. All of my friends in fighting world, thank you so much for
standing on my corner, not only in good times but in bad times. I
would love to show my love to my special friends in music world.
You all are my heroes and great inspiration. Arigato Gozaimasu.
Dr. F

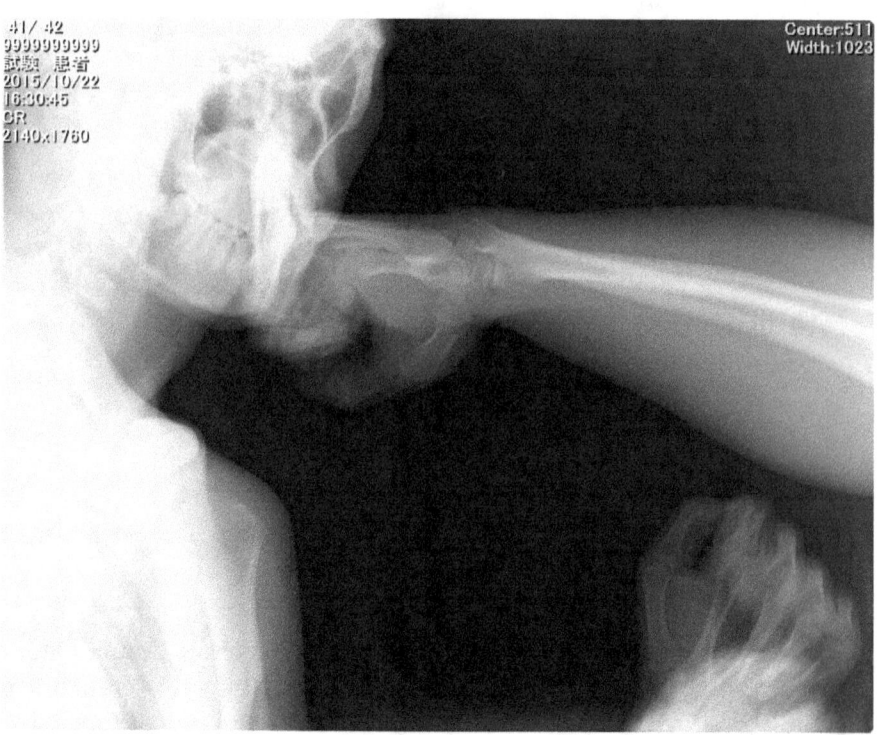

FIGHTOLOGY WORLD TEAM

HIROSHI KATSUI/MAURICIO CARRANZA/
FABIO ROSCH/MOISÉS FALLAS WAHRMANN/
JUAN MA Z PIEDRA/DAVID ORSINI/
DAN NAKAMURA/HON KUEN MA/
MASASHI   SAITO/HIDEO KATO/
JUAN CARLOS AUGE ROS/JASON LAM/
DANIEL PEREZ/JASON DROGUETT/
ANGUS WONG/CHI KIN FUNG/GAVIN SZETO

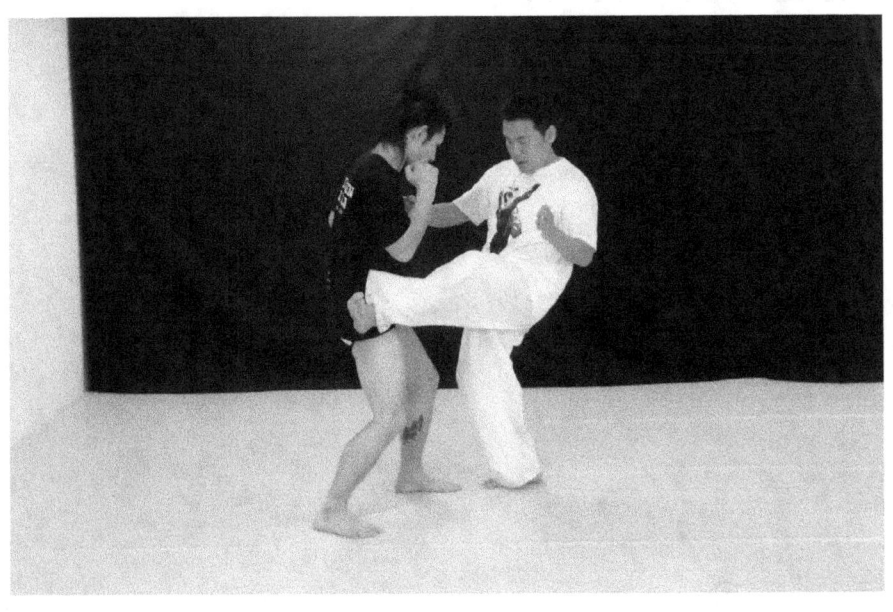

CONTENTS

1:Visual Function

2:Breathing in Fight

3: Proprioception

4: Joint Angle

5: Stretch Reflex

6: Gravity

7: Motor Unit and Impulse

8: Scapula/Upper limb

9: Base Of Support & Movement

【Introduction】

When do people want to be strong? I think there are various answers, but I think that it is time to think "You want to get over present yourself". You know some things that cannot be solved with your own solution, so it is likely that a more certain solution will be realized by getting over yourself. I feel that recognition of the present situation and expectation for myself being strong became the identity of the mind seeking "strength". Originally humans created Martial arts. If human had no fundamental desire of "wanting to be strong" , there should have been no martial arts. Martial arts are not for strong people originally. They are for those who want to be strong even a little, or want to live strongly. The title of this book is Fightology, that means medical science of fighting sports. Martial arts is defeating people and medical science is to help people. At first glance it seems to be one concept that looks opposite, but martial arts is the way for yourself to live strongly, medical science is also a way for mankind to live strongly. Martial arts and medical science are not conflicting concepts, they are indivisible to those seeking true strength. Because martial arts are works to know human beings experientially among interpersonal and medical science is also a study to explore deeply for human beings.

In this book, when pursuing strength, I wrote objective facts and scientific principles that might become clues. It is human beings to do martial arts against human beings. You learn the human body and mind, which should surely link with strength. Please enjoy Fightology research, and create your own style! Dr.F

1:Visual Function

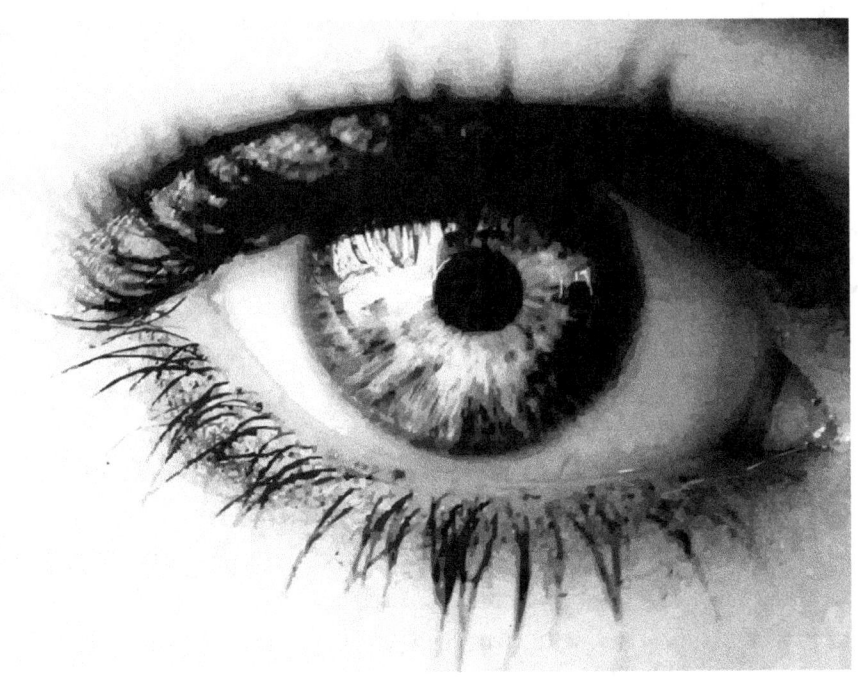

【1-1 Which part of your body do you move first?】

Movement in fighting sports such as striking or grappling, involves moving multiple parts of the body at the same time. Therefore a question is raised, "Which part of your body do you move first?". In this section, I will focus on this particular topic.

An example I shall like to illustrate is most of us is we find delivering combat actions difficult if the information from vision is absent. In fact, we rely on the most part on our vision to receive information from the opponent, to be able to better adjust a position in order to respond to the opponent's actions. As it has been mentioned above most of the information is gained from vision, and we respond to our opponent's actions based on the judgment our brain does of what it receives from our vision. Therefore, if our visual input is absent, our brain fails to process the opponent's information as well as our own movements.

However, I'd like to share a unique experience of mine with you. I had sparred with a blind judoka (Judo practitioner), the sparring began in a condition where we were both holding each other. Surprisingly I was taken down by him repeatedly; he was able to tackle my game once he got in contact with me. Therefore I expect that if the sparring were engaged in a condition where both of us have a normal visual acuity, the level of combat would be even higher.

【1-2 Fighter's eye】

Top fighters use their eyes very well. They not only see a small point to hit, but a large area from several angles, and continue with a fast movement. For example, fighters who are good at counter-attacking, receive varied information from the opponent, while adopting different positions and lines of attack.

Fighters who are good with high kicks control their eyes to feint in the fight. They are able to hit a high kick suddenly after attracting the attention of his opponent downward. To the contrary, I have the experience of focusing on the opponent's facial expression during matches lost. In fighting sports, it is very important to control where we look before a powerful attack. When we change our line of sight, the fighter will be able to control the match. In daily life, human beings are sensitive of being observed, and it can be perceived as confrontational when it happens, like "We had a confrontation with our looks" or "I feel observed". To improve the ability of vision relates directly to the strength, so we should improve our vision as fighters!

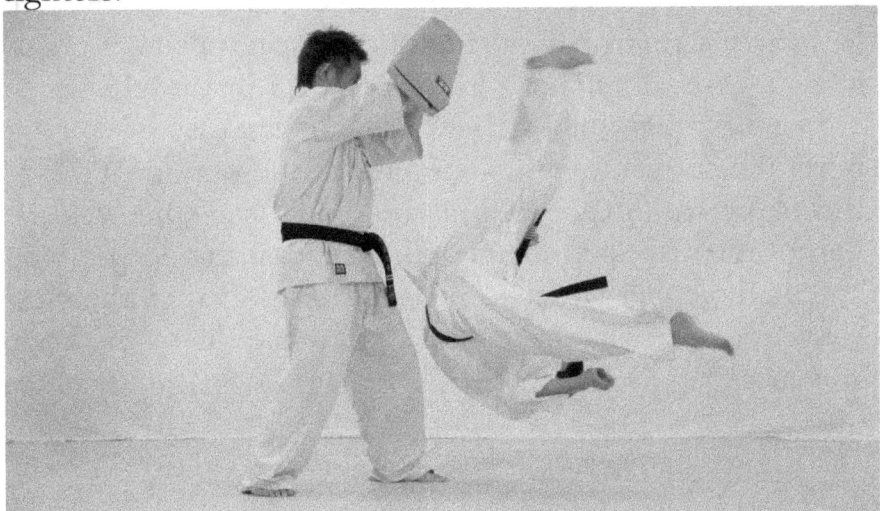

(Karate champ,Daishuke Komiyama's Domawashi Geri)

【1-3 Visual function and punch】

Well, now let's do an experiment. Choose a partner and ask him to hold up a mitt, to start

(A) observe a fixed point in the mitt and then hit it, then
(B) find the same point on the mitt and hit through it (trying to pass through the mitt).

Repeat performing the same hit movements, making changes only on the view point on the mitt. You will notice that the power of the blow will be different in "A" and "B".

If the fighter targets the surface of the mitt, the blow will come to that point, so let's set a goal for ourselves to look deeper into the mitt and throw the hit quickly, this way the whole body will move up to the set position.

The human body will move wherever the eyes' view determines. In the same way the soccer player looks to kick the ball to a point behind the opposing team's goal posts, or like a baseball pitcher throws a fastball that reaches even further back than the catcher's mitt. In the case of combat sports the surface of the abdomen or the opponent's face tend to be the objective, but we should set ourselves the goal for our attacks to be targeting centimeters deeper than that, then we will notice a big difference. Change the view point and it will make the difference in your body movement.

(A-1)

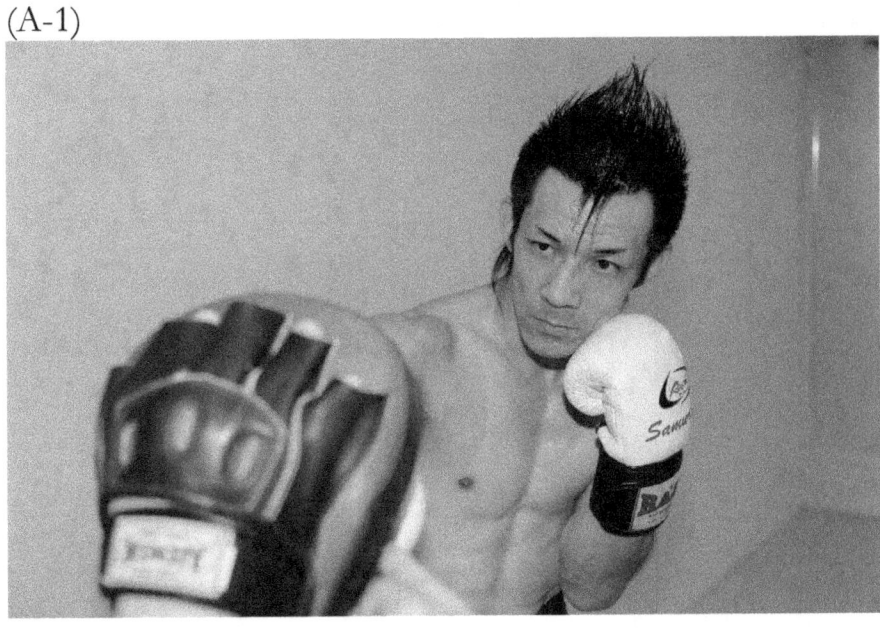

(B-1)

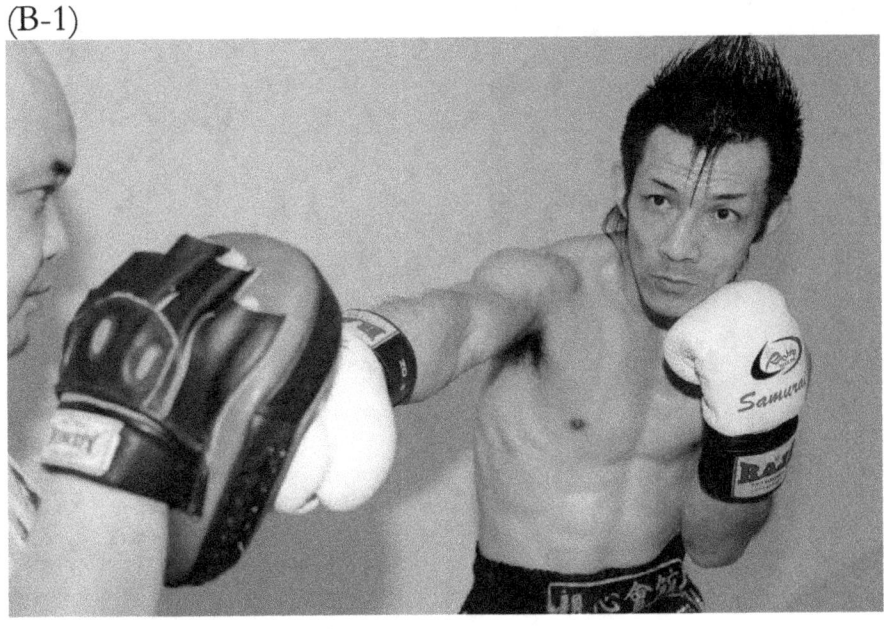

(A-2)

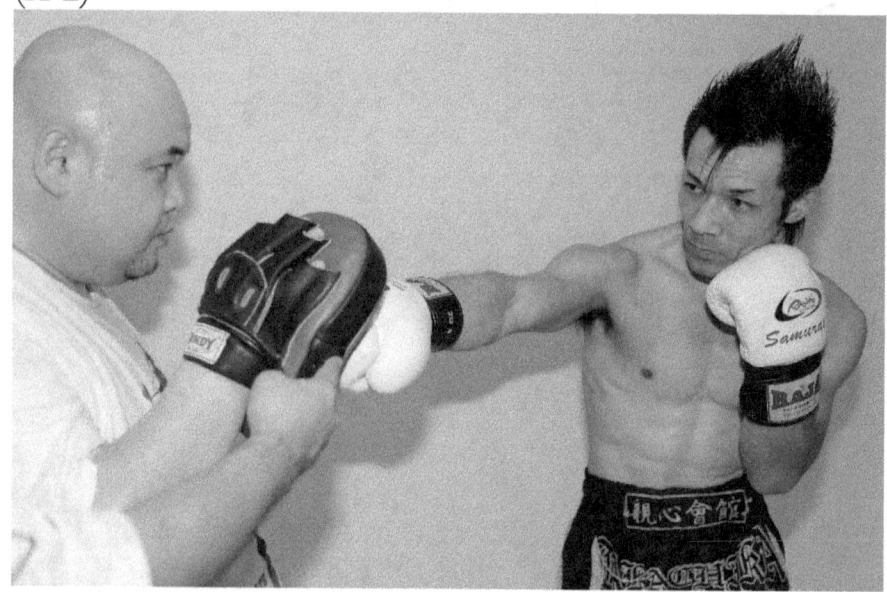

(B-2)

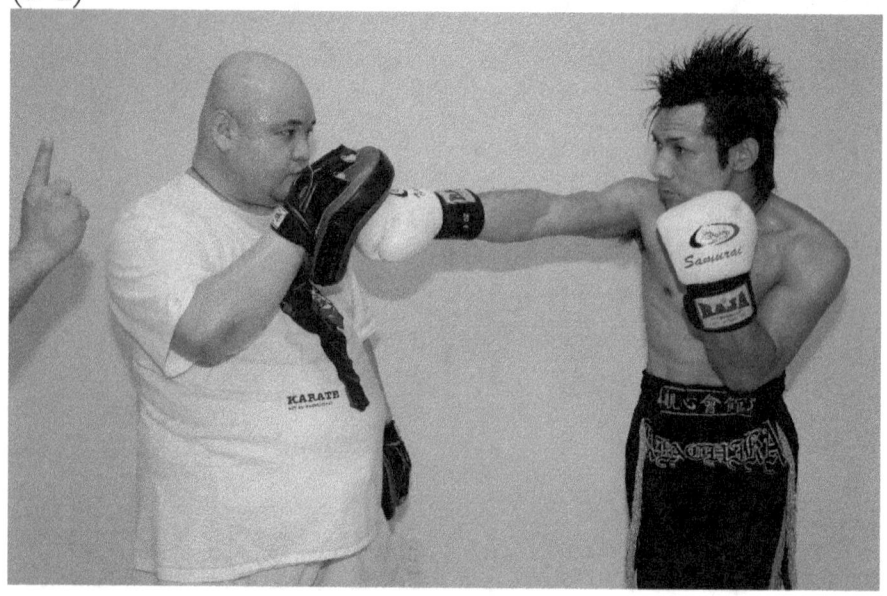

If you understand the difference in power made depending on the viewpoint, then please try to do the technique changing the viewpoint. At first, watch A, and next watch B. Change your goal from A to B. In a slight movement from A to B you change your view point, your eyes and pupils move, the muscles around your eyeballs move, your facial muscles, your neck and your whole body moves towards that direction. In addition, staring at the same goal from the start to the end, makes your speed slow down.When your punch approaches the goal, your brain put the attack on the brakes unconsciously, so changing the view point to high speed makes your body be faster. Please observe in detail KO Fighters, their eyes move real fast, and never stop!

We can take advantage of these principles. When you practice your form and fighting movements changing your viewpoints, you'll be aware of the importance that changing your viewpoint will also change your movements. Please observe deeply high leveled KO Fighters, their eyes move real fast, and never stop! We can take advantage of these principles. When you practice your form and fighting movements changing your viewpoints, you'll be aware of the importance of change your viewpoint will also change your movements.

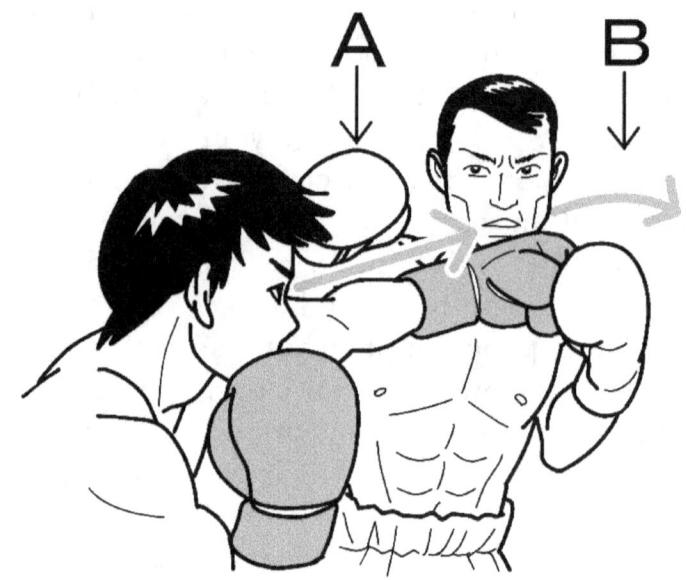

(A to B, changing of the viewpoint)

【1-4 Visual function and kick】
  Now, let's try with a kick:
(A) set a point with your eyes on the surface of the mitt to reach with a kick
(B) imagine/view the same point behind the mitt and do the kick.

  As you could experiment with your punch, the power in (B) is bigger. Try the exercise and change the view point on the mitt. You will notice the change in your strength depending on your view point.

(A)

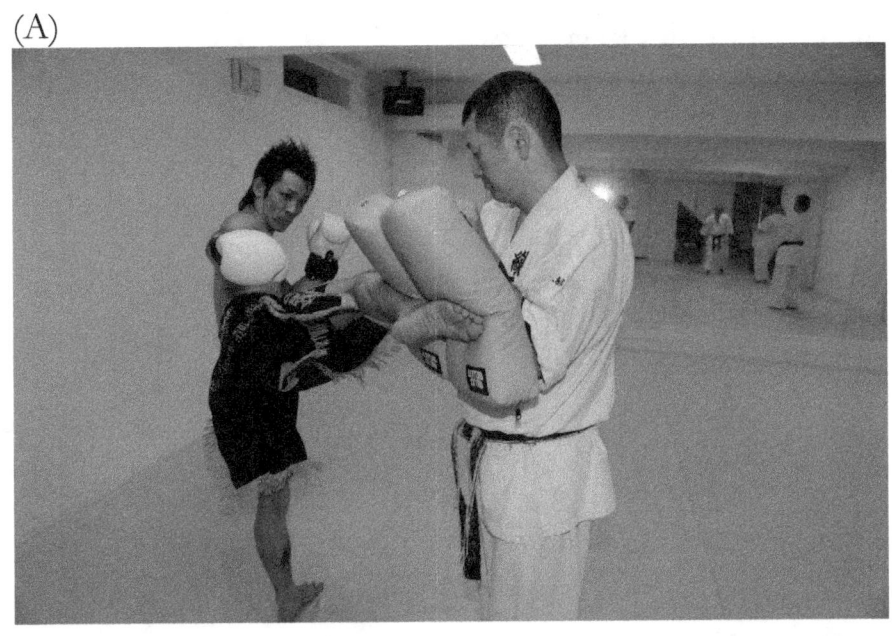

(B)

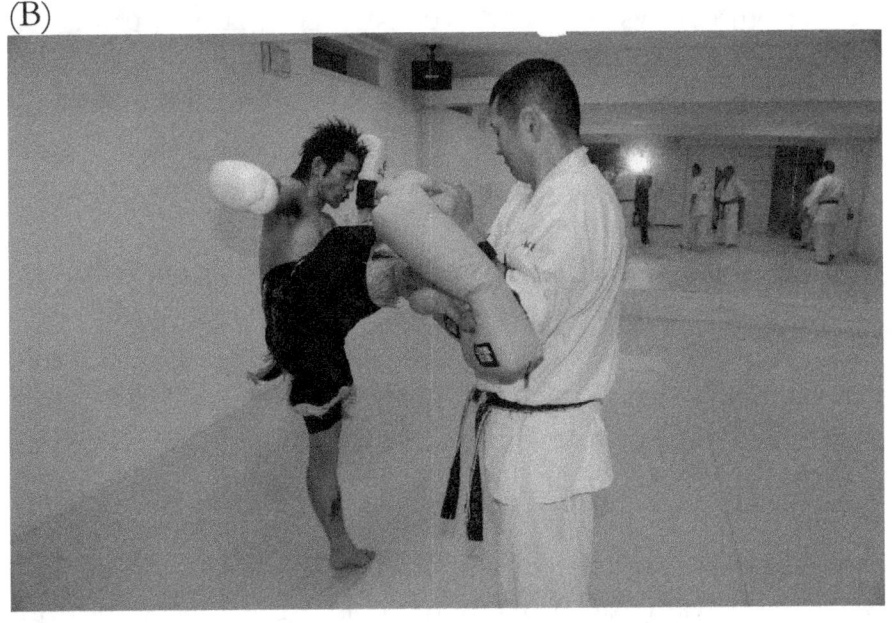

【1-5 Viewpoint to go forward】

"I won´t win if I do not go forward", "you need to make your opponent go back", "I want to exert enough pressure on my opponent and control the fight". A key point during a match in combat sports is to "set a viewpoint" which gives a very good chance to advance.

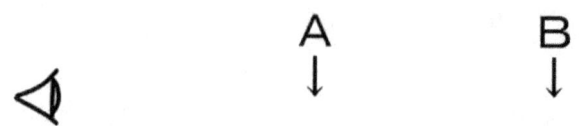

If there is a chance to impact your opponent, even when delivering blows to the chest, compare putting a viewpoint/focus on the chest of the opponent (point A) and do the same punch but setting your viewpoint some centimeters behind the chest of the opponent (point B), the punch delivered when focusing on point B will do more damage to the opponent.

The fighter who has difficulty stepping forward in the fight, usually sets focus on "point A" on the chest. But, when we throw a punch and knee kick, what we are actually thinking is "I want to move the opponent back". If that is the objective then you don´t want to hit the place where he actually is, what you have to do is focus your punches to "point B", the place where you want your opponent to move to. The idea is to transfer the viewpoint to the place where you want the movement to be and do the motion. By adding this work based on the visual information you obtain, the body perceives this and will carry itself to the place where it should be in order to execute the next movement. In this way the trajectory and movement itself of the punch and kick can vary only by changing the location of the viewpoint. By applying this technique you will see a change in the force output that can be exhibited depending on the way of placing the viewpoint, the person holding the mitt will feel the change in the pressure for sure.

Please pay a lot of attention when training trying to set a viewpoint and then combining it with the movement, do not use only your muscular strength to try and make your opponent move back and don't concentrate on creating a lot of power to push forward. Move while focusing your viewpoint to the place where I want to go in the next moment, this way the body will operate accordingly to get you to that place. This may be called "a usable formula" to be common in every movement of a martial art and Budo.

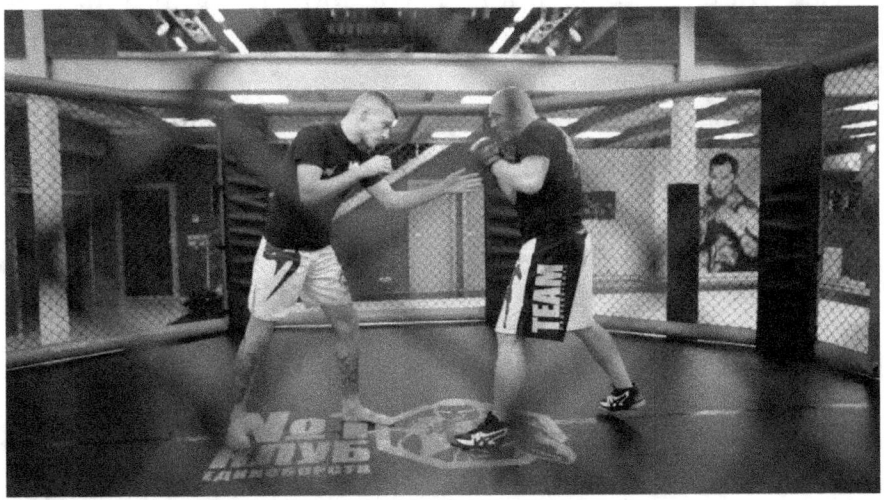

(from Kyokushin WKB,Shihan Fomin's Training)

【1-6 How to catch a moving opponent】

Let's see how to grasp the opponent's movement, and how to use the visual function at that moment. At first, hit the stationary mitt. It's easy to catch the mitt in sight when it's stationary, in my opinion. Like during the match, it is hard to hit the target while the opponent is in fast motion, but at some point when the opponent stops moving it is easy to attack. On the other hand, the fighters who practice with a static mitt could be very good at "Mitt hitting", but that's a different story when it gets to deal with moving opponents during matches in reality. The reason is the difference between the action of observing a stationary object and the action of observing a moving object. If a fighter wants to be successful it is very important to train with moving mitts and changing distance. Where you focus your sight also is an important point when you want to grasp your moving opponent.

Take mitts for an example, if you look at the mitt itself, it gets very difficult to follow the movement of the mitt. For example, let's suppose you want to punch your opponent's chin. If you only focus your sight on his chin, it gets difficult to recognize when his chin moves. Let's make an experiment of grasping the opponent now. The partner holds the mitt and faces the fighter, then move the mitt slightly back and forth, then the fighter must say out loud if he sees the mitt come forward or backward. The fighter then will do two exercises to compare which way is easier and practice his vision by doing the following patterns while the partner moves the mitts:

A: focus your eye only on the mitt
B: See the mitt and everything behind it at the same time

(A)

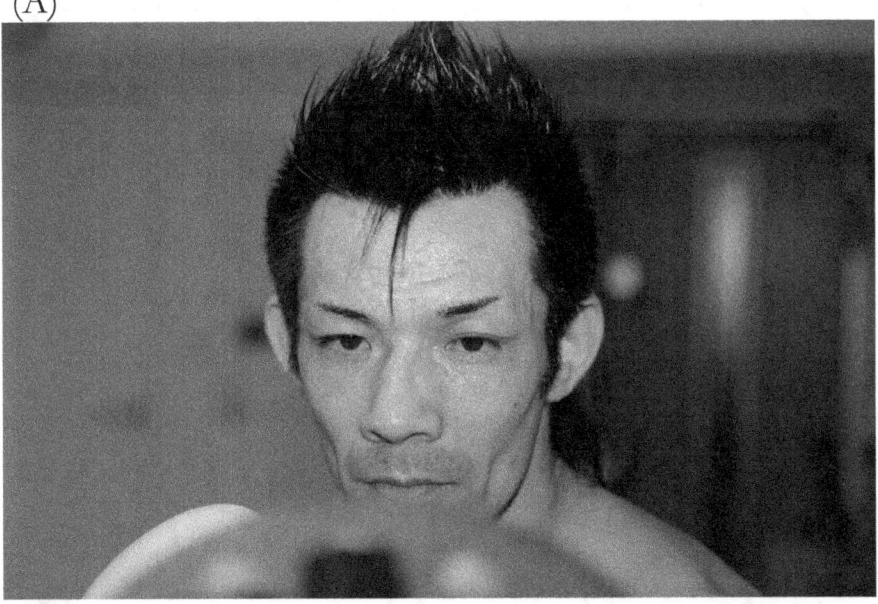

(B)

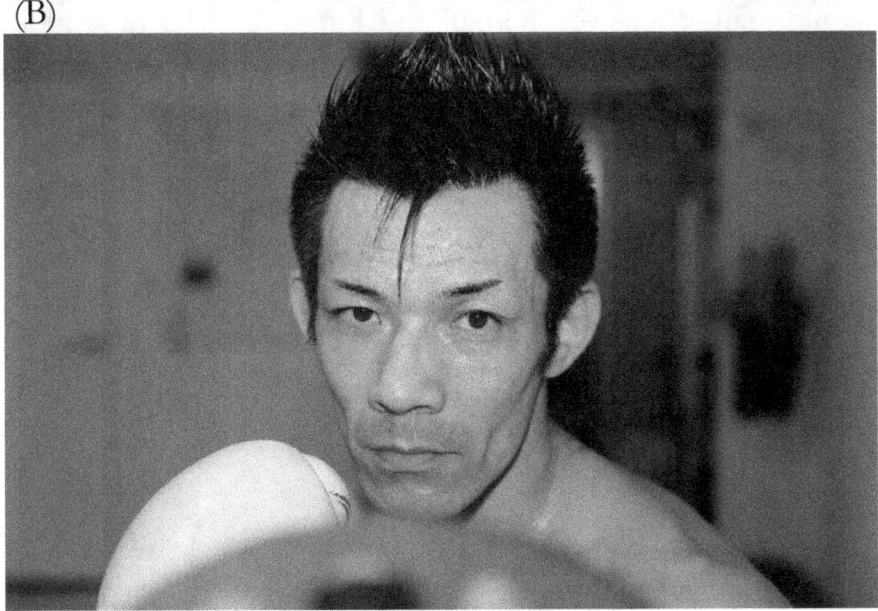

How do you feel? You will probably notice that when doing pattern B it is easier to grasp the movement than doing pattern A. The pattern A, you only see the mitt, so it's difficult to realize when the object makes size difference. This is due to the condition of focusing on only one point.

With pattern B, you realize it's very easy to see the size difference of the object moving, by having information of the surroundings which are not moving. The reason this happens is because you are putting the surroundings in the sight, to grasp the movement by the change in the distance between the surroundings and the object.

It's the same principle applicable to the fact that a point moving on checkered ruled lines is easier to see than a point moving on a white piece of paper. I have many memories when I was playing baseball, I was told to see the ball well to be able to catch it. Every time I heard that I would really focus on the ball and I couldn't catch it and all my teammates would stare at me. I suppose it was easier to predict where the ball goes if I was trying to observe the ball and the scenery at the same time. So it became much easier to grasp a moving opponent, not only seeing him but using the surroundings as information. In consequence, "Watch the opponent well" and "Watch the opponent and the scenery" are similar but very different advice.

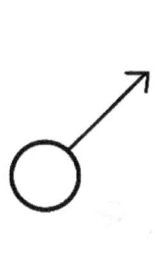

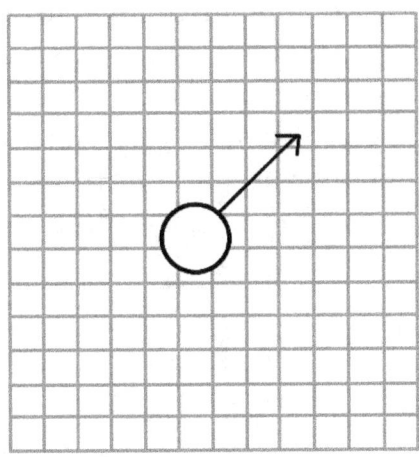

【1-7 Central vision and Peripheral vision. Two systems】

The eye is an element that transmits the visual perception to your brain and ignites your body's movement. Due to the structure of the eye, two systems are functioning. Viewing a narrow area on the line of sight and its surrounding area is called the central vision. The center visible range is called the center field of vision, seeing a wide range and all of its surroundings is called the peripheral vision, but each has a distinctive characteristic. Central vision works well especially in a part that is good at distinguishing colors and shapes, such as staring at the face of a person, (like staring at a point with a magnifying glass or a microscope). Central vision is the system which fits in the situation of looking at some detailed object carefully. On the other hand, peripheral vision is not a thorough view of the object, it is a system that is suitable for identifying movement and position by seeing the surroundings as a whole. Looking at the whole starry sky, seeing the natural scenery, seeing a train coming closer is a good exercise for your peripheral vision. Even in martial arts and Budo, peripheral vision is very suitable to capture the attacks of opponents who jump in from outside the field of view and with rapid movements of the opponent.

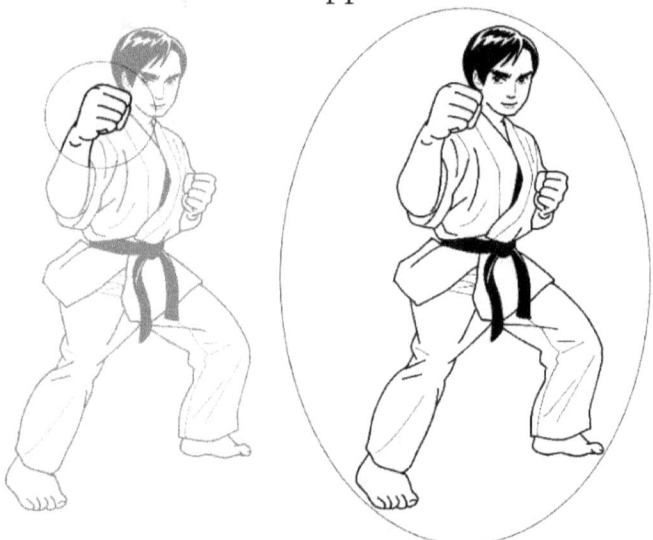

Haven't you ever had such experience in a match?

"I found that the right low kick hit and it worked since my opponent couldn't stand balanced, and at that moment, I kept looking at the part I kicked, then I got a counter attack with his/her high kick."

"When my punch to the stomach produced damage to the opponent, I kept looking at his/her belly and was KOed by his/her upper knee kick."

"My punch with hit the opponent's face and I tried to overthrow, after everything became completely invisible except his/her face."

In these conditions, peripheral vision cannot be used well, there is a possibility that the ratio of foveal vision has increased. When falling into a losing pattern, there are many cases that only a part of the opponent, or the opponents themselves are in sight. While fighting, the fighter who is looking at the whole picture while looking at the other's face is easy to catch the opponent in peripheral vision, so it is easy to respond to the counter and other techniques coming from various directions and unexpected movements of the opponent. But if the fighter sees only one part with the central vision, the risk of getting attacked by the opponent increases as the movement is hard to capture.

【1-8 The focus and the angle】
When I recall the matches that I have won, without mentioning the opponent, I always remember certain seconds of the match and where I sat during the meet, the movement of the referee, the energy of the audience among other aspects of the whole event. This is the evidence that the input from sight information while having a parametric view is very important. When the sight range becomes wide the fighter's mind is calm and can get in the flow of the match and cope with the situation of the fight a lot better.A good sense of fighting is to be able to output techniques while inputting data at the same time. The human is usually narrow-sighted, this explains why sometimes fighters are nearsighted and can have moments when they lose their calm and express that they "lost sight of myself".

By the way, a condition to have heard almost none of the voices of the second in a match is so-called a lot of I lose, and a phenomenon to shut out sound entry. It is in a condition to move while feeling that I do exercise (the output) and is not tired strangely while opening up a channel of the entry all the way. However, I use the stamina immediately and I tired and end when I am going to do only the output with interrupting input entirely. It is mysterious because it change whether you start it whether I output while inputting or output without inputting. I decide to clap a hand with bread by the team where I belong to, and to do a signal to start a sound, and change a focus. It is decided at meeting of a second and the fighter for the time that the fighter will become hot, and viewpoints will begin to gather in one point. So I change a focus suddenly like changing the angle of the camera when he watch the small part of the opponent. It becomes like a multi angle. Furthermore, a second conveys "a glance" or "view" or the instructions using such words and the fighter prepares to change it when I rallied in a game hard and view became small.

Then the fighter incline to the direction "Oh, here is vacant" and "Where the movement of the opponent is seen". A place becoming vacant is seen to the fighter by the guard that look firm from a front face when he change some angles. In addition, it is hard to lead to KO even if the fighter get the blow that he can see. When the fighter is defeated, mostly "it is the blow that he cannot see" .The fighter can make an opportunity of the escape from the scenes which seem to be knocked down by changing of the focus when he almost fell into his defeat pattern or when he was not able to find a breakthrough.

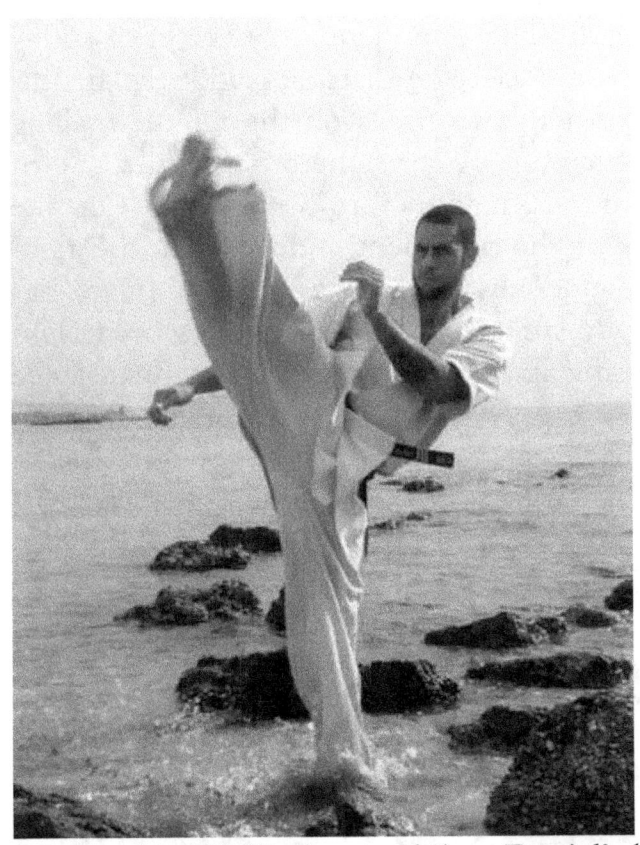
(Kyokushin WKB champ,Shihan Daniel's kick)

【1-9 Controlling the opponent's glance】
Let's observe the movement of the opponent's eyes.
Make a group of 2 people, then use a finger as a focus
point in order to let your partner focus on it. When the
finger is getting close to the partner, the eyes of the partner
are directed towards the center (this movement is known as
adduction). Next, if you pull the finger away from your
partner, his/her eyes are departing from the center (this is
known as abduction). Convergence reflex means the
reaction of both eyes adducting when the subject is

approaching forward. The opponent's convergence reflex occurs if you have reduced the distance suddenly. In this moment, the vision tends to focus on the middle making the sides more difficult to be seen, therefore the hit rate of high kicks and hook punches are very high. On the contrary, the eyes of the opponent abduct when the fight distance extends suddenly. Since the angle of view has become wider, body strikes such as front kicks or straight punches are easy to hit the target once the fight distance extends.

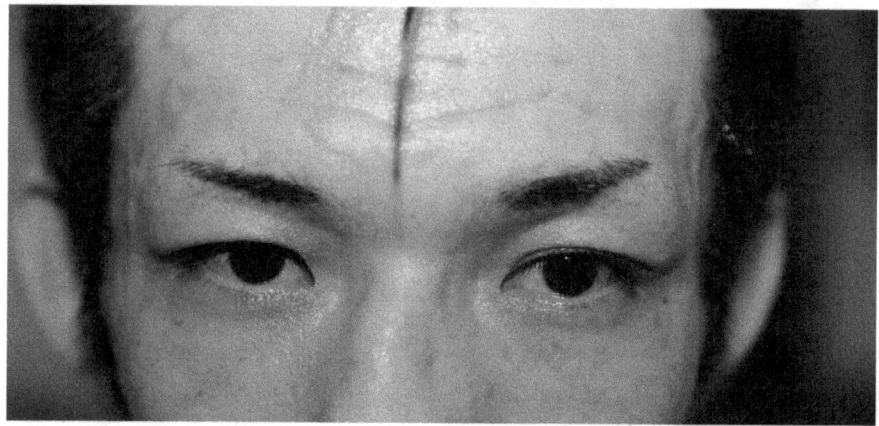

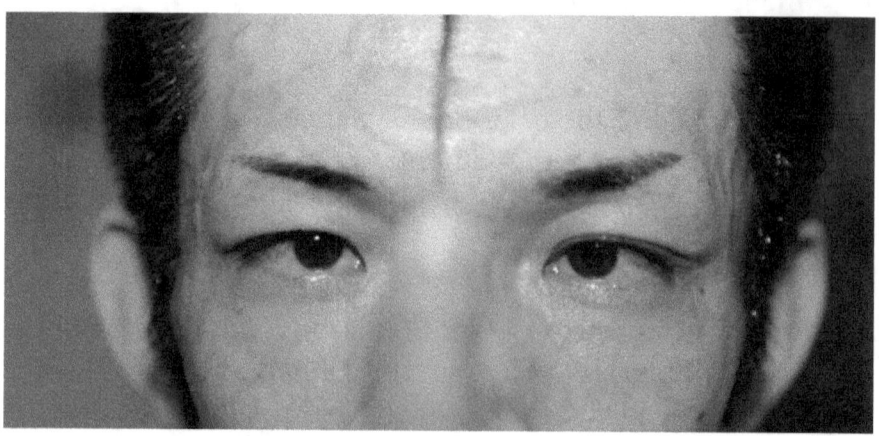

There are a lot of fighters that explain their combination and attack techniques choice because those are "easy to perform" or "it is a good pattern". On the other hand, the first-class fighters apply techniques which are hard for the opponent to respond to.

【1-10 Catch a moment】

Now let's do the training without optical information. The fighter must close his eyes. In this moment, optical information is not available. Where is the mitt? Where is my opponent standing? At what distance is he and what is the angle of his position? Those are some key points that you don't know without your sight information. With the fighter's eyes closed: first, the partner holding the mitt changes his position several times moving around the mat/ring. Then the person with the mitt makes a signal to the fighter, saying "go" out loud, and then the fighter immediately opens his eyes and performs the technique (kick or punch) against the mitt in the direction where he heard the voice. This will allow you to improve selectivity by making you process information from your sight faster, hence making it easier to grasp a sense of space and distance, making it easier to find the angle and technique that fits the situation.

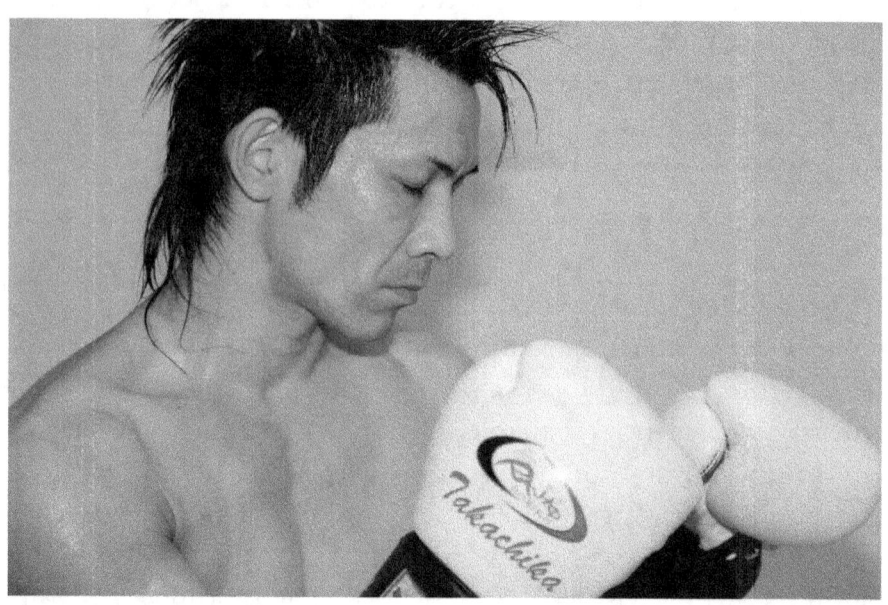

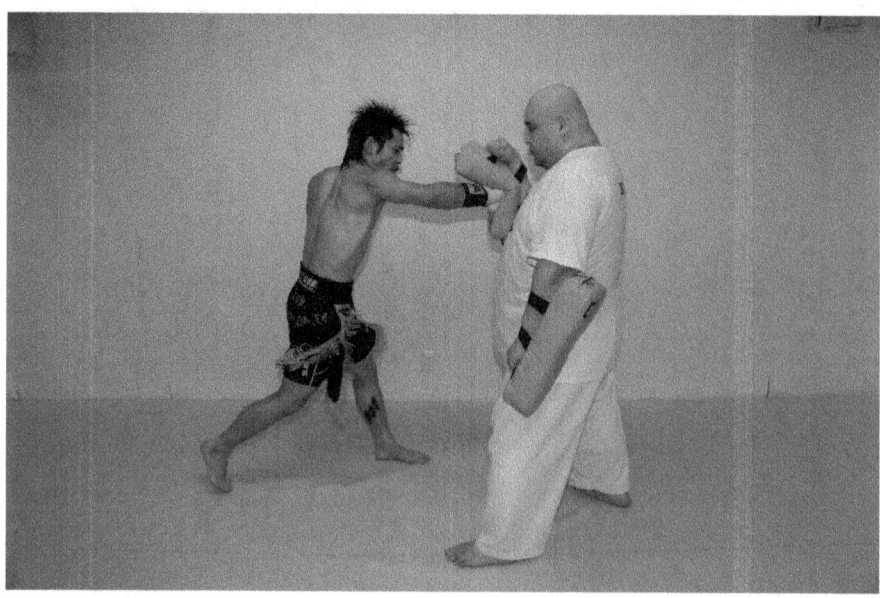

Each round of a kickboxing fight lasts three minutes, three minutes for karate as well, and five to ten minutes in

MMA. Although it may seem like a lot of time, you should train to fight instant to instant and to do this you must exercise training without vision performing drills like the one mentioned above.

Visual information, including drills between training partners and oneself should be analyzed instead of as a "moving image", but rather as "continuous still images overlapping" (the "instant to instant" technique), training to be able to immediately respond to the previous still image received through your sight. If you make a mistake, then emphasize on the reaction speed, and try to instantly combine your next technique with your visual information. This training will improve your ability to seize the moment or instant during a fight.

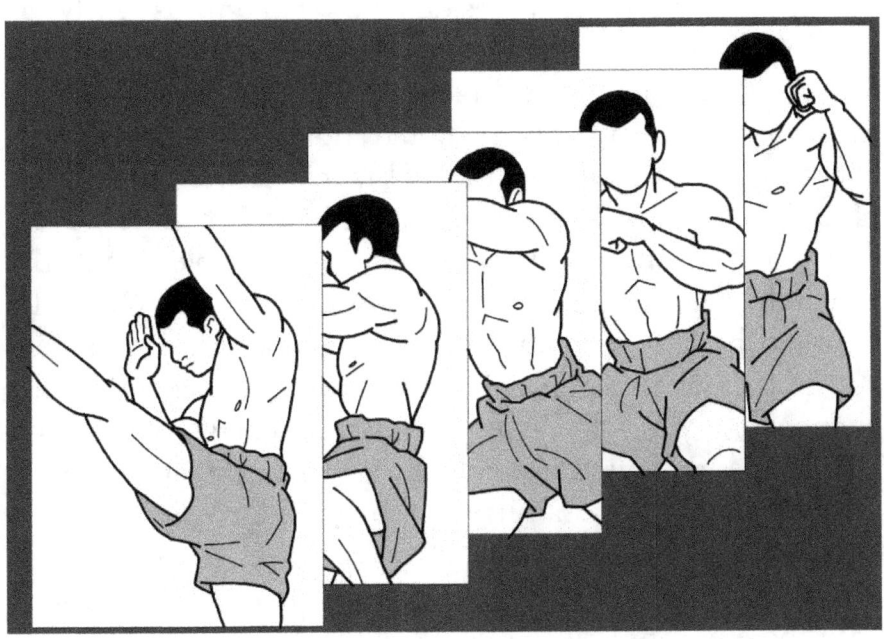

【1-11 The meaning of stadium and ring examination】

A good practice for competitive fighters is to always conduct an examination of the stadium and ring / tatami before the fight. Top fighters input sight information into his/her memory by viewing the stadium from different viewpoints such as the outside of it, looking at the ring from the audience seats and the whole stadium from the ring. The performance of a fighter who is accustomed to fighting in small stadiums decreases once he fights in a large stage. This is because the background has changed from what he is used to which confuses the brain especially fighting for the first time in an unknown stadium, the unknown background will affect performance greatly. Therefore, it is very important to pre-work with the information input, get inside the stadium as early as possible and get comfortable with the stadium and the scenery that you will encounter during the fight. I decide the points that my team should notice during the ring checking period. During the fight, if a fighter can't keep himself relaxed, the fighter can shift his or her view to the 2nd floor of the audience seats (for example) once the viewpoint has changed, the information changes. When the fight has boiled down and you are in a deadlocked position, you should try to change your viewpoint like changing the channel on your TV from news to comedy. When you change your viewpoint and change the information you receive you may find a different/better way of moving and fighting.

It is different to fight in a place where you´re familiar with the environment than a place that you are not familiar at all since there are differences in scenery, such as the mat and the ring, other sounds, temperature and humidity, to

34

name a few. Once the fighter adjusts to the new environment, by inputting the information through his/her five senses, precision of the movements improves. Top fighters are able to process all the information that is being received as a visitor and covert the place into his/her home during the stadium and ring check. World champions sit in several audience seats before the event starts and imagines the playout of the match.

Fighters control their state of mind by changing their point of view and imagining themselves fighting inside the ring and in different of places within it. Like I said above, image training is vital to have the strength of not missing the chance of defeating the opponent until the last moment, even after going through one or two extensions.

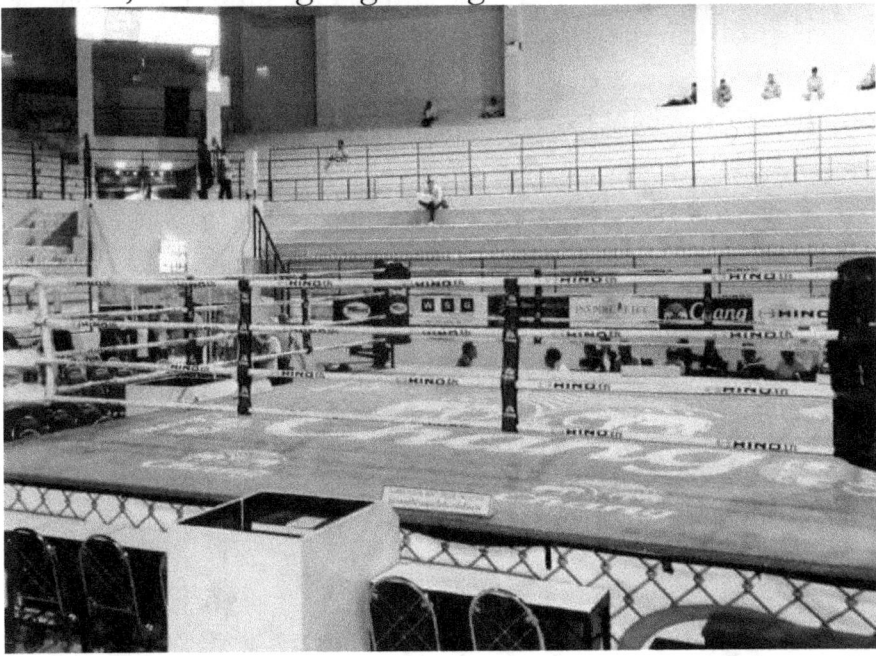

【1-12 What is the eyesight secret hidden in kata?】

The first movement you do when performing a kata is to turn your eyes toward the direction you will go in the next move. When you change the direction to the left side in a basic kata like Taikyoku or Pinan, you move your eyes first. First, the eye is in motion then the head follows and after that the spine rotates. That´s a process based on eyes and spine rotation. The message behind the exercise is that the sight is the very first movement of the kata. The same applies to the movement when wanting to change the orientation, to perform a smooth movement it begins by moving from the eye. (There is also a kinematic meaning of kata, which is to look for ease of motion when performing a difficult movement) It is said that a kinematic chain is when movement that occurred in some one part of the body affects the other parts. How to produce the kinematic chain is of a great concern to improve performance.

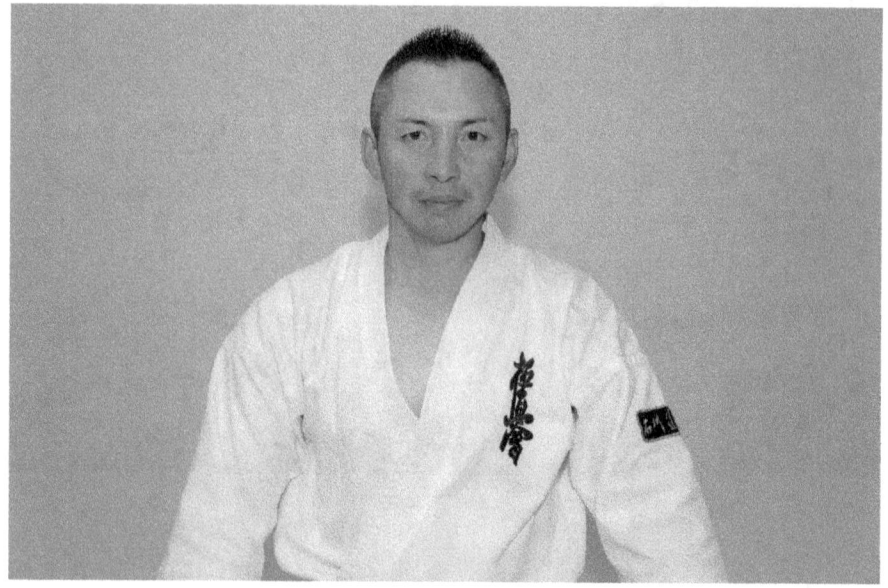

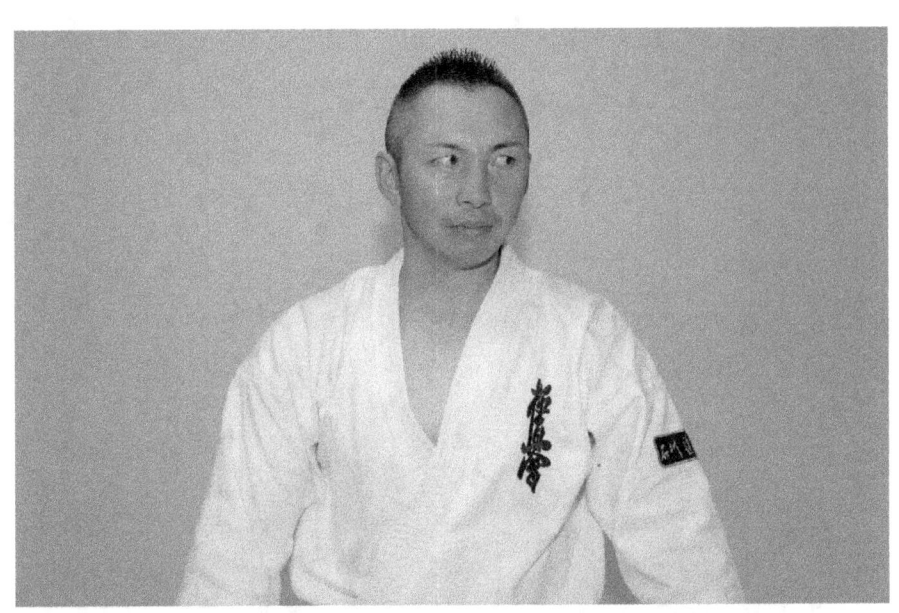

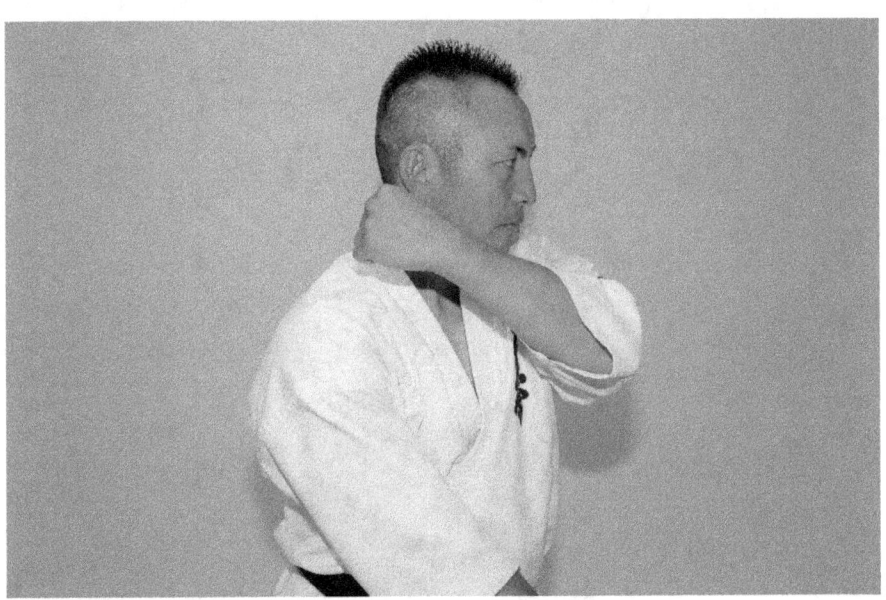

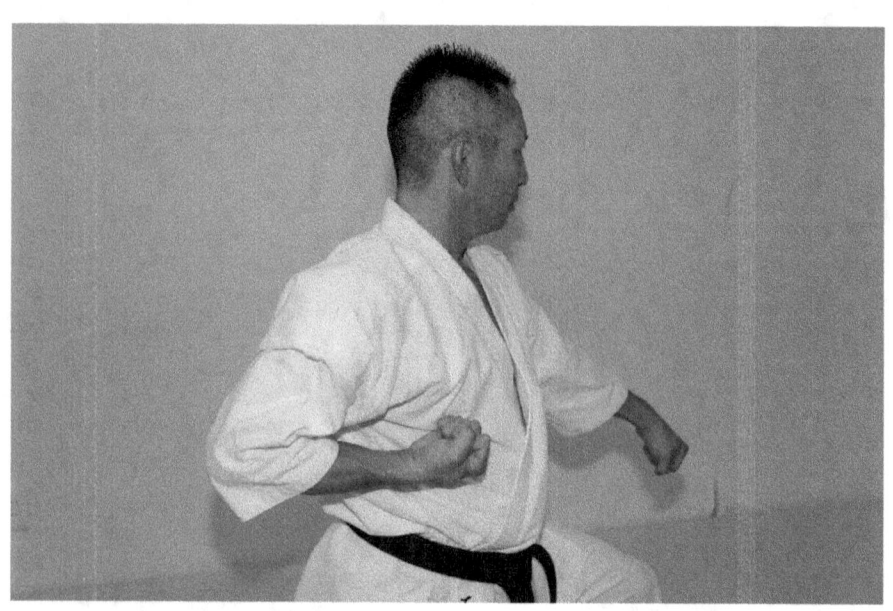

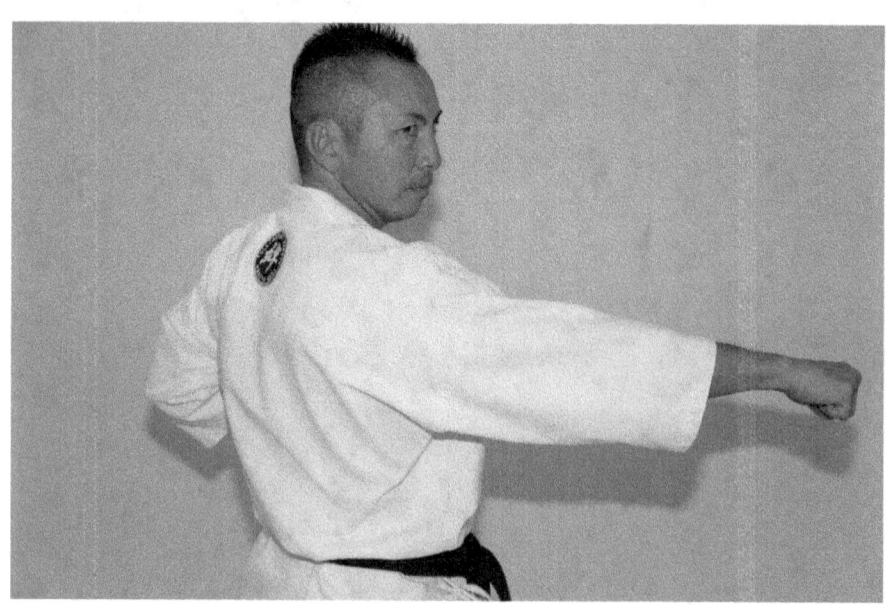

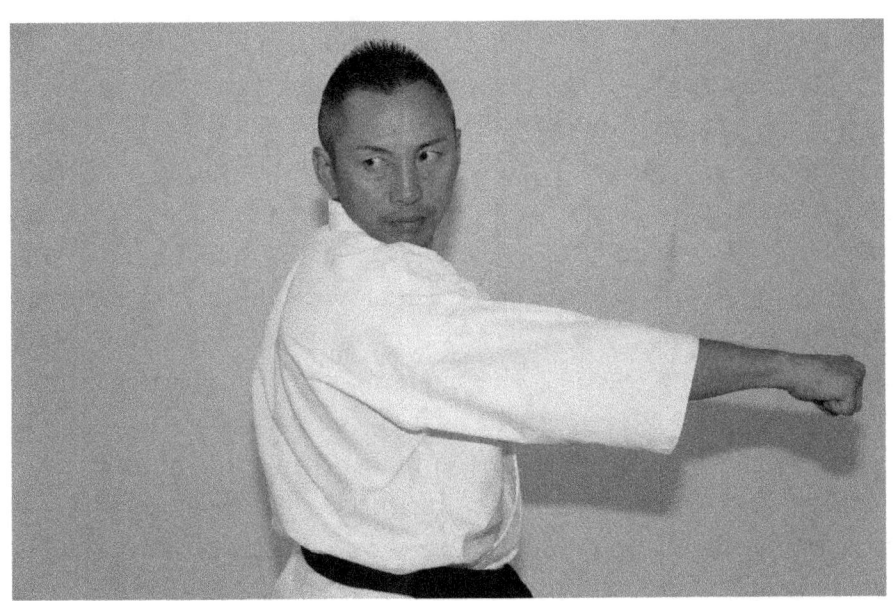

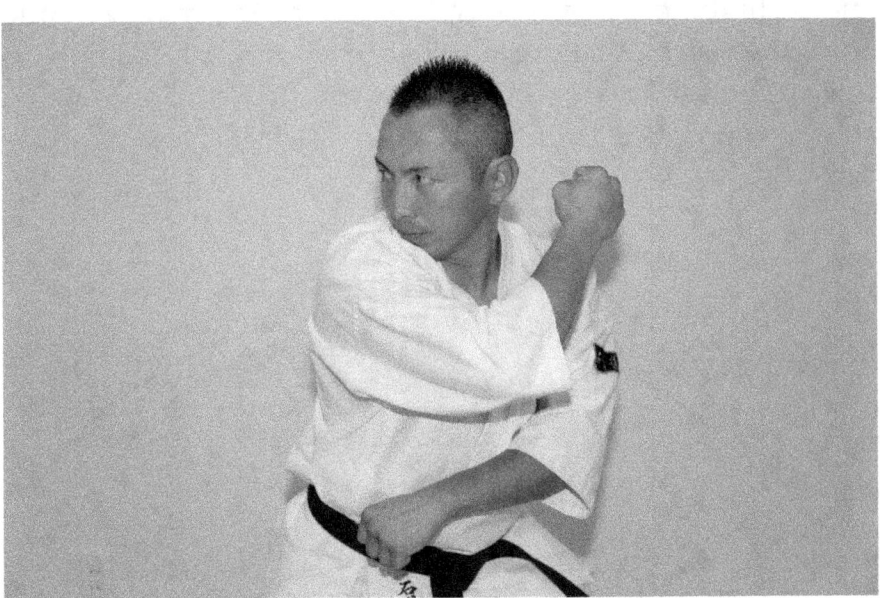

(Kyokushin shihan,Akira Ishikawa)

In fact, slow or dull movements of fighters become faster if first you move your eyes faster. It's easy to do a high kick when you first look at the floor before kicking: the body will move in a direction opposite to the force of gravity, which will make it easier to raise the high kicks. Predecessors who created kata cleverly hid a variety of secrets to become strong into the movements of the katas. How to become strong has been kept a secret, only taught to family or close people, it´s like a code, that is not understood if seen from the outside (only the person who knows it can understand). Finding the essence of the performance improvement through kata in a martial arts and Budo is a very interesting work. I feel that your eyes and sight function were used as a sensory system in the conventional martial art, Budo and sports. In addition to this, why not try to move the eyes first as an essential starter to produce a kinetic chain?

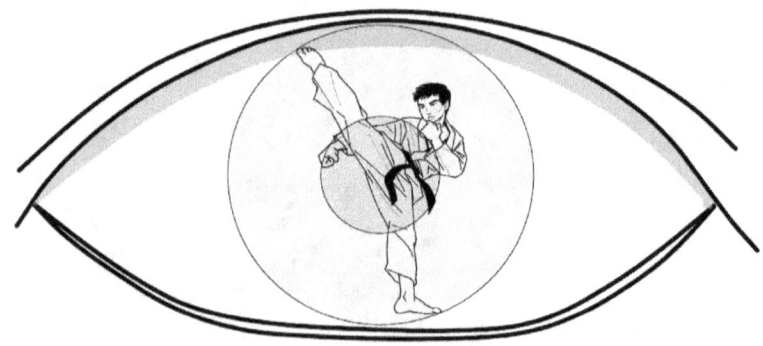

2 Breathing in Fight

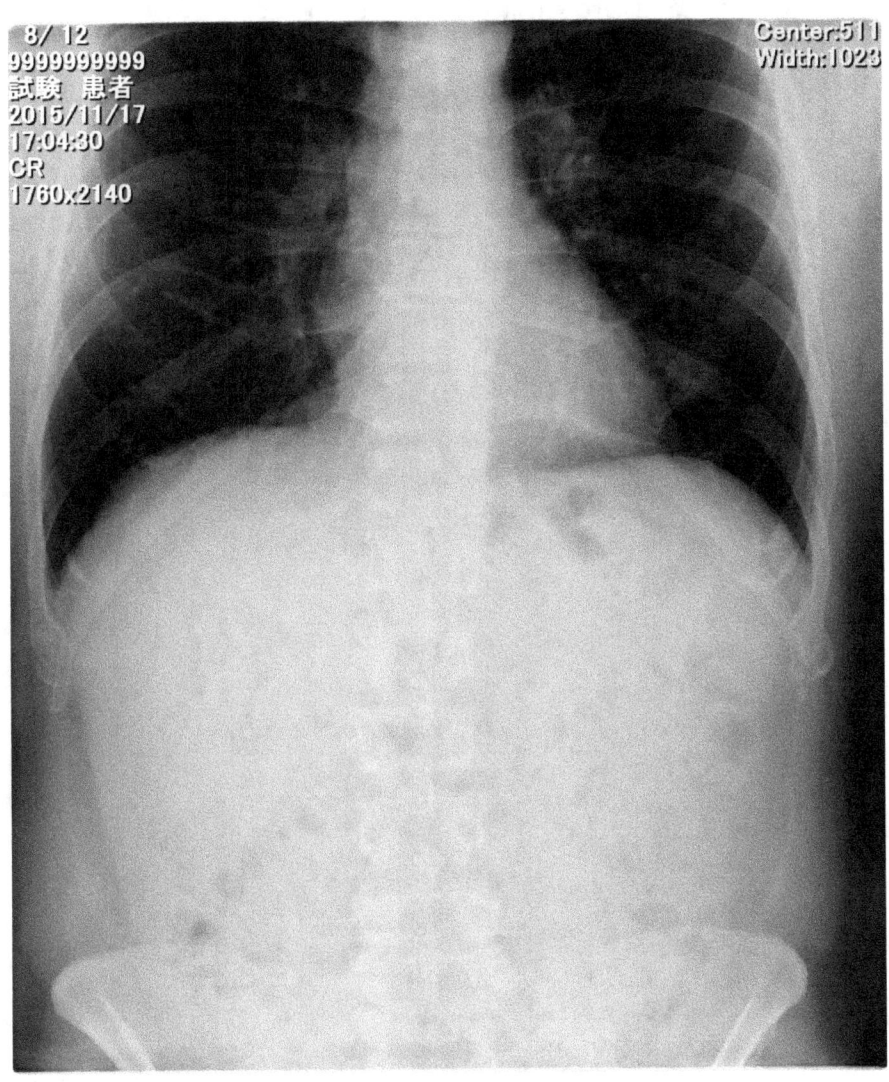

【2-1 Role of breathing】

Breathing is essential for human being to sustain their lives. We have approximately 60 trillion cells in our bodies. And those cells takes oxygen to produce energy for themselves to work. Oxygen is taken in mainly by the lungs and it is combined with the hemoglobin in the red blood cells. The oxygen is delivered to each cells to the whole body. In exchange for it, the hemoglobin and red blood cells receive carbon dioxide and the waste material which are generated in the cell. Hemoglobin returns to the lungs by the bloodstream again, and the carbon dioxide and waste material are exhausted outside the body as expiration.

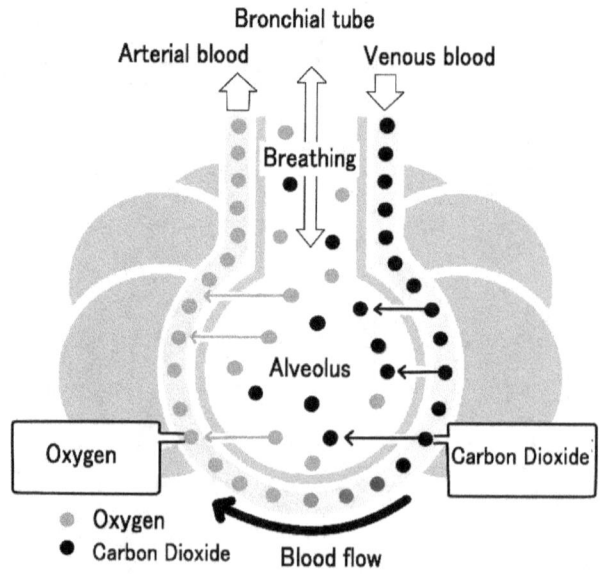

The living body is maintained, because of oxygen and a carbon dioxide emissions by through breathing called "gas exchange" that is carried out smoothly. When breathing is jeopardized from a state of respiratory failure, like pneumonia, heart failure, suffocation, and asthmatic attack happens when oxygen is not able to pass through the body. Therefore, in the human body there is a given sensor of feedback, where oxygen and carbon dioxide density is monitored strictly.

The information about the breathing is accumulated in real time by the respiratory center of the brainstem and that respiratory center coordinates the most suitable breathing number of times and depth of breathing automatically and unconsciously. So we may think breathing is "a commonplace" thing and we are "not conscious of it" in daily life, and it is natural for us to think so and for us to be that way. In the healthy person's everyday life the most efficient breathing is unconscious breathing, we should say.

When it takes exercise load that is higher than a daily life level, you must take suitable way of breathing for the exercise level. For example, if you try to reach the summit of Mount Everest, you must know the effective breathing way in the place where oxygen density is low. If you try a long-distance (10 Km) swim without taking rest, you must know the effective way of breathing makes you keep swim longer. In the same running race events like 100 meters race and the marathon, the suitable way of breathing is different because it is different how long you need to use muscle between a 100 meters race and the marathon. The suitable way of breathing in a martial arts and Budo differs by the kind of competition, or situation. Let's think about these two cases in Boxing.

1: Breathing for a long fight (12 rounds) reduces the stamina of the opponent gradually.

2: Breathing in trying to make one-blow K.O. in the Round 1.

The suitable way of breathing is different in these two occasions, and the way of breathing in trying to overwhelm the opponent by tons of punches is different from the way of breathing in trying to beat him by a counter blow. Which is the suitable way of breathing in the fighting? How should we do in the certain situation or occasion of the fighting? Here, I would love to show you the relation between breathing and the exercise in martial arts.

【2-2 Breathing and speed】

During shadow training, think about your breathing while performing four techniques: one-two punch combination, left hook followed by right low kick. For a fighter who has difficulty being conscious of timing, the breathing in this exercise, having the following pattern help you understand better: Usually it goes, exhale in one, and inhale, then exhale in two, and inhale, exhale with a left hook, then inhale and exhale in right low kick. In this way of breathing, the attack and breathing are paired one to one. On the other hand, a top fighter techniques change the timing of breathing during the fight:

"Exhale in one-two punch and left hook, inhale and exhale in right low kick."
"Exhale in one-two punch combination, inhale and exhale in left hook and right low kick"
"Exhale during the whole exercise (one-two punch combo, left hook and right low kick)"

One

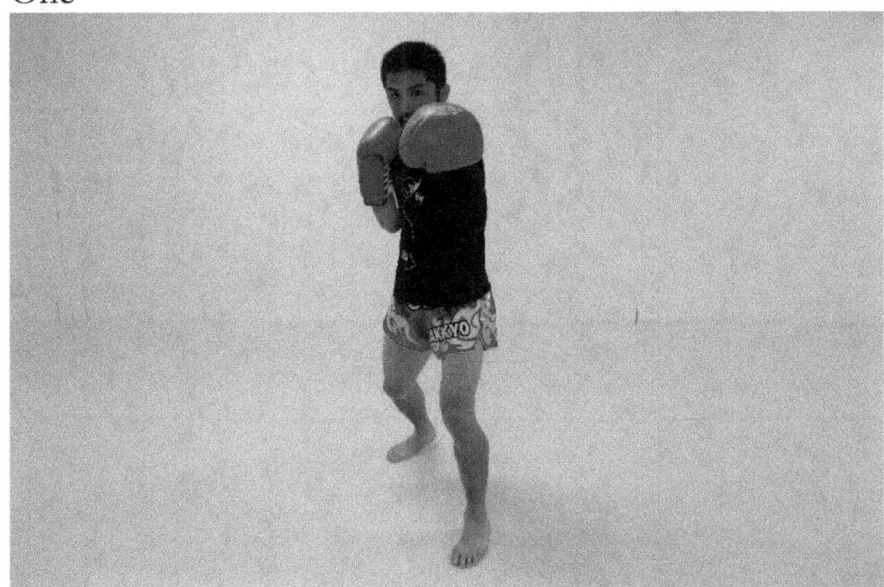

Two

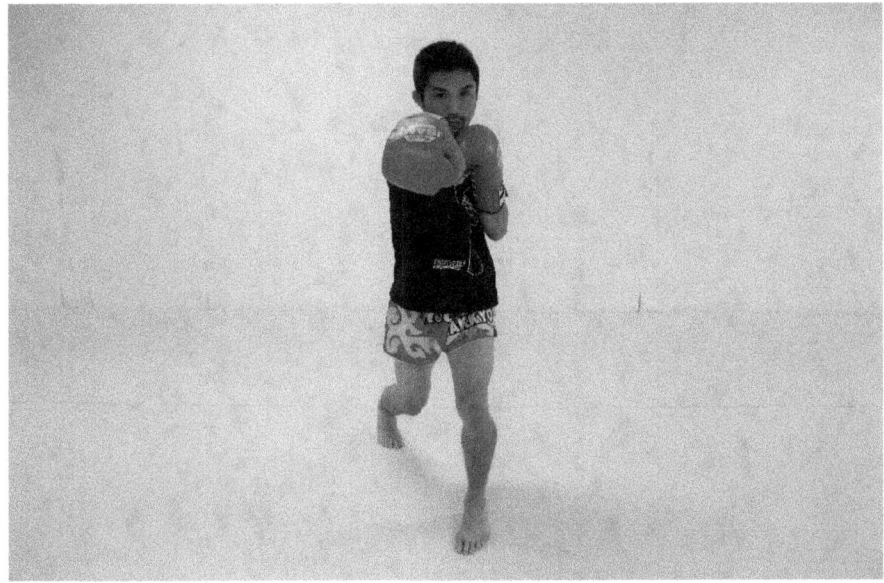

Lefthook

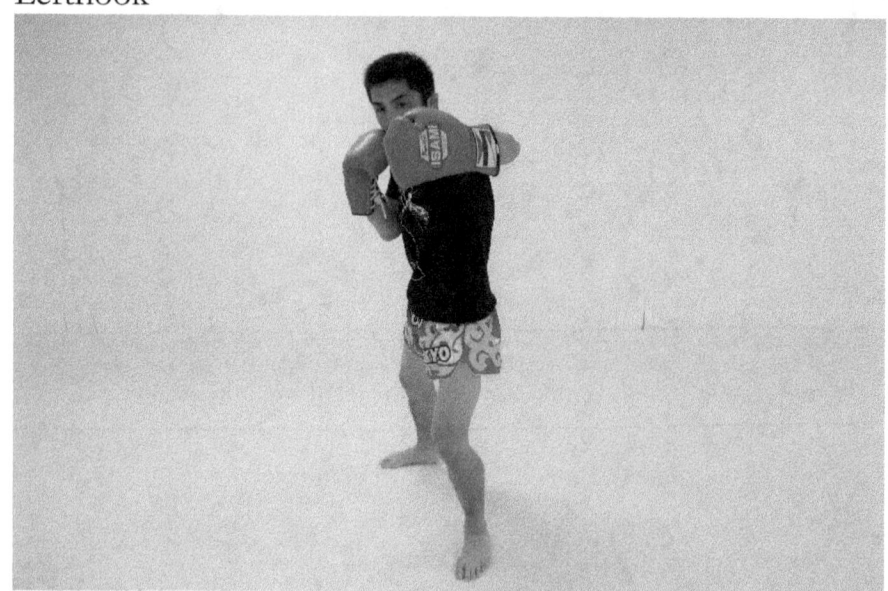

Right low kick

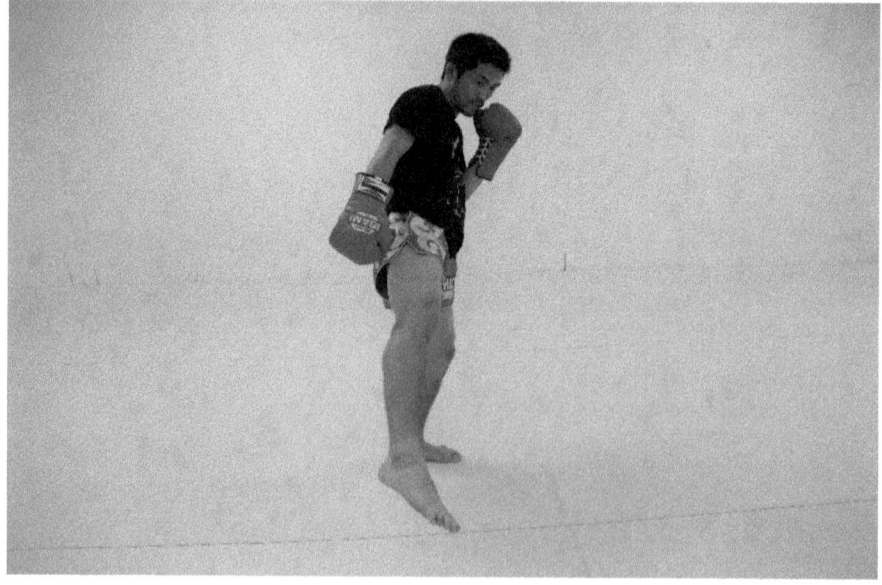

As you notice the work of techniques that are executed with usual breathing practice are long but the work of techniques that a top fighters breathing are short. If you can use as many techniques as a top fighter will use during your one cycle of exhale and inhale, the speed of the strike will surely increase. Breathing is concerned by the respiratory muscle group in the body, the diaphragm is the maximum respiratory muscle of the human body and it exists to partition the chest and the abdomen. When the diaphragm contracts, the thoracic cavity also contracts (negative pressure) and you inhale. When the diaphragm relaxes, the air within is exhaled. If the attack and breathing are paired one to one, while the diaphragm moves one time, you can never use two or many techniques. By changing the timing of the breathing, like two, three techniques or more during one cycle of exhalation and inhalation, you can have an advantageous breathing skill in cases when you rush into the opponent, when you are going to K.O. him by repeated blows, or just when you want to disturb the attack rhythm of the opponent.

When you want to achieve speed and power in one big blow, you must do the opposite. When you are going to give a big single blow in karate demonstrations, like in breaking a baseball bat, breaking a pillar of ice, or breaking roof tiles, you will do with a loud shout. If you want to give a strong and fast blow, you need to be conscious of "striking while you exhale at the MAX volume in the shortest moment as possible as you can" with the intention of letting out all the carbon dioxide in the lungs and respiratory tract. When you exhale, the diaphragm moves all the way from the bottom to the top. Usually when Muay-Thai fighters are kicking mitts and opponents, exactly same breathing pattern, like exhorting and shouting a loud "ahh!" yell. This means the movement is completely in sync with the breathing. We get to know that they are "exhaling" because of the sound (their loud yell). So, now we understand why they say that a man who can yell in a loud voice in his training will get to be a strong fighter. And then, we can also say: If the children today who seldom have chance to yell in a loud voice at school and public place yell in a loud voice in dojo or gym, they can get to be stronger in martial arts and also growing up to be in good health and tough.

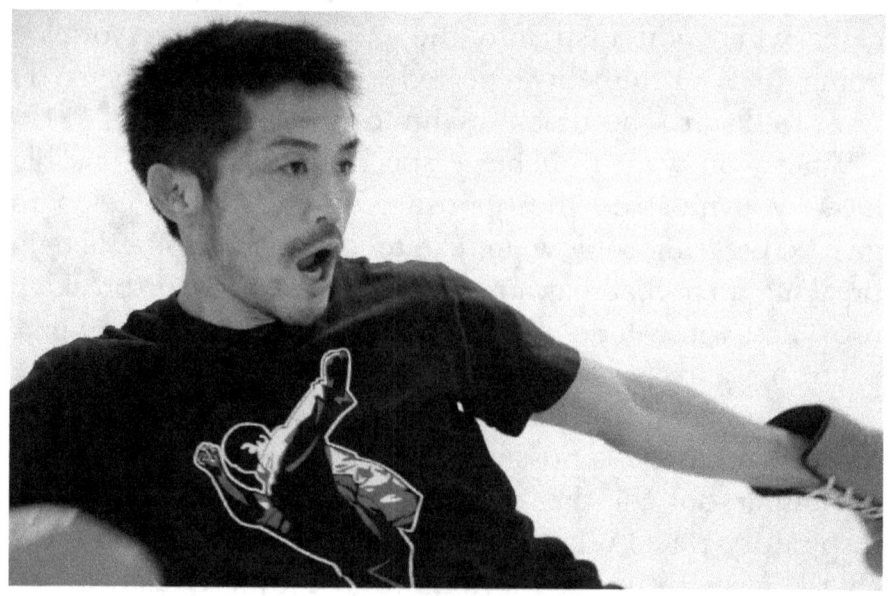

Exhale

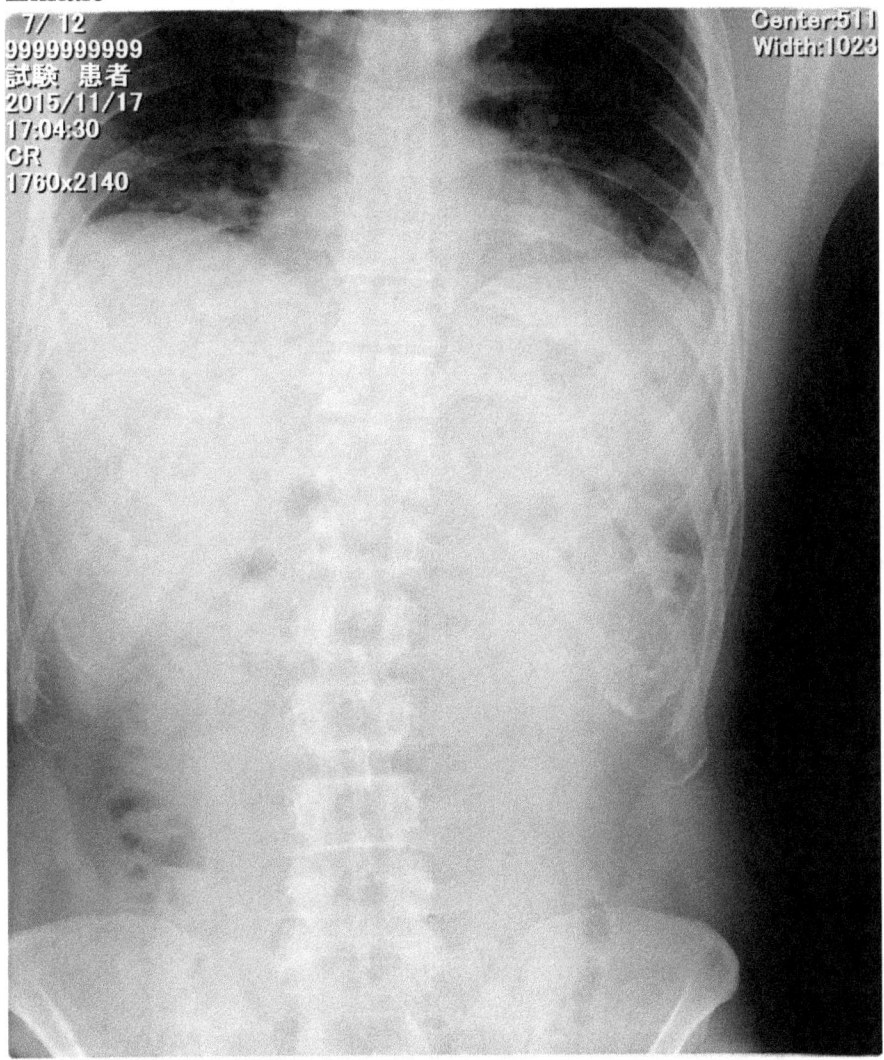

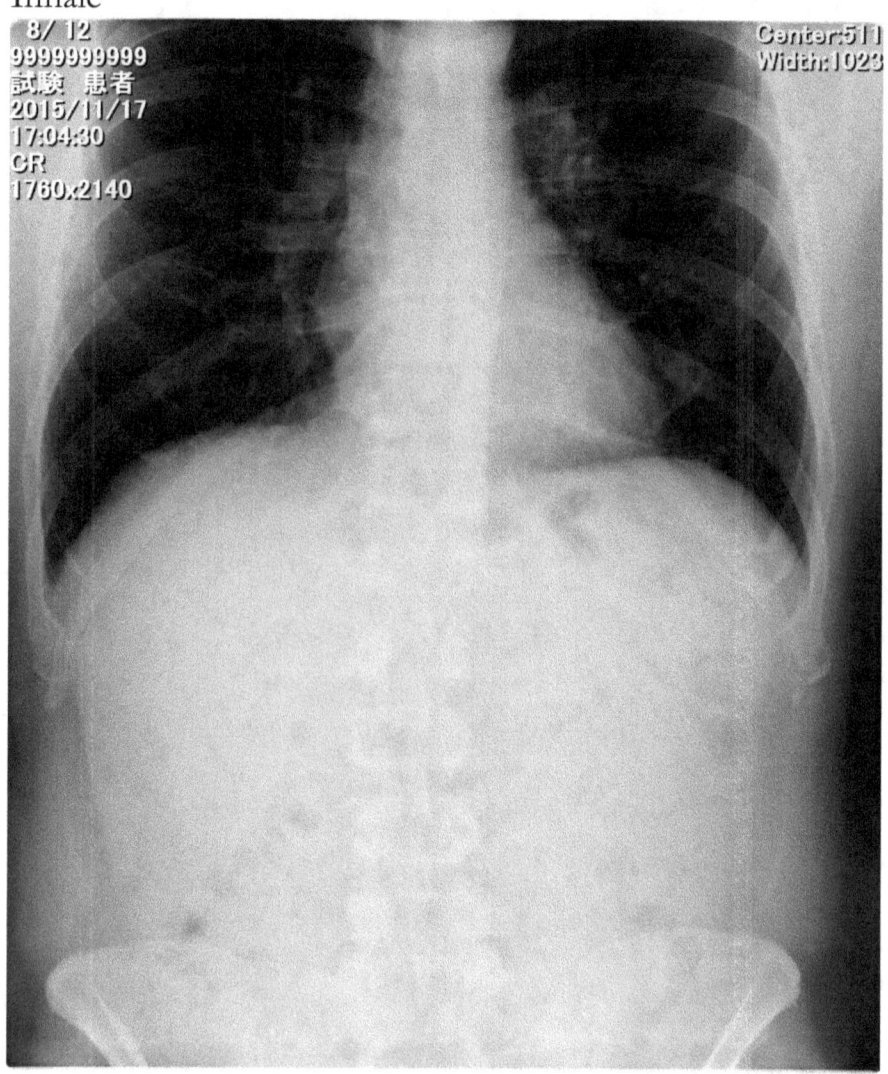

Inhale

8/ 12
9999999999
試験 患者
2015/11/17
17:04:30
CR
1760x2140

Center:511
Width:1023

【2-3 Breathing and power】
There is a report that athletes who have lower back pain tend to have atrophy of multifidus muscle in the lumbar vertebrae when is compared with athletes who don't have lower back pain. The multifidus muscle group is, a small group around lumbar vertebrae, and antagonistic of a muscles group which consist of deep abdominal muscles. Antagonist muscle means that it is paired muscle that does an opposite movement. For example, in the upper arm, triceps brachii muscle is paired with biceps brachii muscle, and the pair is involved in flexing and training extending the elbow.

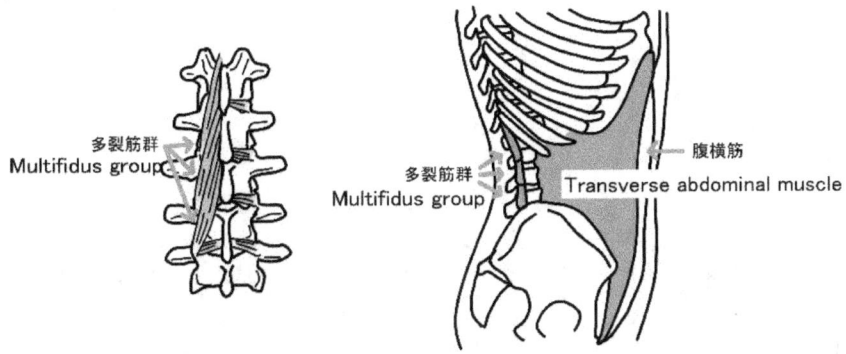

An opinion proclaims that "the lower back pain athletes group that have atrophy of multifidus muscle have a weakness in transverse abdominis muscle which is an antagonist, at the same time it causes lower back pain in sports movement. A study group of a certain rehabilitation medicine tried to prove this opinion, attaching an electrode to skeletal muscle group and transversus abdominis muscle to examine called electromyography (EMG), and they found a very interesting result. They found the fact, surprisingly, before the big lines such as an arm or the leg muscles shrank, the transversus abdominis muscle also shrank. The transversus abdominis muscle has a shape that surrounds the lumbar vertebrae like a corset, and abdominal pressure strongly increases when it shrinks. It also plays a role of protecting the lumbar vertebrae, proved that a turn "to protect low back → to show muscular strength" met human physiology.

【2-4 Experiment by the punch】

Here, let's try some experiments! In a group of 2 people, one fighter throws a right straight punch and stops in the place that it hit. His/her partner pushes back. At the moment, please compare these:

A) Punching while breathing in (inhale)
B) Punching while breathing out (exhale)

A)

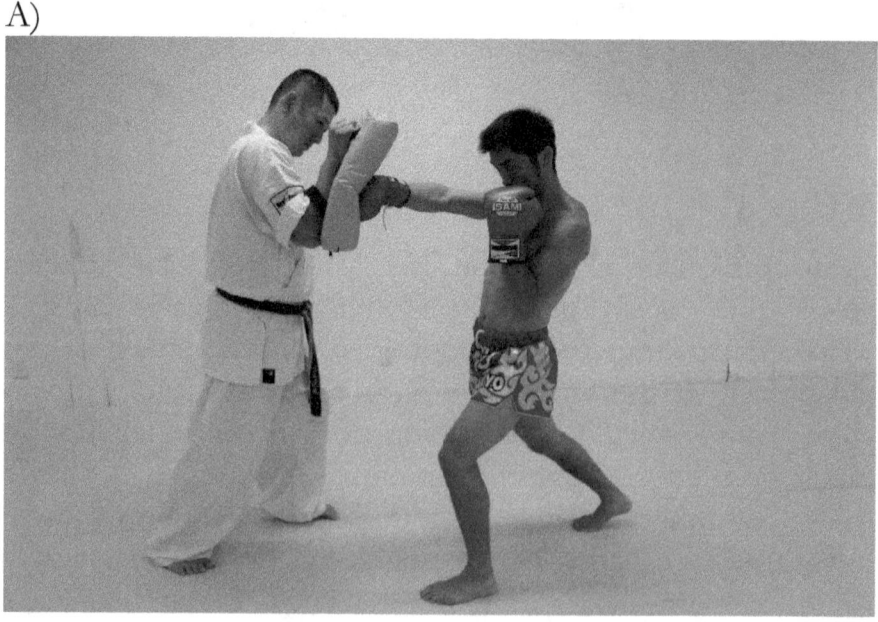

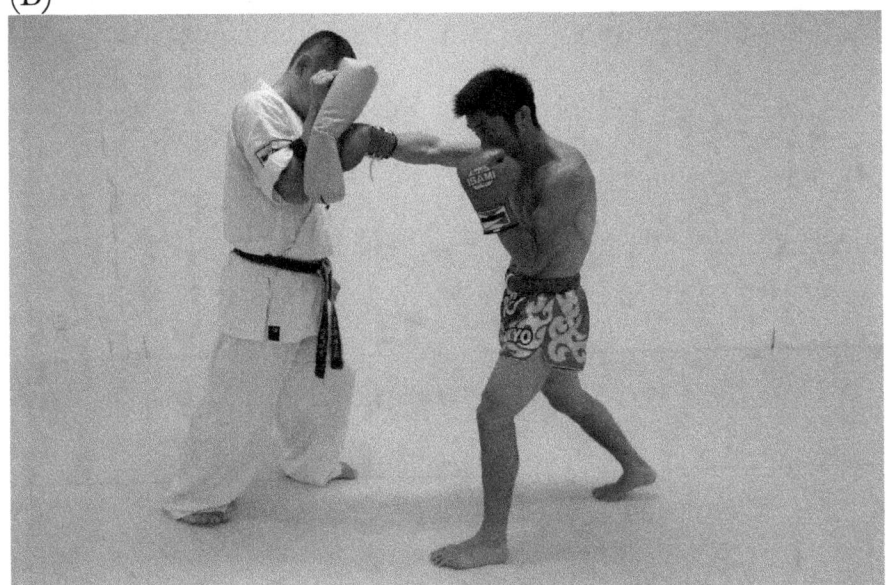

Probably you should feel the stronger punch with much more power generated when you let your transversus abdominis muscle strongly shrinks and retract the stomach while breathing out. It is recognized as an essential breathing method in competition, including weightlifting and powerlifting, when momentary power is required. At this point, some athlete said, "I feel that the muscular strength of the upper body and the muscular strength of the lower part of the body become one". If there is someone who does not feel that the force is occurring with respect to the musculature in both the upper and the lower part of the body. Please check the lumbar vertebrae area and see how to use transversus abdominis muscle and breathing. You will know that power will improve considerably after you check and correct it right.

Please breathe out so the transversus abdominis muscle will shrink, and let's aim at the improvement of the performance and the improvement of the fighting career.

Not only the blows but also the moment to lift up an opponent by Judo, Jujitsu, MMA, Wrestling, and so on.

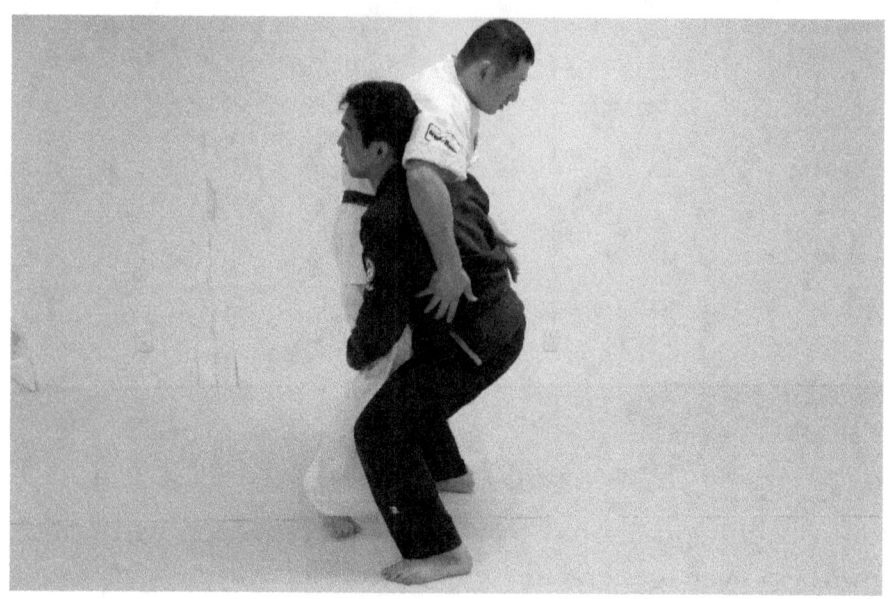

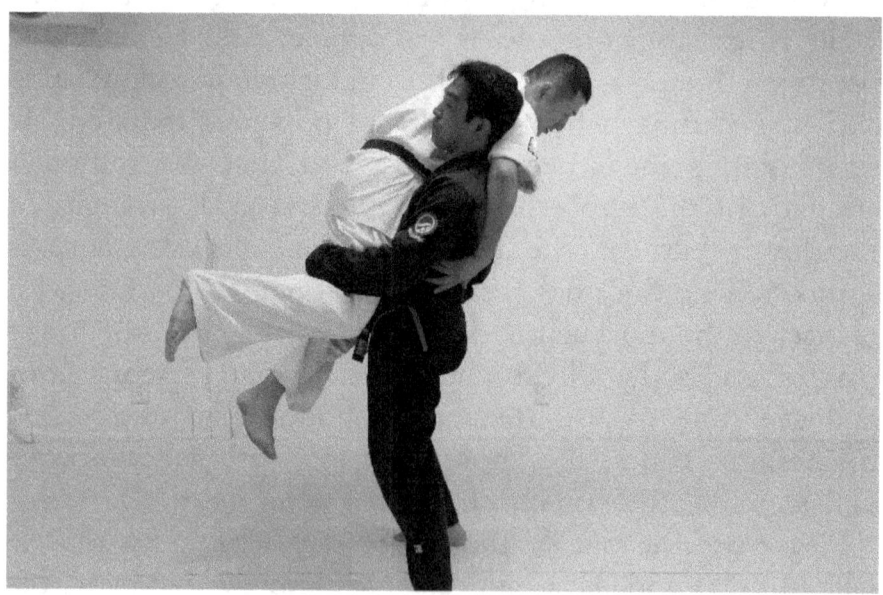

【2-5 Experiment by the kick】
A) Inflate your stomach while breathing in and hit with your knee
B) Retracting your stomach while breathing out and hit with your knee
A)

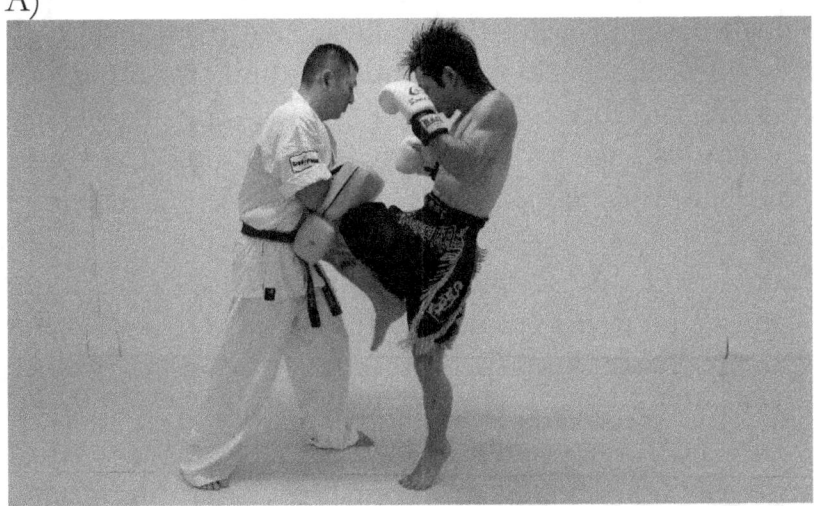

B)

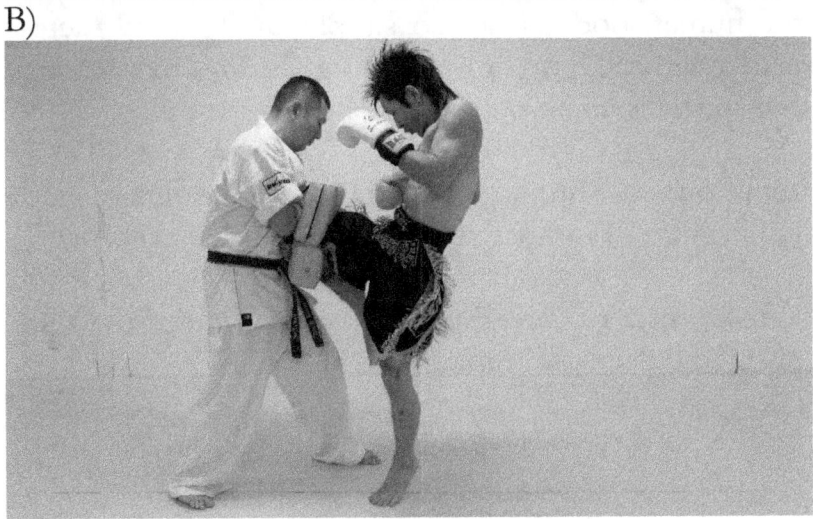

You may try it with front kick or axe kick, whatever. You will find that you can raise kicking leg a lot higher with ease. The reason why is that it becomes easy to put up your leg without an abdominal muscles interfering, because the internal organs come close to the lumbar vertebrae side (the back side) when the abdominis muscles contract. Those who are not good at high kick, high front kick, high round house and back spin, tends to think that it is just because he is "lacking flexibility" or he only has "hard body", but can try kicking high while letting transverse abdominis shrink consciously, you will see a different result.

Speaking from muscular tissue point of view, it is right that "muscular strength and power rise if you make your muscle big. When some people say "If the range of your joint movement is wide, you can kick higher" is an opinion just from the joints point of views, it's just one of a lot of elements of high kicking. Of course those are important, but the human body is not so simple, and several factors are related with each other in harmony. So you may say that fighting sports is an all-out fight of body and soul.

Breathing out → Shrinkage and transfer abdominis muscle → Stabilization of lumbar vertebrae → Muscle exertion.

Let's make use of breathing power to understand the complicated linkage of human body!

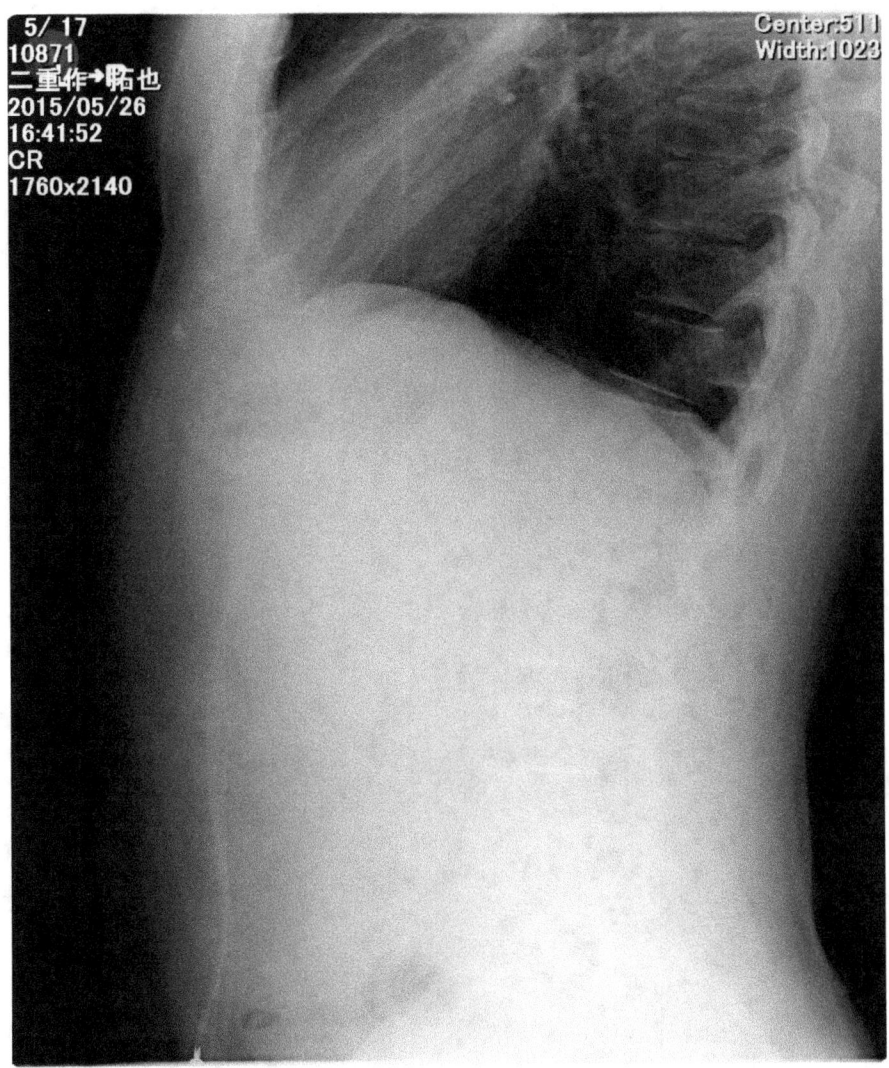

Inhale

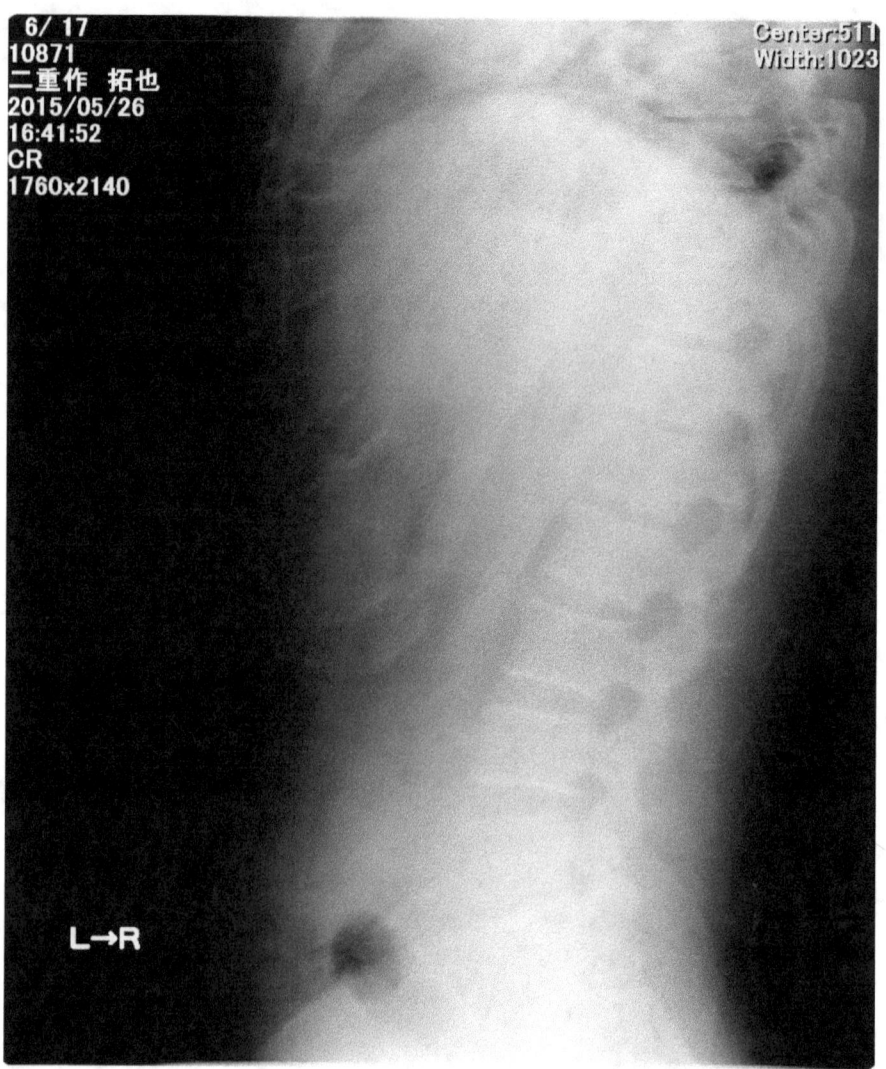

Exhale

【2-6 Breathing and stamina】

When we want to develop stamina, a big effect will be made when we become more conscious of our breathing.
"How much time can you move with only one breath?" (I assume this as an index).

Let's do some shadow training as fast as you can, and keep on exhaling while doing the exercise. When you finished exhaling, stop the exercise and see how long you did the exercise. The quantity of oxygen you are able to take in with only one breath is limited. So, the purpose is to be able to keep on moving with that little oxygen. The human body changes when it has an oxygen deficient condition. In this circumstance, the oxygen concentration is low. The body produces in the kidney a hormone called erythropoietin. The erythropoietin works on the bone marrow which is where blood is produced, and effectively increases red blood cells, this increases hemoglobin that carry oxygen throughout the body, so in conclusion oxygen has a better transport that goes throughout the body.

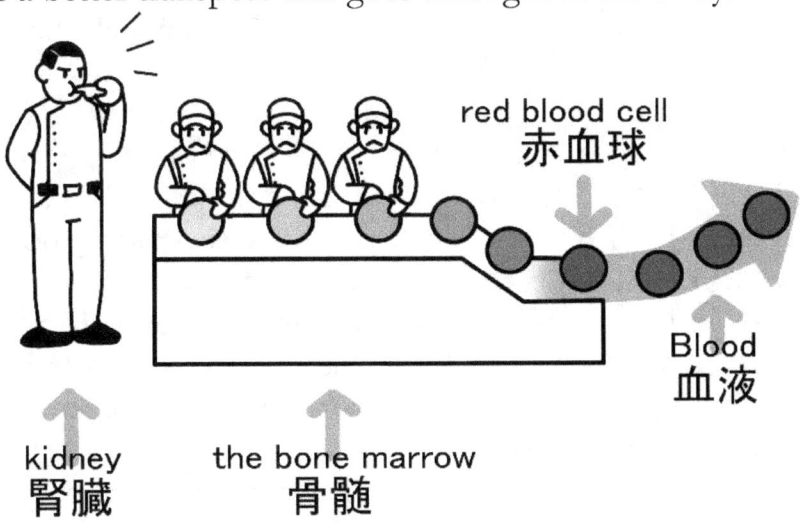

red blood cell
赤血球

Blood
血液

kidney
腎臓

the bone marrow
骨髄

59

To produce a similar effect, Olympic marathon runners lodge and train at a high mountain to expose themselves to low oxygen concentration, this is called "high-altitude training". Martial art fighters also do this kind of training that simulates "high-altitude training" by wearing a special mask. Any exercise that reduces the number of times you breathe in as much as possible prolongs the time of the exercise and also connects to stamina training to get an effect similar to that.

【2-7 Developing stamina project】

Mr.Makoto Nishiyama, graduated from the Tokyo University which is the most difficult university to enter in Japan. He is a businessman, a father, and a pro kickboxer at the same time. He was an excellent pro kickboxer and had three Championship belts in his in hand, which were All-Japan's titles, the WFCA's world title and M-1 champion title is of Muay-Thai. He also won by KO in K-1 world max 2010. One day he fought in a certain match, he was OK at the beginning, but his stamina disappeared in the midst, and lost by points after full five rounds. Afterwards he came to me and we designed the revival project.

First of all, he sat down on a chair holding 3 kilogram spindle in both hands, and then he started shadow boxing very quick, on and off, repeatedly. I recorded how long he could continue it when he inhaled, and I stopped counting the seconds when he finally exhaled. We tried this training every week. He was able to shadow train for only 12 seconds at first, gradually he was able to maintain more than a minute. As the length of the time of one round at a

kickboxing match is three minutes, means that he was able
to keep moving during one round only with 2~3 inhales.
Of course many factors affect the real game results, so I
know that things doesn't always go straight nor does always
contribute to the results. Nishiyama, had no confidence
with his stamina before, but he overcame it with this simple
training that shows him what he needed by objective data
and also make it clear for any fighter to do. Finally he got
win by K.O with upper knee kick in the final round, and he
got the world title. In the following match, he kept fighting
full five rounds against the opponent who was a ranker of
the other denomination and he won the victory again by
points.

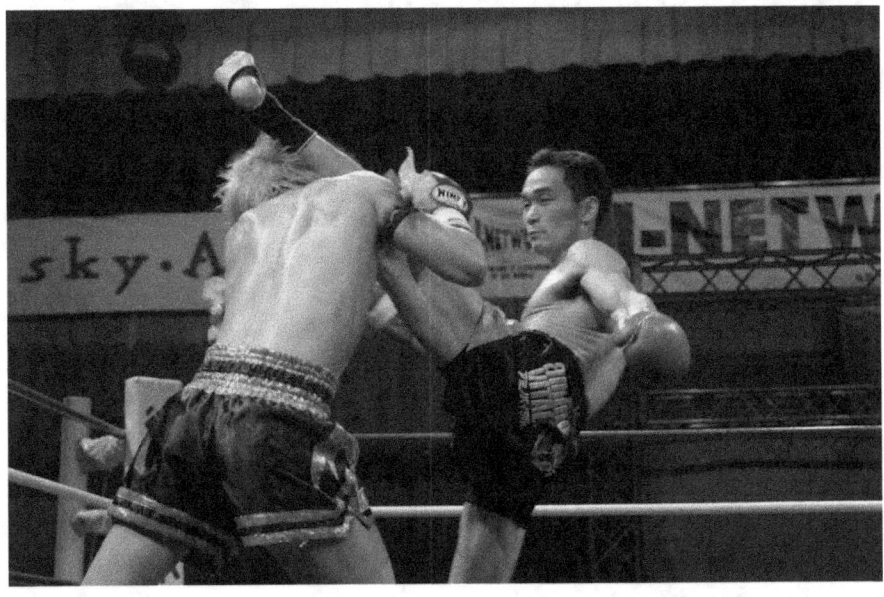

When a fighter doesn't have confidence in his stamina, if
the match turns to be a war of attrition, it is natural for him
to feel insecure. I think this is the most important fact for
every competitor to acquire enough stamina and be

prepared so they can keep fighting full time against an opponent. We can't tell when the match will be over before we fight the match. In addition, working out with a straw in your mouth is effective way of imposing a load on breathing. Breathing with a straw, make respiratory tract resistance grows high, and you can impose a load on both at the time of inhale and exhale, then your respiratory muscle is strengthened.

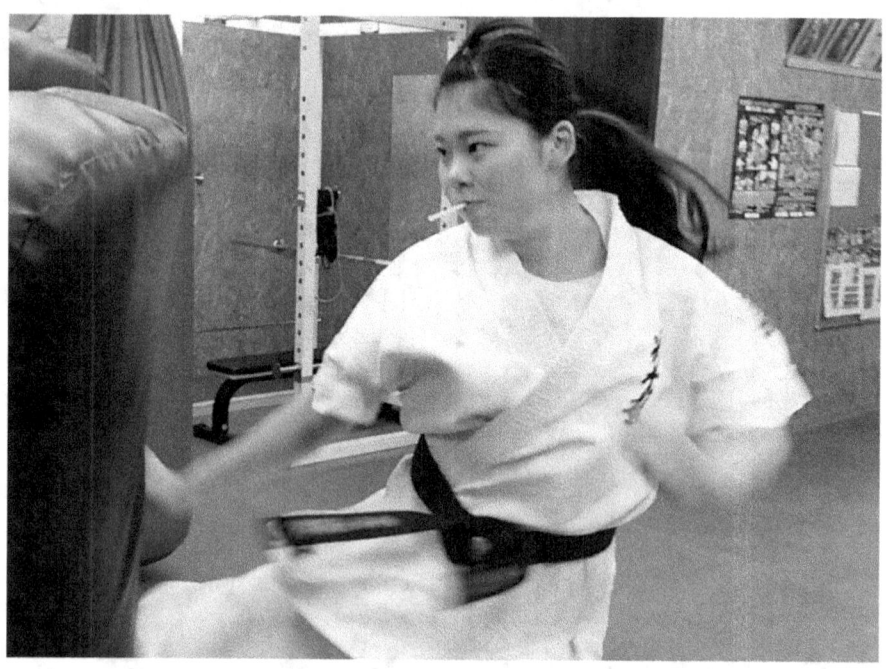

【2-8 Resistance in water】
Swimming is a very effective way to exercise. The water pressure exerted on the rib cage and abdomen can be a training of the respiratory muscle group. Since loads other than gravitational direction are applied underwater,

resistance on the "Movement itself" is one of the merits which is difficult to see in other cases.

For strengthening the cardiorespiratory function of combat sports athletes, who participate in events like events such as running and jogging are mainly adopted, but when injuring the lower body, or during rehabilitation, injuries worsen if you forcibly run, It will rather weaken. In that case, if you introduce underwater walking or swimming, sometimes in training in the ocean or river, training is not limited to stamina, as well as prevention of worsening of injuries due to reduced load on the lower limbs.

In fighting sports and martial arts, contacts with partners are constantly present in the exercise system, so tearing of microscopic muscle or tissue.

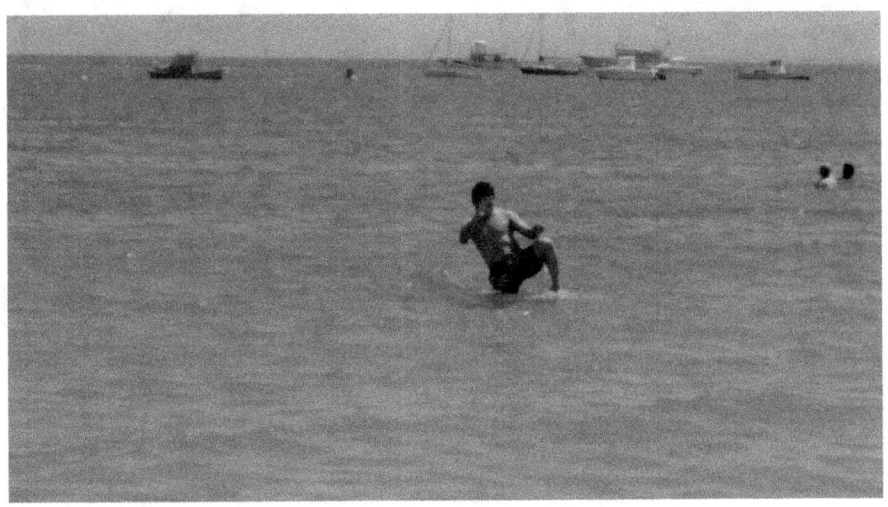

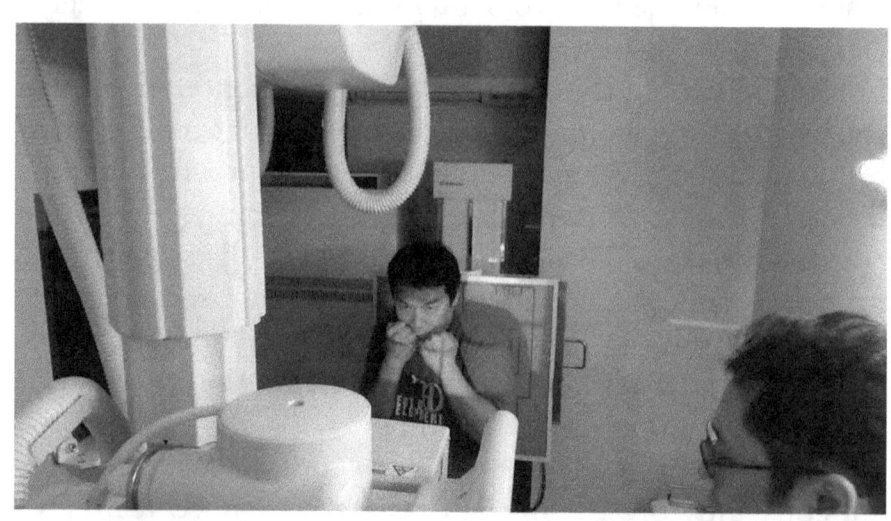

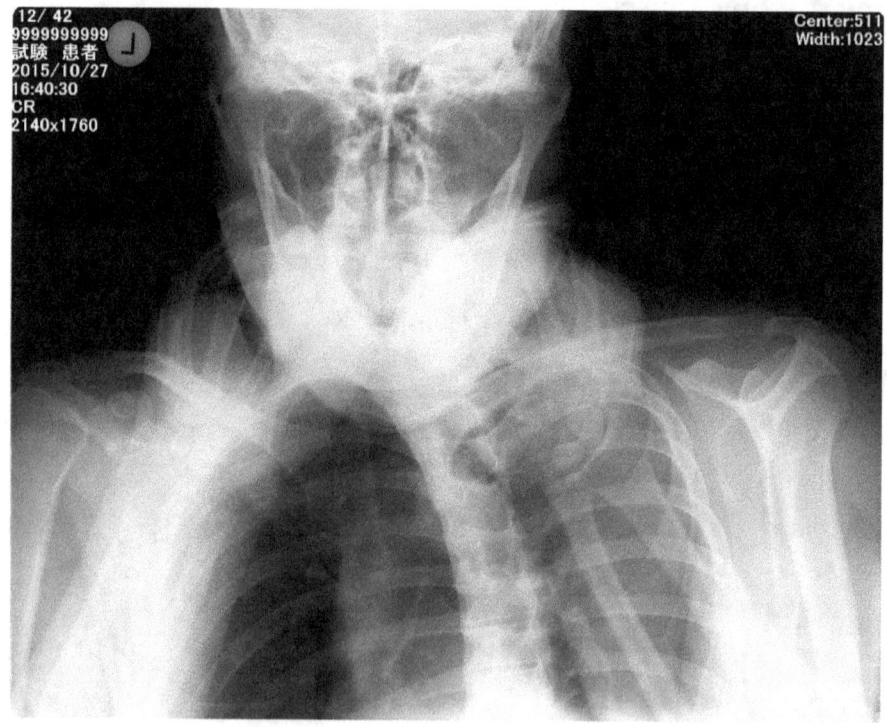

12/ 42
9999999999
試験 患者
2015/10/27
16:40:30
CR
2140x1760

Center:511
Width:1023

3 Proprioception

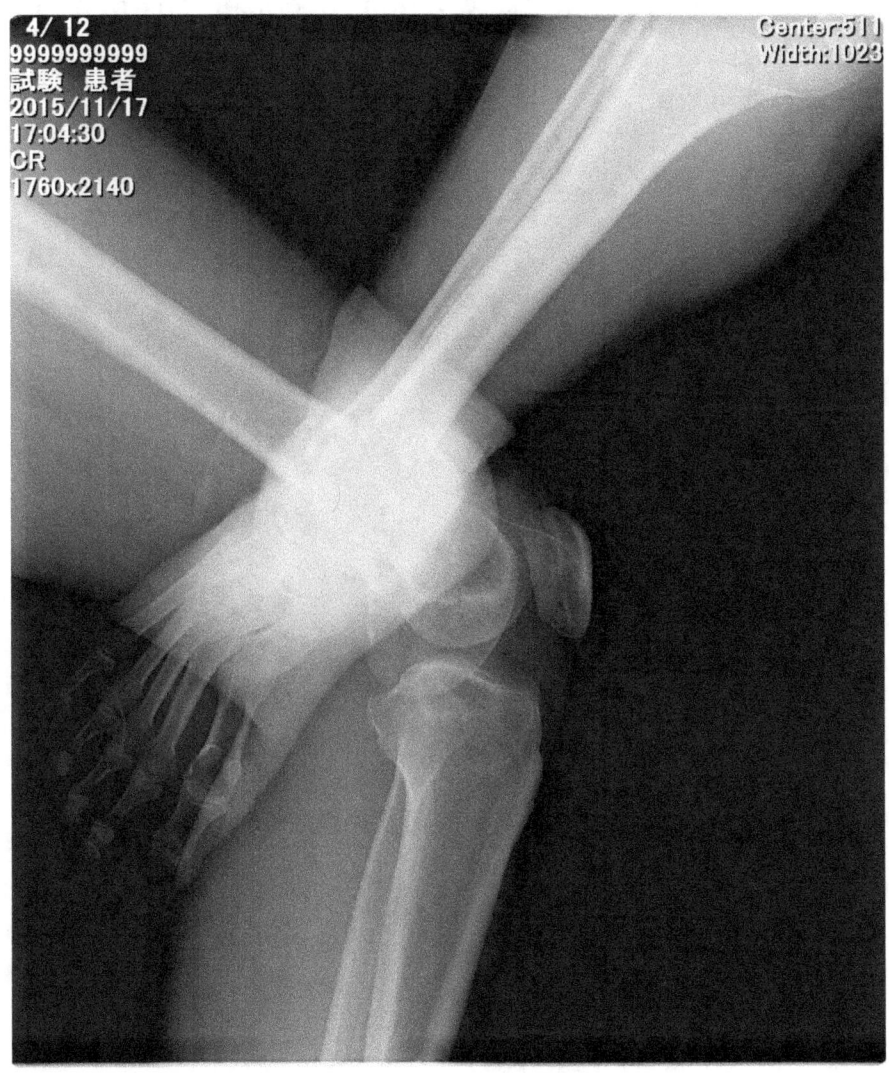

【3-1 Proprioception and performance】
The input of information, except sight, is very effective for performance and safety improvement in fighting. Proprioception sends information such as the position of bone, the angle of joint, the pressure of muscle, to the brain for processing. The term proprioception comes from the Latin "proprius" it means "one's own", and "capio", means "to grasp." This term refers to a person's unconscious perception of movement as detected by the nerves in the body. Proprioception allows a person to perceive the information of their own body.

For example, try this:

1. Close your eyes.

2. Let both arms hang at your side.

3. Bend your left arm at the elbow up 90 degrees.

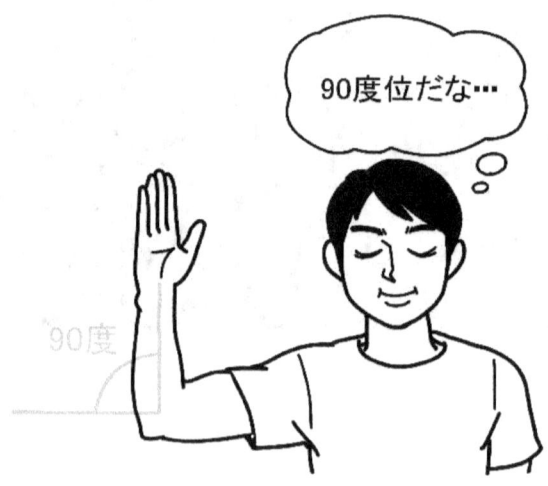

I think that you can perceive or sense that your flex is at about 90 degrees without having to look. It will be less difficult to do that at approximately 120 degrees, or 45 degrees performance with your eyes closed. Proprioception, is the sense of "To what angle the knee bends", without inputting the information from the sight sense." The vector of force is at the direction from left to the spine", "The muscle tension of the calf is high."

A strong fighter is intuitively aware of this sense, and able to move in a way that allows them to keep superior balance. A strong fighter is able to counter strike even with minimal information from the sense of sight. Even in sparring, the information received through proprioception from the moment in which he touched the partner in the grappling or ground fight, is a result of training countless hours. In a real fight or match, sometimes sight is limited by a partner´s attack or bleeding. The fight continues, so fighters should train with this in mind:

1) Improving the ability to process sight information.
2) Improving the ability to be able to move when sight is limited.

【3-2 Close eyes and apply external force】

I would love to introduce an example of a program that gives students a path for concrete proprioceptive improvement. One beneficial training exercise goes as follows:

1. A fighter stands with closed eyes and,
2. A partner pushes him/her in various ways from the outside.
3. A fighter uses his senses to adjust.

This training develops a fighters ability to look for a stable state, while flowing motion for power, and well-being, while using external force adversely against the opponent. For example, the partner pushes the same shoulder, but sometimes rapidly, or slowly. The partner changes the direction of power, or pushes the shoulder twice or three times, always adjusting movement and timing.

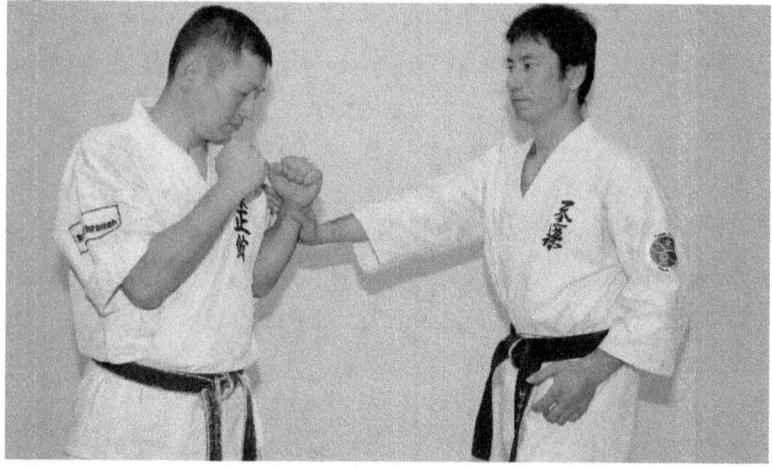

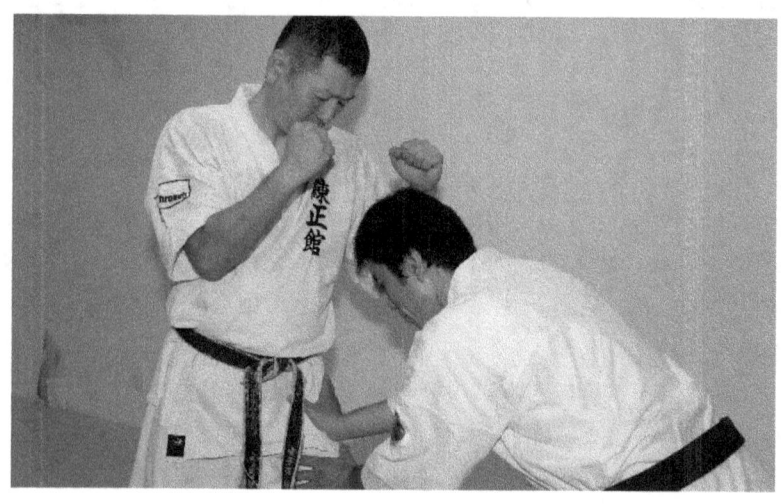

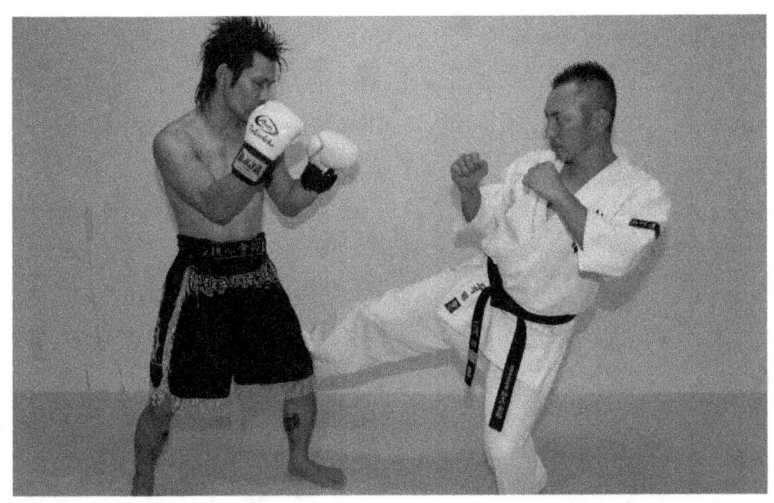

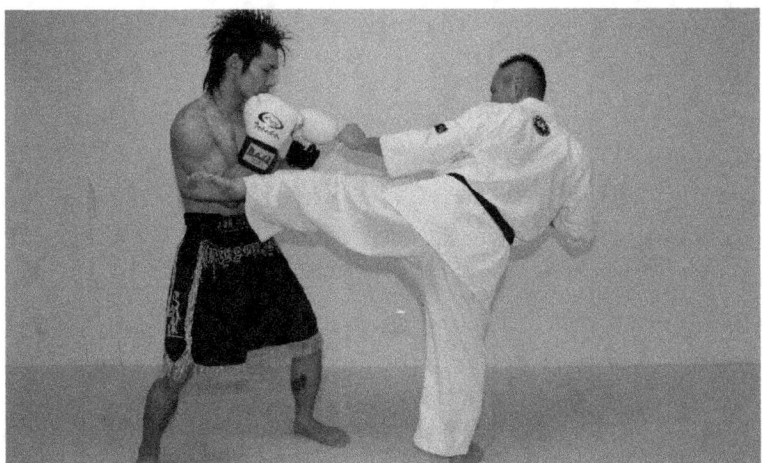

The first-class fighters only block against a kick of an opponent for an instant. They understand the role and the intention of the kick, First-class fighters can tell the intention of their opponent. They know when a kick is a fake or a lure, they know when an opponent is spent and his kicks weaken, they know when an opponent is only going for points, and they know when an opponent is truly serious and gunning for a takedown.

These can look like the same kick to a less experienced fighter but they are all very different situations. A first-class can make the right linkage between information from the proprioceptive nerve system and his/her memories of fights. Learning "how to react to the external forces from an opponent" is an essential theme of martial arts and Budo. As good fighters progress to becoming first-class fighters developing this ability is an effective way to proceed. Please change the external force in the empty hand into a kick and change it into a part of the tackle and the throw.

【3-3 Moving from an unstable state】

From the state standing firmly on the flat floor, hit the mitt and the sandbag, kick. I think that this is done in every dojo and gym. Of course, these exercises are very important in the sense that you know the stable condition. However, it is a waste if you stay there. What is more important from that point is building a "neural circuit that can move even in an unstable state". In the actual match, the battle progresses in a situation lacking stability such as low kick being kicked and legs shaking, shaking the brain by getting a punch and collapsing the balance. So, if you are only practicing to attack only from a stable position, you will learn a program that will "move after restoring the collapsed balance to a stable state". As you pursue how to move the body at the next moment of instability, neural circuits including proprioceptive sensation will be constructed more and more. Starting from a tricycle, it becomes a bicycle with training wheels, then remove the training wheels, and then even be able to ride an unicycle. You cannot see it from the outside, but it has the strength to get it for the first time seeking such instability. After experiencing an unstable place, if you experience a stable place, the quality of your movement will change at all. This can also be said to be a load for getting stronger.

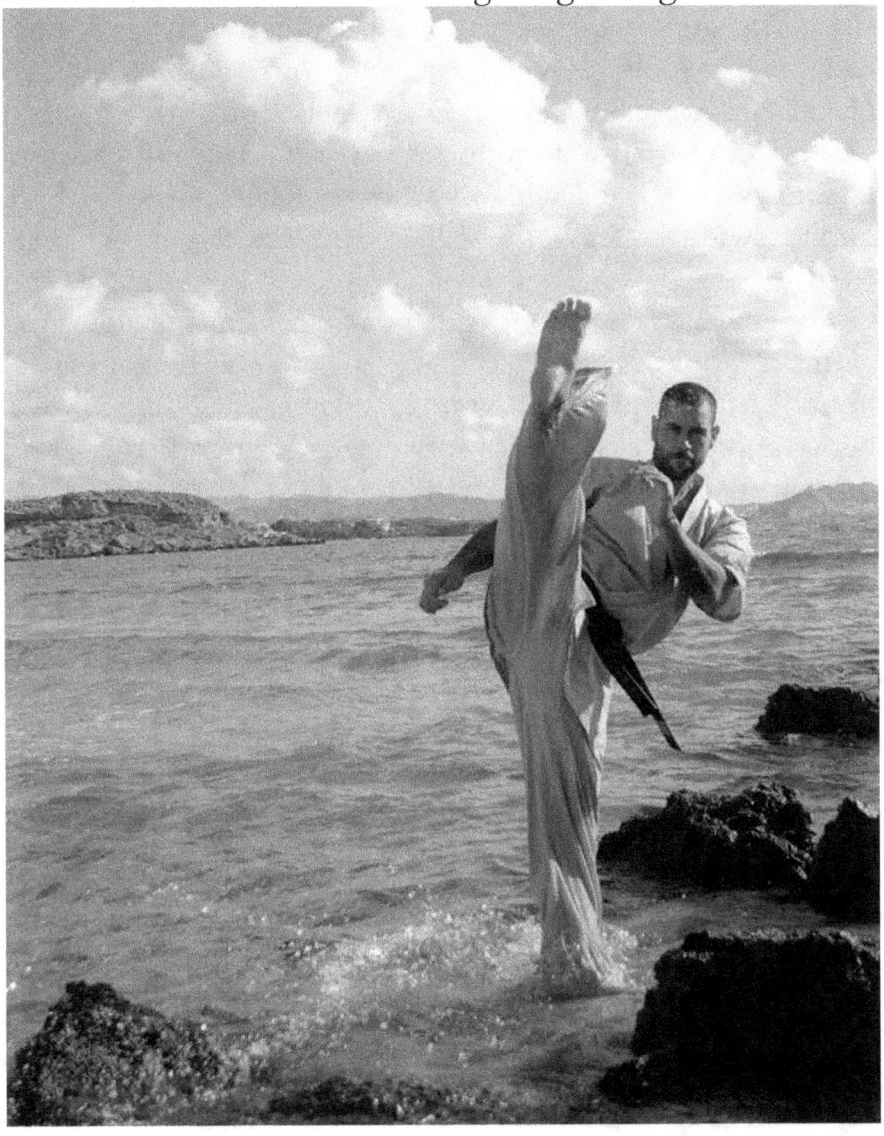

In the case of mixed martial arts, the deployment will change in the style of A standing technique, B throwing technique, C grappling technique, so even one blow must be able to deal with various aspects very much. Various situations are predicted with the same punch and same kick, such as blows when moving from standing skill to ground, blows when the opponent gets into throwing, and blows to capture the moment when rising from the ground position. It is an era where you cannot win unless you are familiar with the movement that connects the aspect of A → B, B → C, C → A, as well as the exercises of A, B, and C respectively. How long can you make an unstable time within 2 hours of practice time? And in the remaining 22 hours of life, how much you can increase the relationship between inputs of proprioceptive sensation and streak out, this part becomes "invisible difference".

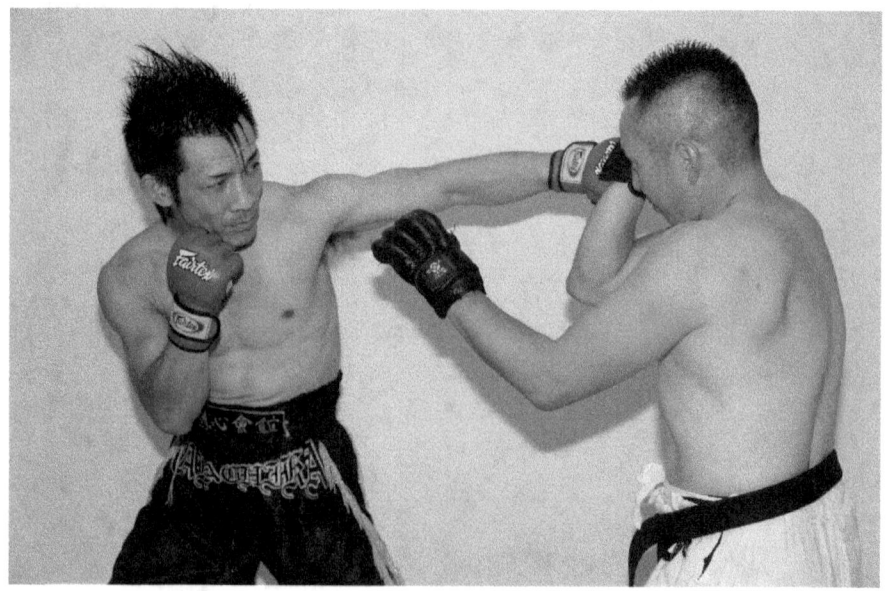

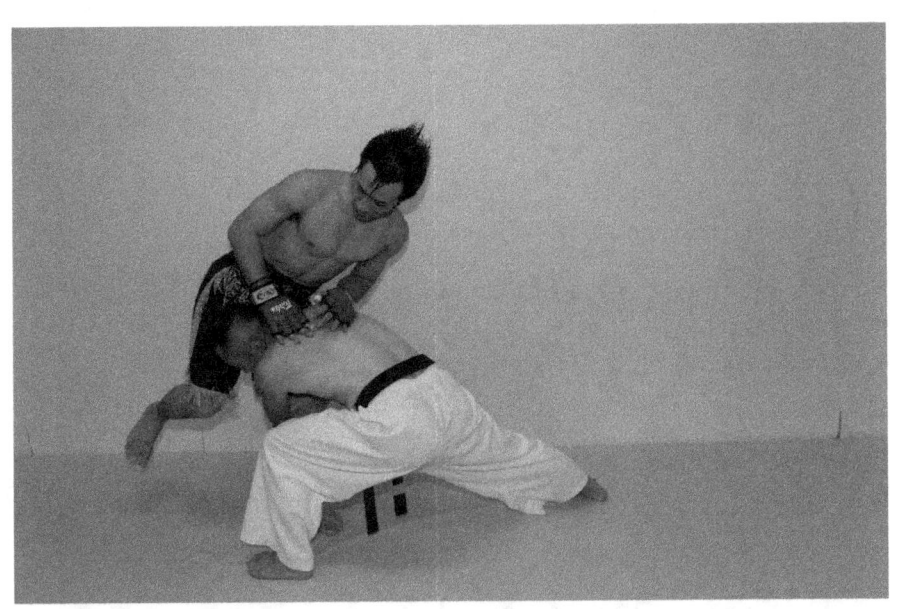

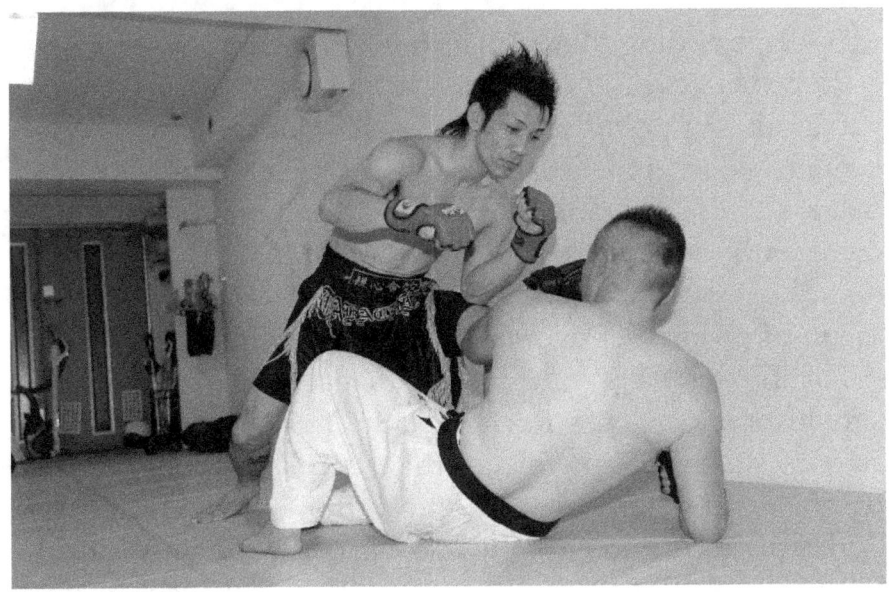

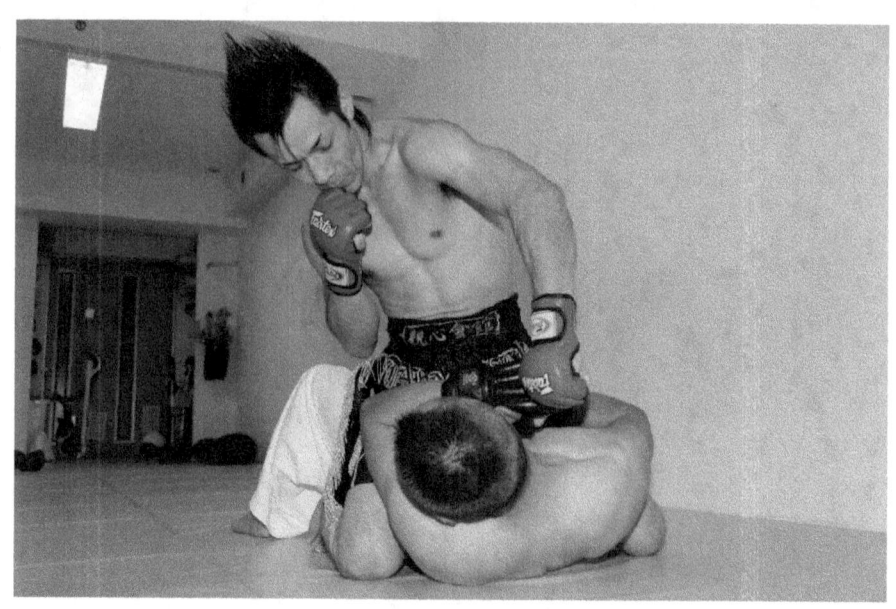

【3-4 Eye closing Muay Thai clinch】

Proprioceptive sensation training creates various variations by shutting out visual information. While keeping safety, practice the regular practice. Just that alone makes a considerable load. For example, clinching is commonly done at kick boxing and Muay Thai gym. By doing this with closed eyes it becomes a very effective menu of proprioceptive sensation improvement.

The fighter side will close both eyes. The partner side should open the eyes to protect the fighters' safety. Please start as slowly as possible so that there is no injury due to batting and hit the forehead. The partner should move their bodies to a position which is easy to receive and lead the state where the fighter is easy to move. This can be done not only with standing skill clinch, but also in a standing state like grappling or sumo wrestling.

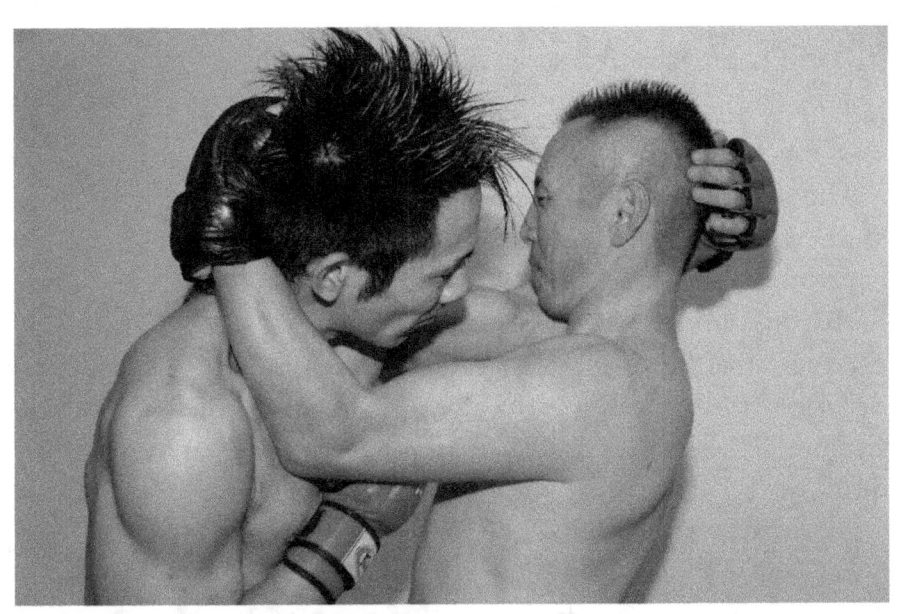

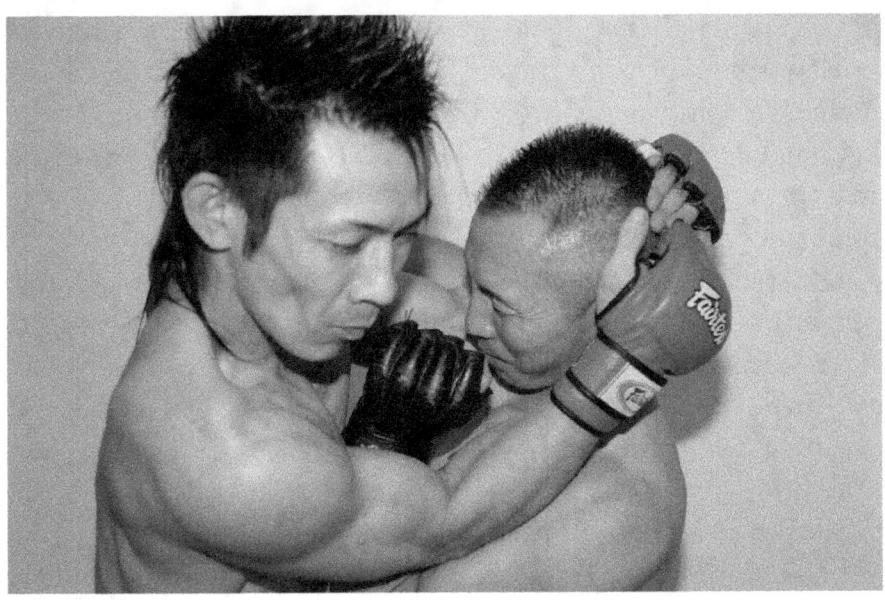

【3-5 Proprioceptive sensation improvement program with balance ball】
·Balance · Defense Standing Techniques

The fighter creates a state of knee standing so that the shin strikes the ball and holds it with a fighting pose. If you cannot get onto the balance ball successfully, please start with the state where you first ride the ball and do shadow boxing of only the upper body. Those who can do shadow boxing on the ball getting gently lightly attacked by the partner. The fighter will maintain a balance or perform a defense in response to the opponent in front while recovering from unbalanced state. Just by doing the defensive movement, the center of gravity always moves. There are fighters who say "Do not move the center of gravity" and "Let me stay still" with this program, but it is not an image of such movement but rather it is done by an image "to find a position that is likely to be stable while keeping on moving" works better. (It is the same principle that it is more stable to balance while moving the body than to completely stop on an unicycle.)

The partner who pulls off the attack, let's profit this opportunity, make different kinds of blows rich in variety. Both the kicking side and the defending side will throw away the consciousness of "let's do it well", you should challenge and fail more and more, make a neural circuit including proprioceptive sensation from falling to the ground repeatedly but safely.

When creating a neural circuit, the number of success is not important, but the number of trials is. Please try to increase the denominator (the number of trials), not the numerator (successful number of times). When the number of successful times increases, please stage up to a more difficult load.

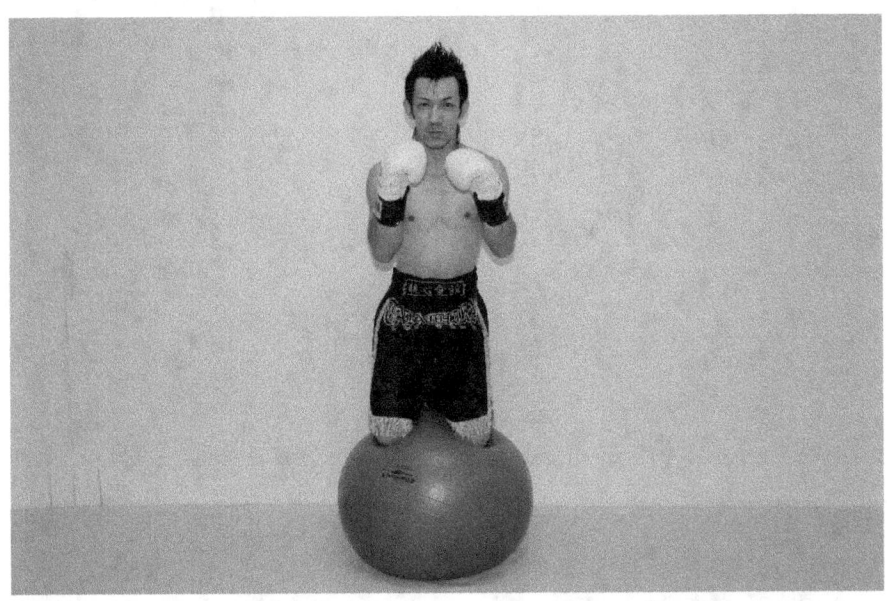

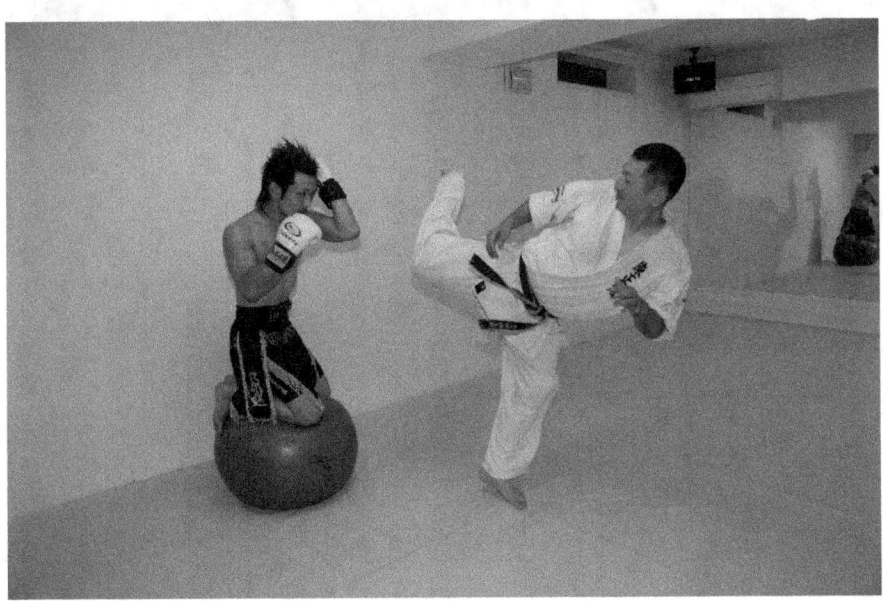

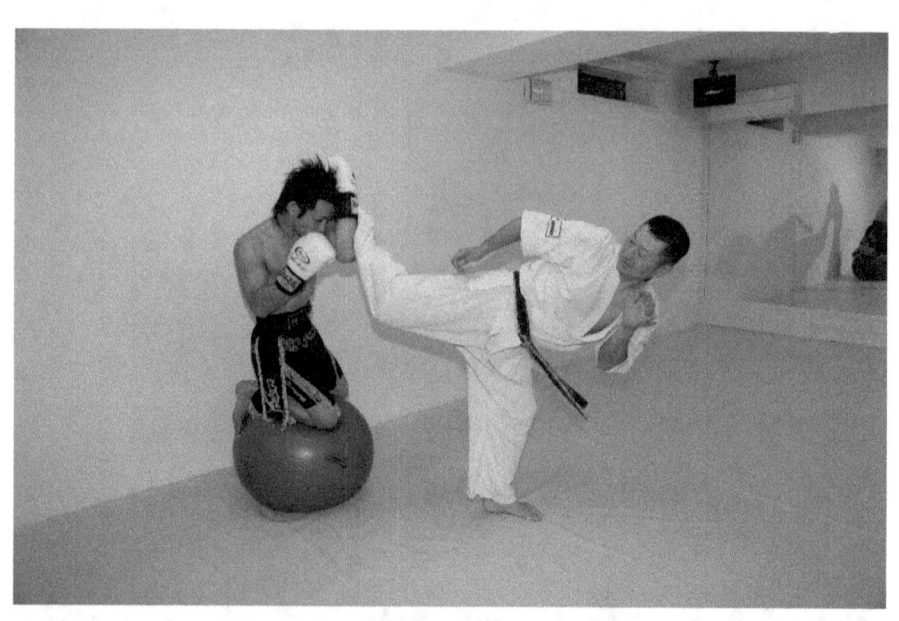

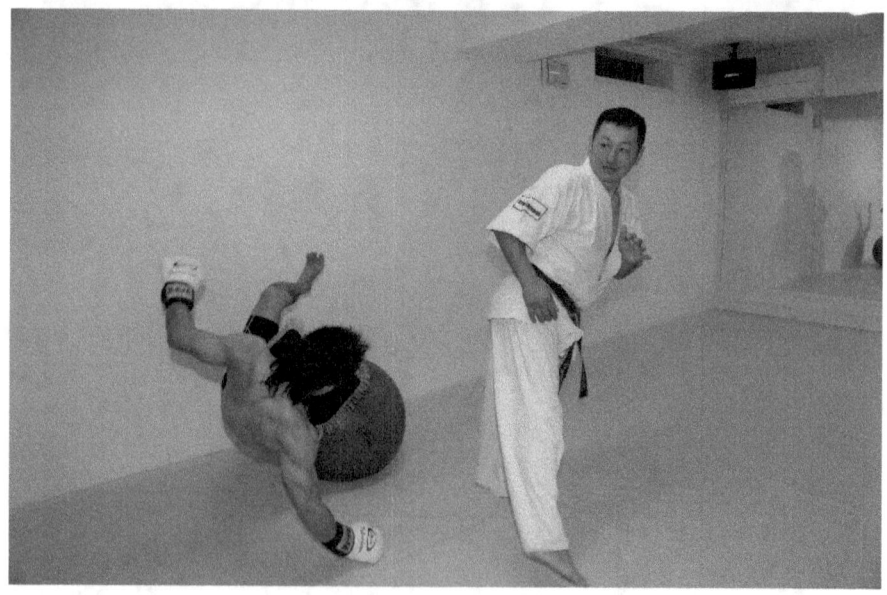

· Balance · Defense MMA chapter

It is a way to train proprioceptive sensation in mixed martial arts. The fighter lies on his/her backs against the ball and make their backs touch the ball. Then ground only one foot to the mat. The partner stands in the direction of the foot, kicks toward the fighter, and the fighter performs defense using jumps on the free side leg and foot. Not only the muscles of the arms and legs but also the end of the proprioceptive sensation nerve exists in the back and spinal streaks, tendons and ligaments. Very small muscle fibers such as multifidus muscle groups are gathered around the spine and play a role as a sensor to constantly monitor whether unreasonable load is applied to the spine. Being balanced on the back and the back of the body is essential technique in fighting sport and martial arts with ground techniques, and reinforcement of the proprioceptive sensation around the spine also leads to back pain prevention, so it is important as a program to improve athletes life.

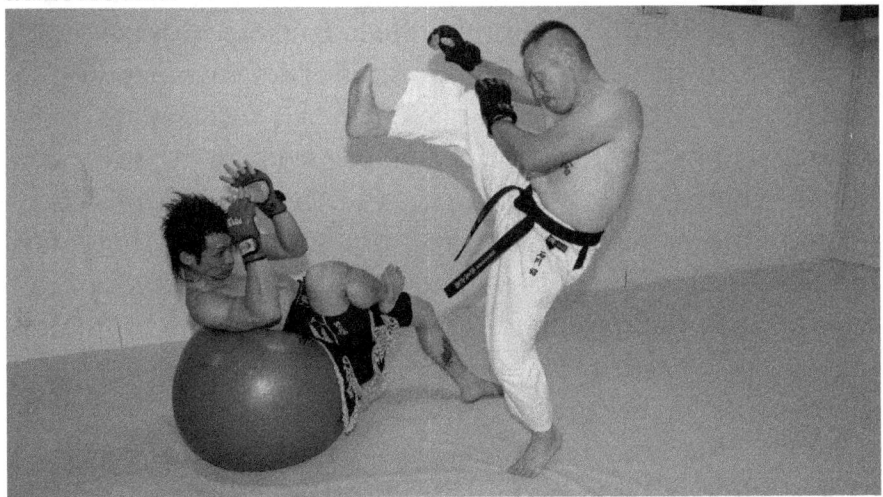

· Balance punch

Like Balance Defense, create a state of knee standing on the ball and will punch in the mitt that the partner holds. This is also a program that you can learn how to use the correct use of your body during punching, while proprioceptive sensory enhancement. When exercising, the main striking muscle is called to be the protagonistic muscle, but even in fighting sports or martial arts, even the same straight punch as it looks, the protagonistic muscle is different depending on proficiency level and type. A fighter who strikes with the shoulder joint as its center will fall down from the ball by reaction when he/she hit the punch. This is the condition of the so-called "hand-hitting" that the triceps and deltoid muscles of the brachial tendon have become the protagonistic muscle. If you are fighting against a pressurey fighter, a heavy opponent, or an opponent who is superior to your physique, you will pull back if mainly punching with the shoulder joint like this.

To hit without pulling back, use the hip joint in a direction to extend from the flexed state. Movement of extension from flexion of hip joint is efficient movement in weight movement of human because it is movement to use when walking or running. Let's use this as it is for the punch which is the hand-hitting. For those who are new to begin with, try reaching to hit 5 times. Please try it till you can throw more than 10 punches with full power. Fighters who tend to have punches only as hand-punching, fighters who hit only with the upper body, there are cases to show the improvement by integrating this program.

Set the theme yourself to find where to position your hands, where to position your head is the best, how to move the spine, which timing you should move the hip and shoulder joints, and so on. Balance ball is one of the goods that can be used as a strengthening method that will make you conscious of invisible proprioceptive sensation.

(1)

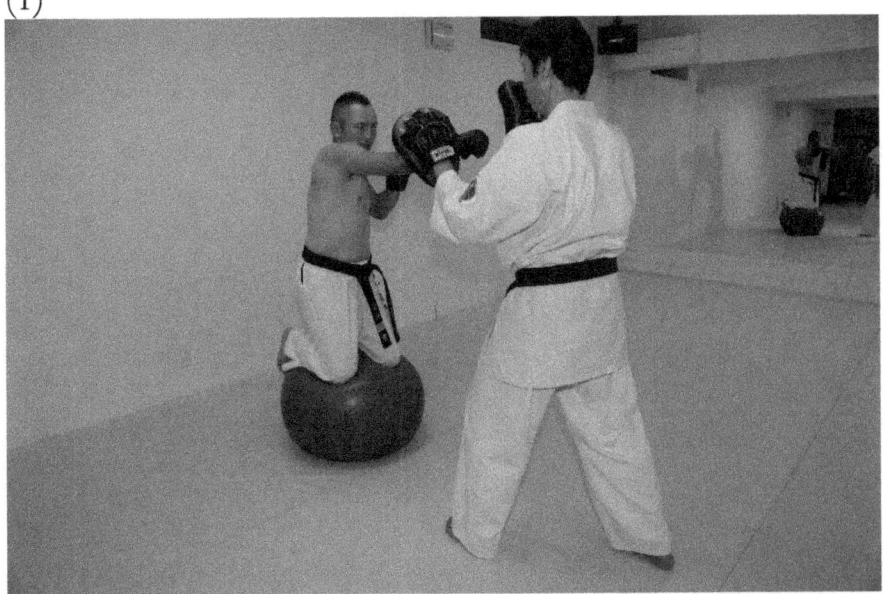

(2)

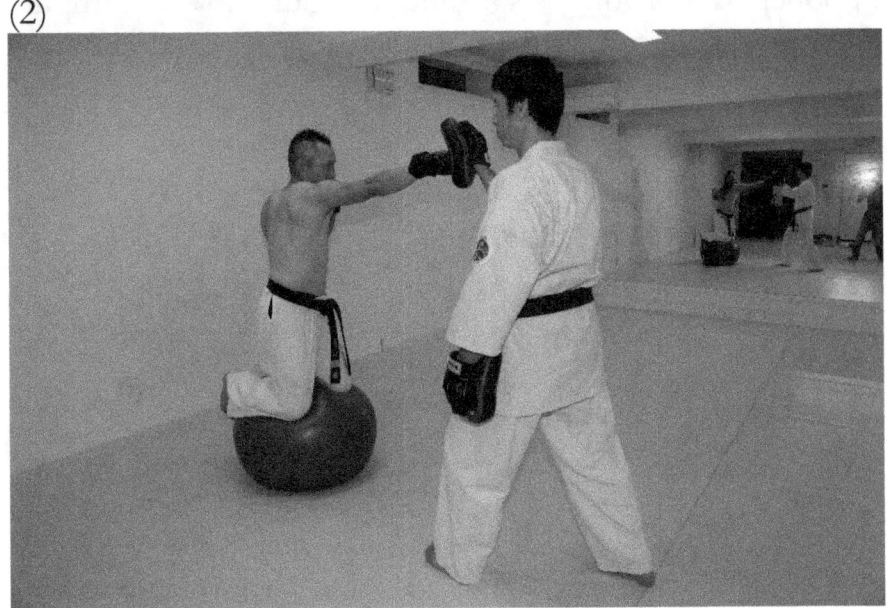

Balance punch (1), (2) comparison (1) is the center of the upper torso, (2) is the punch using the hip joint)

【3-6 Use joints and muscles as organ of information input】

Muscles and joints are indispensable for "exercise", and at the same time they are a group of "sensory organs". Especially in the ligaments on the joints, there are many unique sensory nerve endings exist, and keep sending the information of the length and pressure of the ligament, to the brain. The muscle also sends information on the tension and relaxation to the brain at the rear time, and information on which the exercise proceeds smoothly. First-class athletes of fighting sports and martial arts can use muscles, bones, joints, etc. as weapons when contacting opponents, not only as "Output" but also as "Input" organs through proprioceptive sensation.

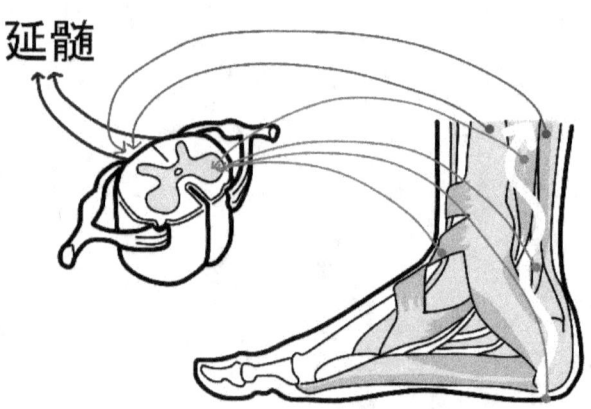

For example, some fighters instantly make corrections such as "I could knock down if I hit another 2 cm outer side", even if your hitting point was misaligned when they kicked a low kick. This is because memory and proprioceptive sensation are linked as to which point you hit makes the most damage at a routine basis, you can perceive the lag. In addition, there are also people sense the opponent, determining the direction in which the opponent is going to move, etc. to make the opponent under his control, with tiny touching part of his body even within just an instant. Although muscle strength and endurance are very important elements in fighting sports and martial arts, they are part of the loop of "inputting information from sensory nerve → information processing in the brain → output in the muscle via the motor nerve" Muscle strength and endurance without sensory input sometimes even interfere with performance. (They say spurious muscle cannot be used for fighting sports, that is because it is not strengthening this loop.) Not only for the fighters who are aiming at the performance improvement, but also for the fighters who are confident in their endurance but not able win a fight, the fighters who feel they are not talented, and fighters with many injuries and breakdowns, I am introducing "improvement of the proprioceptive sensation", wishing them to obtain the feeling of "a new sensation" like a first long distance ride with a bicycle.

【3-7 Training in nature】

In the 1990s, a group with shocking strength appeared in the world of fighting sports where modern scientific training occupies the mainstream, such as weight training and speed training. "Gracie family". It is a family that made the foundation of the current mixed martial art, and Brazilian jiu-jitsu.

Gracie Jiu-Jitsu is developed from Japanese ancient jiu-jitsu which was before controlled to be Judo, that traveled to Brazil, the country in the southern hemisphere. It has a technical system that can handle even the most challenging tournaments of almost anything, like with no restrictions on rules, besides bite, groin attack, and blinding, and had the strength without loss in the past. Rickson Gracie, the representative of the family, who was undefeated for 400 fights, emphasized training in the sandy beach, river and forest, and had the unique strength of manipulating his own supple and tough body freely. Many fighters run or dash on flat tracks and paved roads, but Rickson ran the mountain roads on which large and small stones are all around and unpaved convex roads. Since the ground contacting surface of the sole changes at random, varieties of stimulation are input to the proprioceptive sensation, and the neural circuit is strengthened. Even in training in the river, you can shift your weight while balancing against torrent external forces, and you can obtain the feeling that you cannot get easily in a swimming pool. Instead of hanging with a symmetrical iron bar in the gym or park, he was hanging the obi belt upwards and hanging in an unbalanced condition, and instead of lifting the barbell where the position of the center of gravity is easy to determine, he lifted some rocks and trees in the nature, while grasping the center of gravity of the opponent(object) instantaneously, he was strengthening the neural circuit and muscular strength.

By positively putting himself in an unstable environment of nature where it is difficult to obtain the stable situation, you can respond to changes, not by the direction that you enlarge your muscles and hit them with power, but I think that he was training the way which enhances movement and made a moving neural circuit including strengthening the proprioceptive sensation. Gracie family which the family members are eating with a consciousness that cooks formal natural ingredients themselves and takes in "life" into themselves without using supplements and protein, and seeks the original strength of man. The extremely healthy life cultivated in their nature was the source of strength of them.

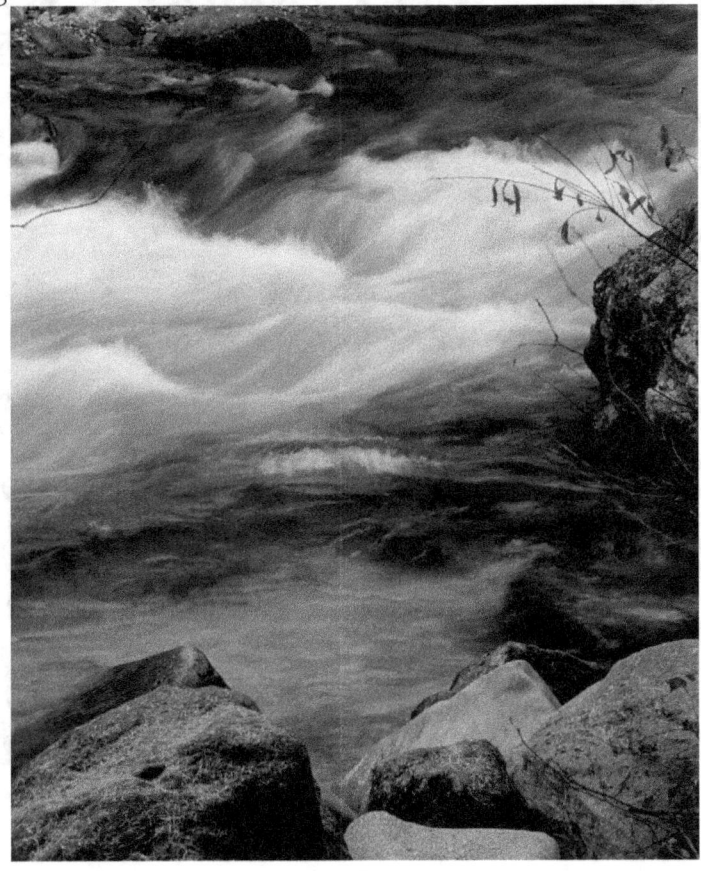

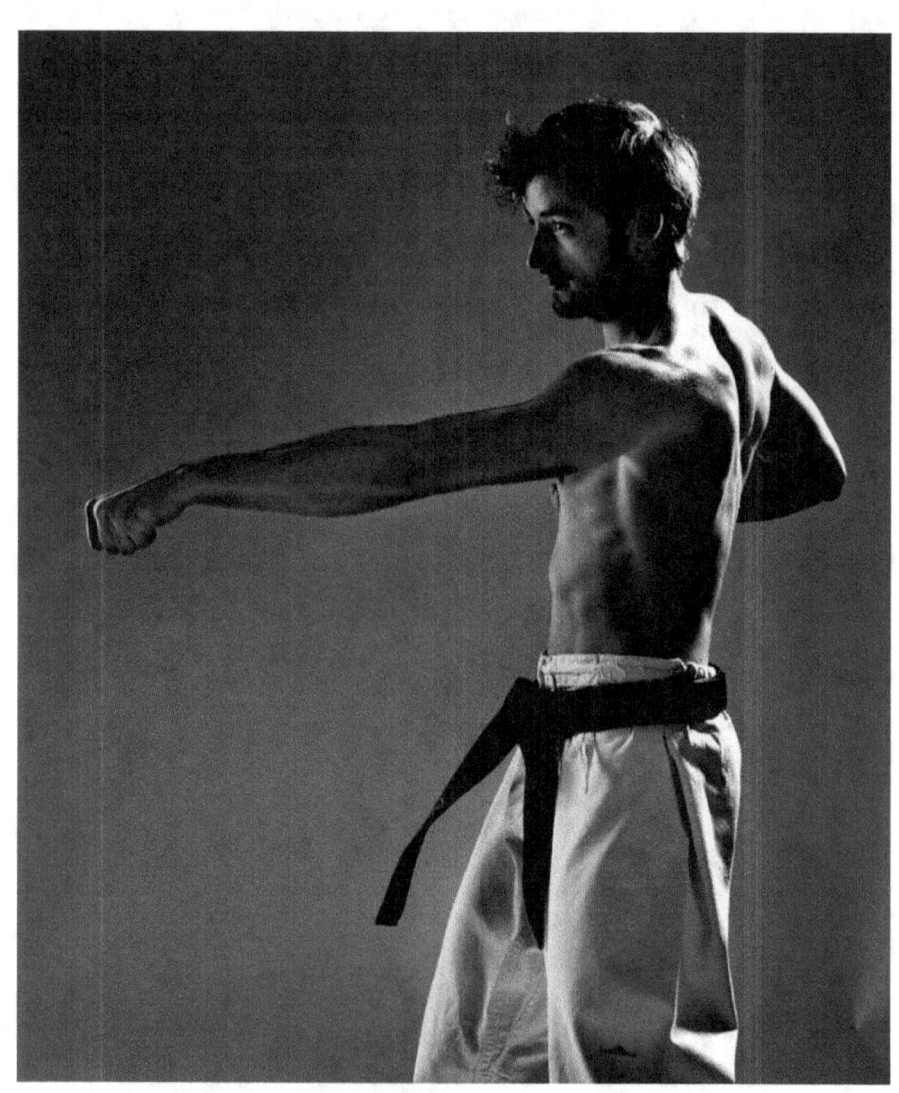

4 Joint Angle

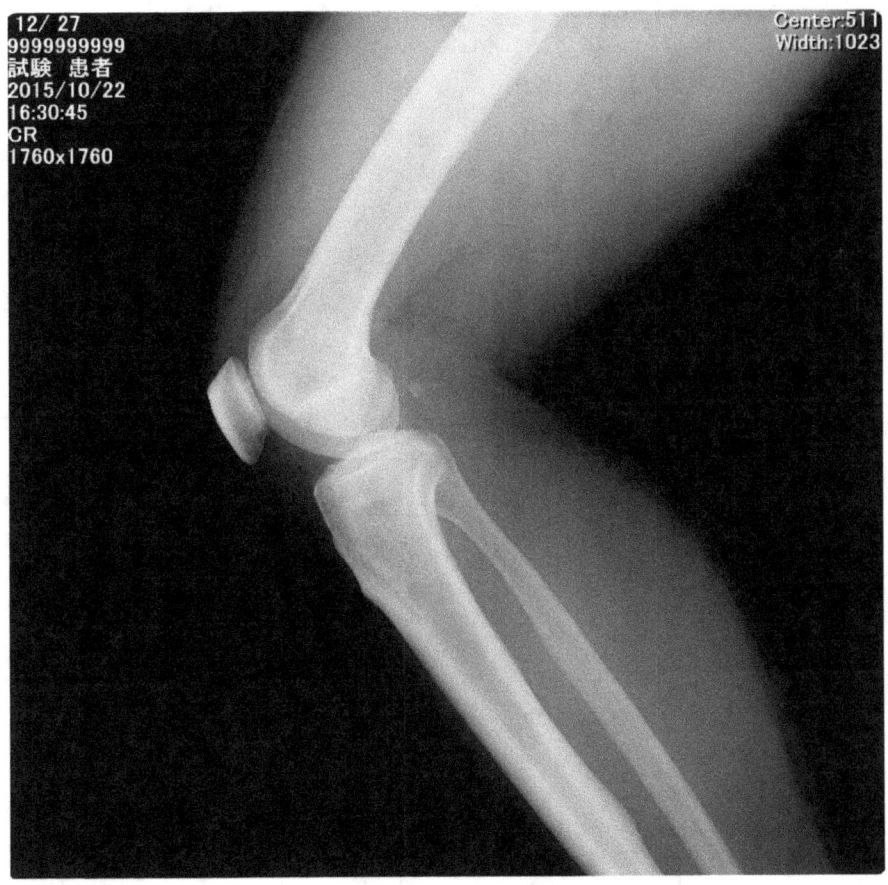

【4-1 About joint angle】

Human being's joints have the angles which could produce the force most comfortably with. For example, the angle of the elbow. For the elbow joint, we define "0 degree" at the angle when you raise both arms straight forward horizontally, and the upper arm and forearm are in a straight line. From that, shrink the bicep muscle to bend the arm to achieve 30 degrees, we call it 30 degrees flexion position. And so as bending 45 degrees then it's called 45 degrees flexion position. Generally, when we talk about the angle of the elbow, we may think of the angle which is made from bending forearm and upper arm with the hinge by the elbow. (In fact, I myself thought that way before I knew the medically correct joint angle measure method.)

The elbow joint 90 degrees is not the angle between the forearm and the upper arm, it is the state that it is bent 0 degrees to 90 degrees. At the 45 degrees flexion position, the angle between forearm and upper arm is 135 degrees. When the angle between the forearm and the upper arm is 30 degrees, it is expressed as 150 degree flexion position.

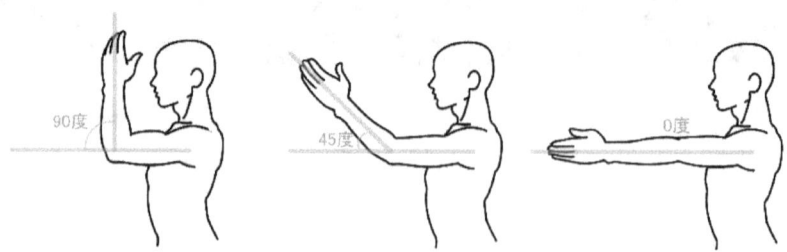

Even in the fingers joint, the second joint from the fingertip is generally called the second joint, but the first joints from the index finger to the little finger are called

"DIP joint", the second joints as the "PIP joint", and the third ones are called "MP joint". In the case of the thumb, because there is no PIP joint, the first one is called the DIP joint and the second one is called the MP joint. Like these examples above, there are many cases where common names differ from professional but worldwide common names and meanings. Here, in terms of giving priority to accuracy, I will describe it based on the above definition.

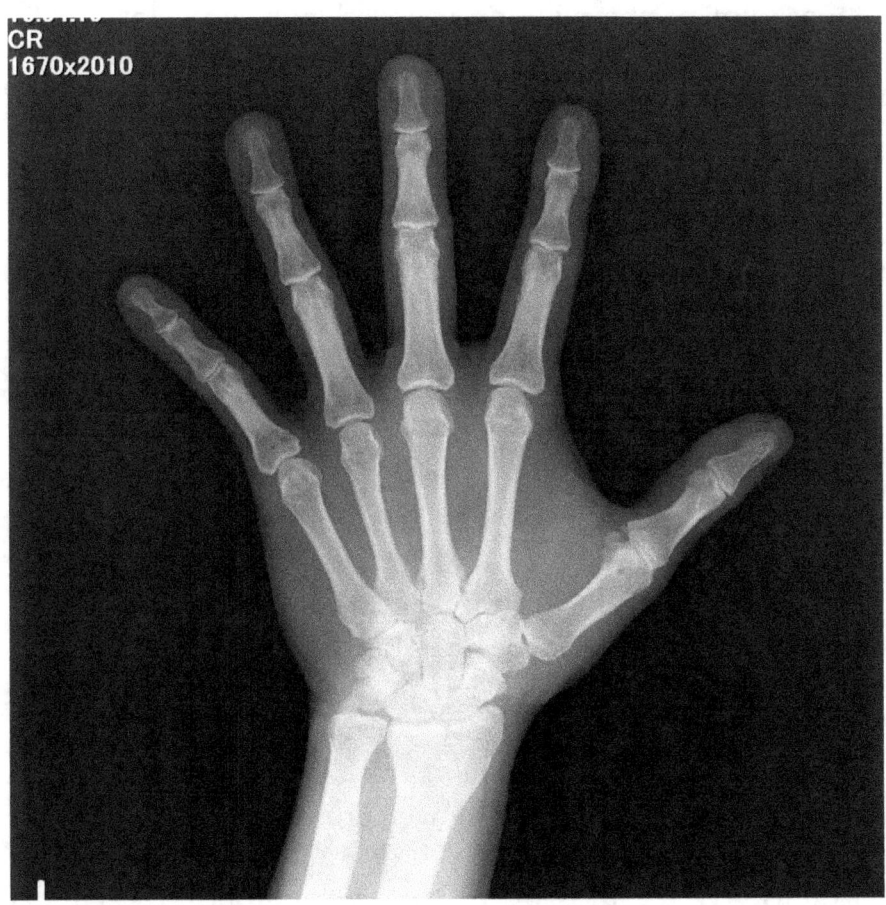

【4-2 What is the strongest angle for bending the elbow?】

The story returns to the joint angle of the elbow. When you go to a supermarket, you may see that, housewives are walking with the largely inflated shopping bags or plastic bags hanging on their arms. At this time, isn't the joint angle of the elbow about 90 degrees flexion position? At the sports day, we do tugs of war. Arn' t the angle of the elbow joint of the winning team athletes also close to 90 degrees, and are the elbow joint of the being dragged and losing team athletes close to zero degree? Thus, when bending an elbow joint, (of course, there are individual differences), an angle of about 90 degrees is the easiest to demonstrate the most powerful muscle strength.

The angle of the elbow at the moment when the upper and hook hit in boxing, the angle of the elbow when grabbing the opponent's gi at judo, the angle of the elbow at the moment of pulling away the opponent's wrist from the armlock (juji-gatame) in jiu jitsu At the moment of pulling down the opponent with the wrestling tackle, the moment of rolling the opponent with Muay Thai clinch, the joint angle of the elbow is 90 degrees or close to it. Looking more finely, it is ideal as an movement, if it's from the smaller than 90 degrees flexion (which the angle of the forearm and upper arm is large), to the state "It becomes 90 degrees when hit". It is not "Hitting/submission with 90 degrees" but "When hit/submission it becomes 90 degrees" as the consequence. From the anatomical structure of the elbow joint, 90 degrees flexion position is made to give the most force, and consumption of stamina is also small. Therefore, you do not feel much that yourself is giving strength of the muscle power as much as the force which is being demonstrated. If you want to generate the same muscle strength at the 45 degrees joint flexion position for example, it requires quite much muscle strength at basic physical strength, and the energy that generating the muscle power could get multiple times more, so it makes you very tired. When you perform a technique involving movement to flex the elbow joint, if you change the timing to the moment of 90 degrees joint flexion, the power of the technique may increase only by that.

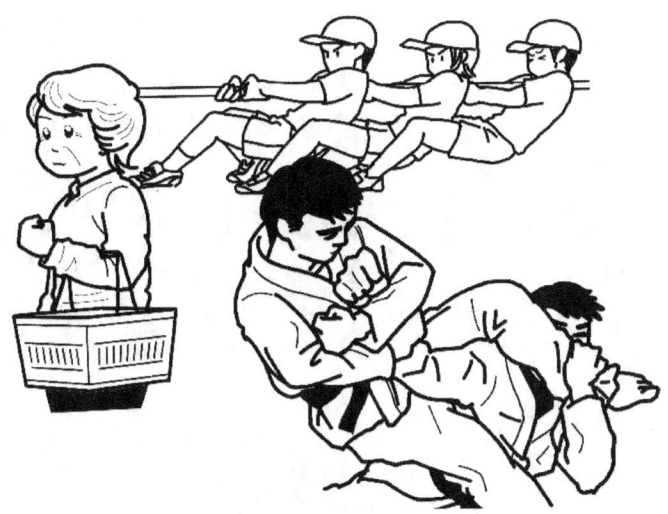

【4-3 Joint angle at extension of upper limb】

Next, let's think about the movement of the elbow, from bent to extended. So called "Extension" Straight punch, pushing opponent with clinching technique, the breaking of ice pillars with a knife hand strike in Karate's demonstration, etc. It is a movement of the upper limb which is very often seen, at the time of extension, the angle at which the strongest muscle force can be shown is around 70 degrees as it is said. As an experiment, do a push up and pause at the moment when your elbows are bent. If the angle of the elbow joint is around 70 degrees, I think that posture can be kept comparatively easier than other angles. It is often close to this angle when a pitcher releases the ball, or when you try to open a heavy door by pushing.

0°

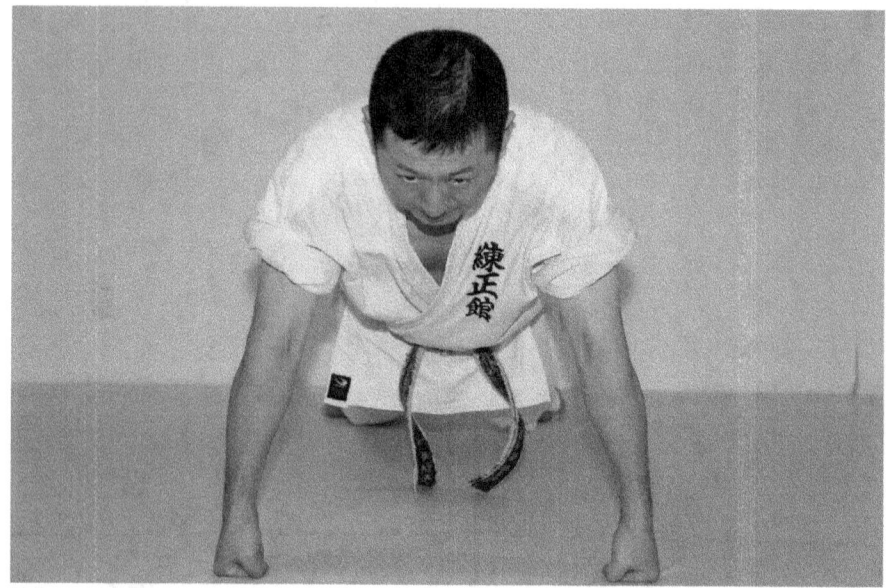

70

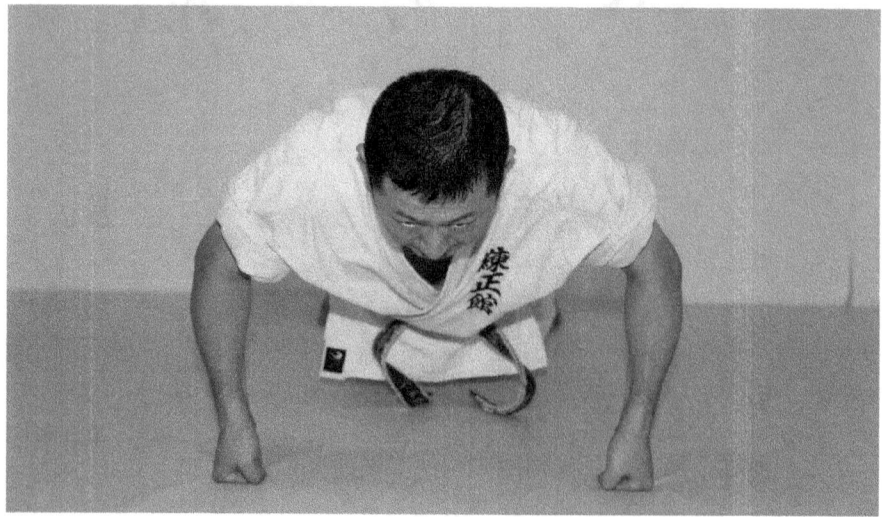

90°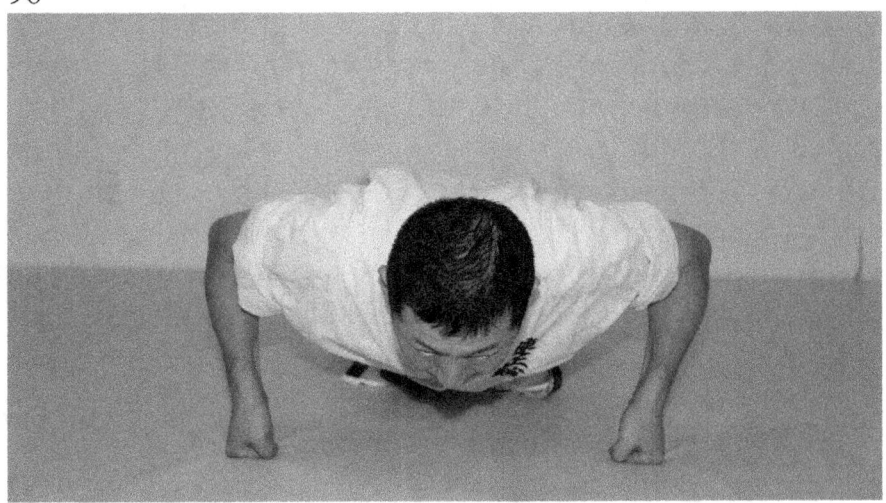

120°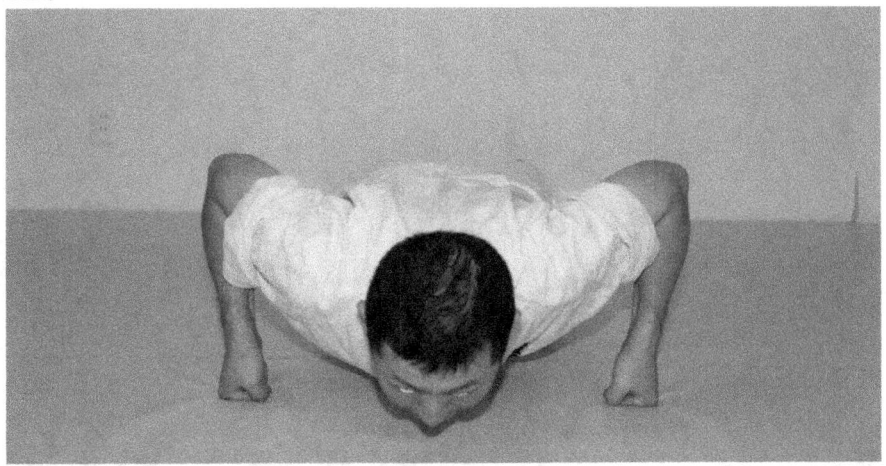

When striking a straight punch at a short distance, it is very convenient to know this angle. On the contrary, some players are restricted by the word "straight", and have only the straight punches with completely extended elbow. The punch with fully extended elbow (the joint angle of the elbow is zero) is very effective as a straight when starting from a long distance, but if you have only this pattern when it gets close distance, since you only have the choice of pull back and hit or let the opponent pull back then hit, you lose your way and you will miss the chance. Knowing the joint angle of the elbow and adding into the technique makes it possible to use different straight punches depending on the distance.

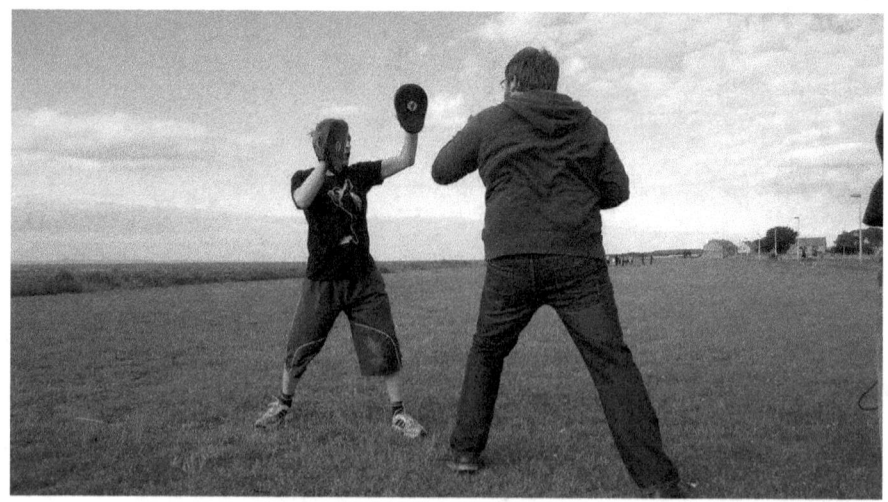

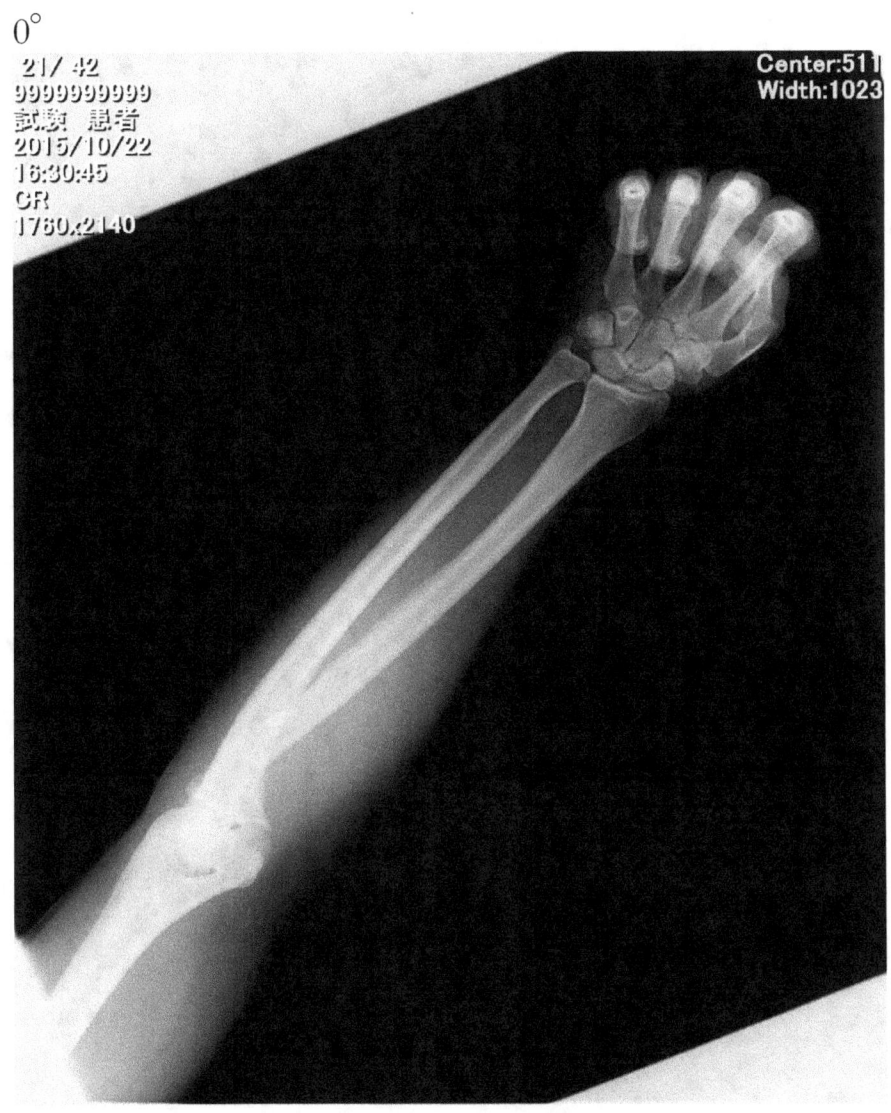

70°

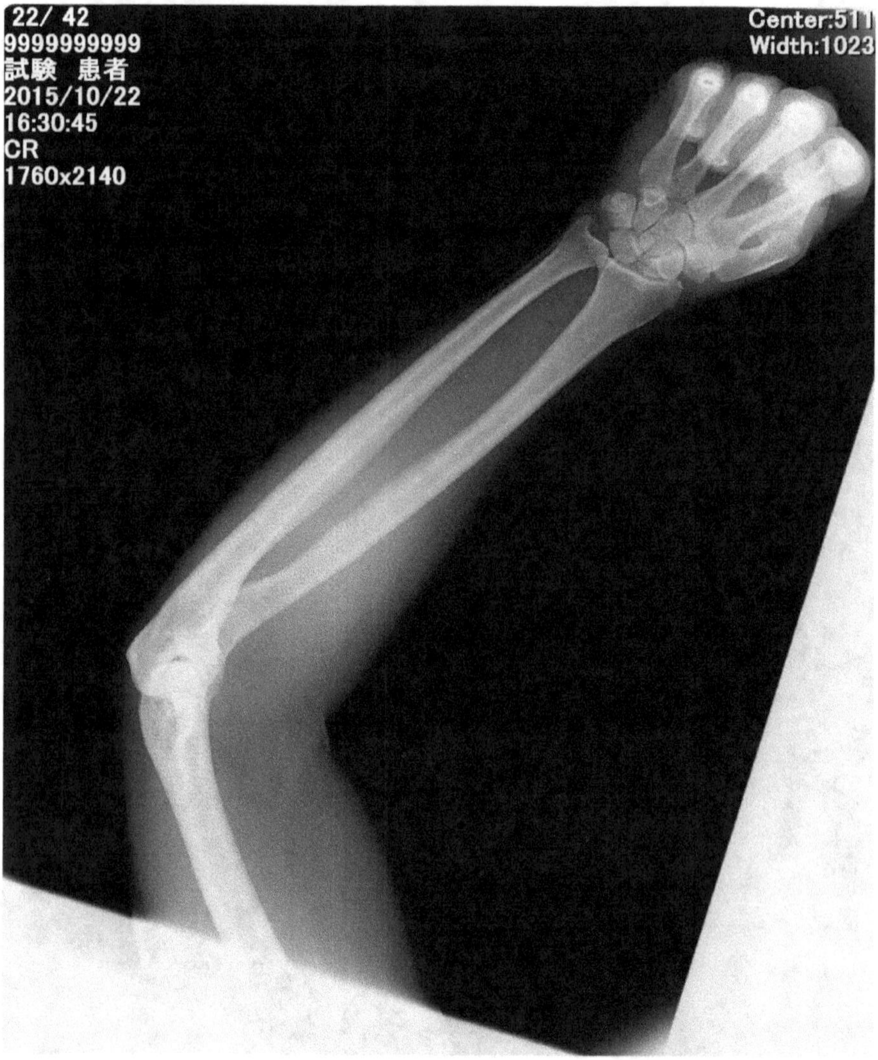
22/ 42
9999999999
試験 患者
2015/10/22
16:30:45
CR
1760x2140
Center:511
Width:1023

【4-4 The effect of combining pronation and supination】
Your thumbs are facing the ceiling (up) when you rise only your forearms by bending your elbow from standing straight. In that moment, your forearm is in the neutral position. From this situation, the direction to rotate the thumb toward the palm by pivoting at the middle finger (the direction of the palm towards downward) is called "Pronation", and to the opposite direction, rotating the thumb towards the back of the hand, is called "Supination"

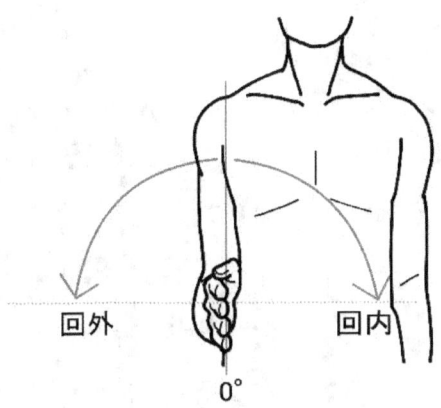

回外   回内

0°

If you add the supination to the bending movement of the elbow (flexion), the flexing power of the elbow joint will become even bigger. In many cases, the palm of your hand is facing yourself and the back of your hand is facing towards your opponent in boxing's uppercut, karate's shita tsuki, pulling movement like neck clinching and throwing techniques, armlock and leglock and so on. Those cases also increases the output by the flexing power of the elbow joint + supination. Conversely, it is effective to combine in the pronation to the extension movement of the elbow. With jab and straight punch, the movement of the throwing technique to push the opponent, the defense movement from the opponent's hits and so on, we can expect the display of the greater muscle power if we add extension and pronation together.

Neutral

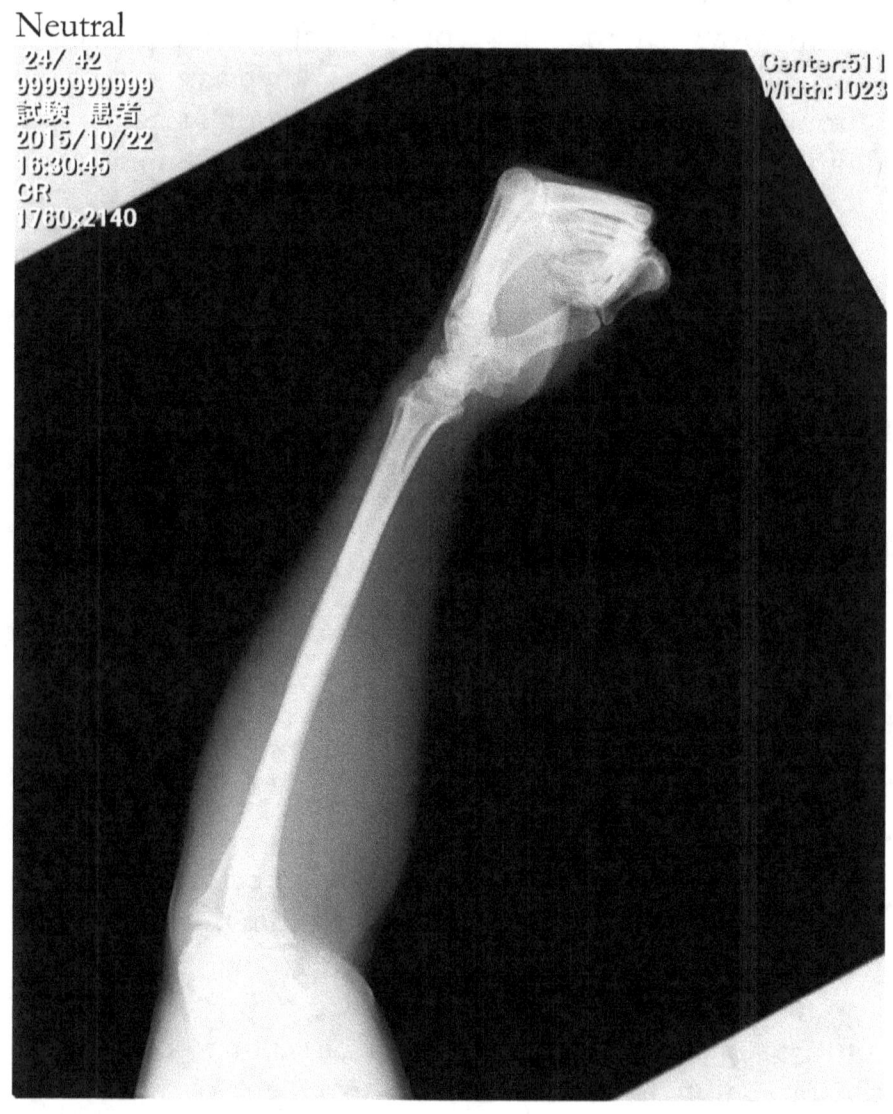

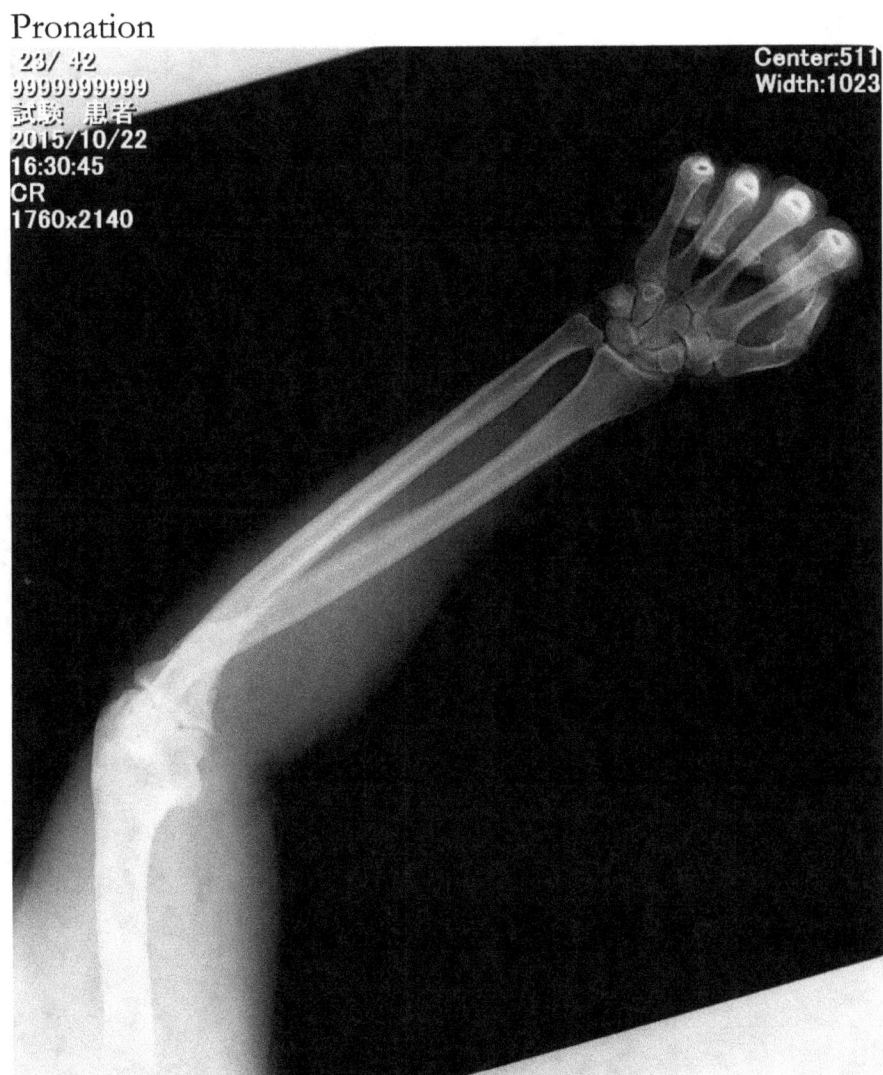

Pronation
23/ 42
9999999999
試験 患者
2015/10/22
16:30:45
CR
1760x2140

Center:511
Width:1023

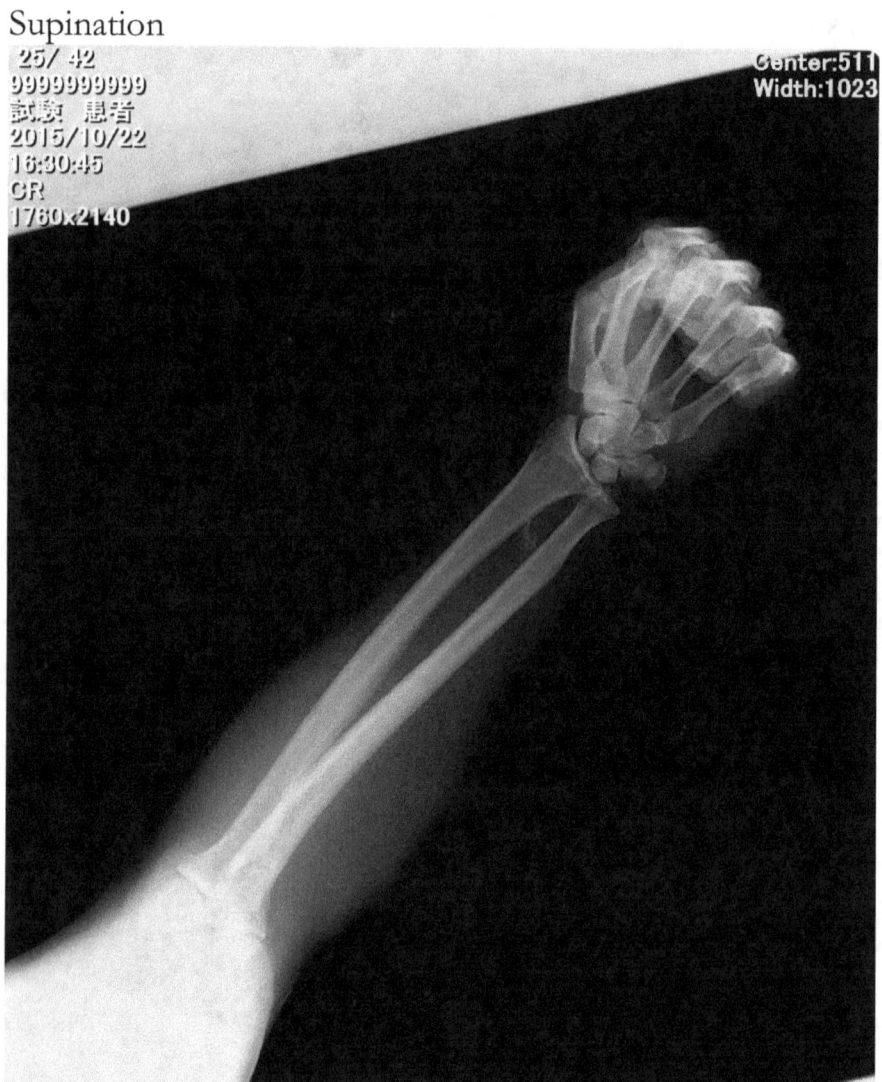

Supination

25/ 42
9999999999
試験　患者
2015/10/22
16:30:45
CR
1760x2140

Center:511
Width:1023

【4-5 Knee angle】

Let's focus on the knee angle this time. When stretching a flexed knee joint, what angle is the strongest output of the muscle? Let's experiment this by making a pair. The athlete lies down with his back on the floor and bends his knee. The partner applies resistance in the direction to extend the knee (extension direction). Stretch the knees and set the angle at which the lower leg and thigh are aligned straight, it is the zero degree. Now, apply resistance with 4 patterns as 30, 60, 90 and 120 degrees. I think that the most power outputs at 60 degrees or close to it.

For example, when you kick your opponent's thigh with a low kick, if you hit at an angle close to 60 degrees, you will easily damage your opponent. Some top fighters use 2 kinds of low kicks differently, Low kick (A) to bring out their opponent's reactions, and low kicks (B) to knock down the opponent. When the distance to the opponent is far, with the angle smaller than 60 degrees, attracting the opponent's reaction, stepping in to the distance where they require for knocking down the opponents, then greater power generating 60 degrees kicks to damage the opponents. From the opponent fighters, only low kicks (A) with a small angle of the knee joint from a distance will be input, so they will react to that kick. At the moment the correspondence to (A) is completed, suddenly switching to kick (B) with different distance and angle, the opponent's reaction will be delayed and the defense will not be in time.

30°

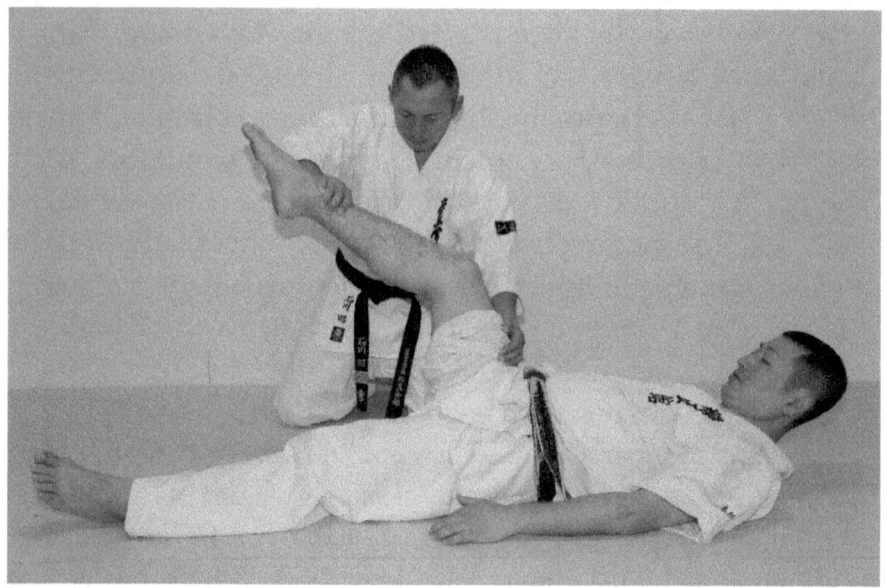

60°

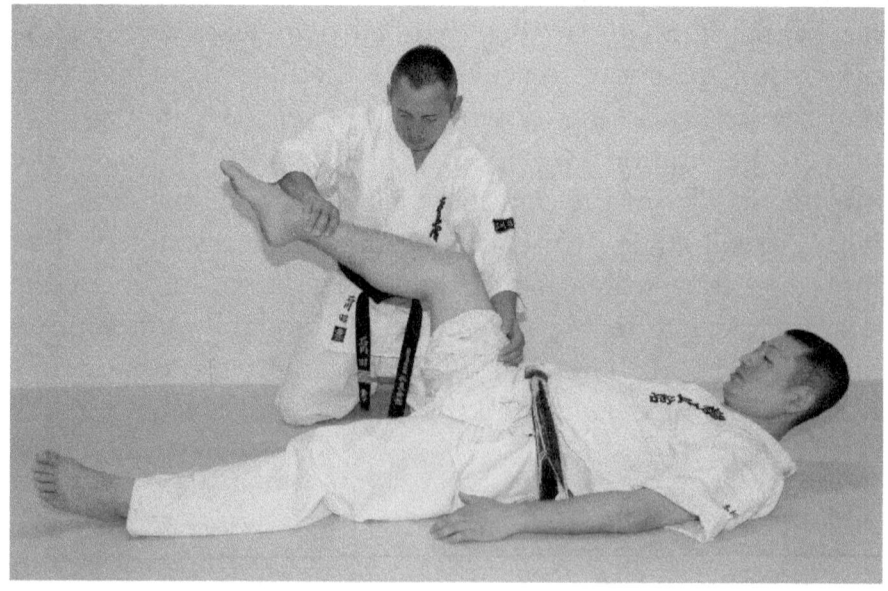

90°

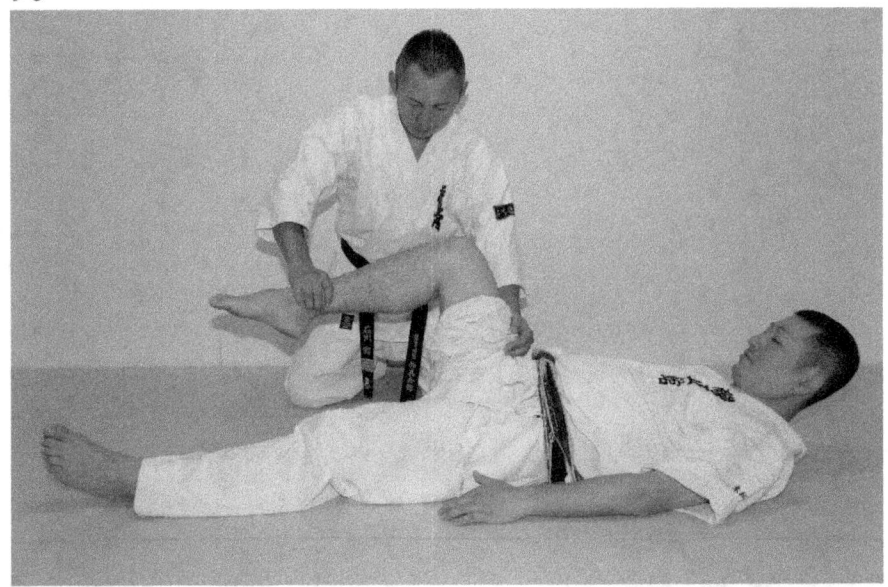

120°

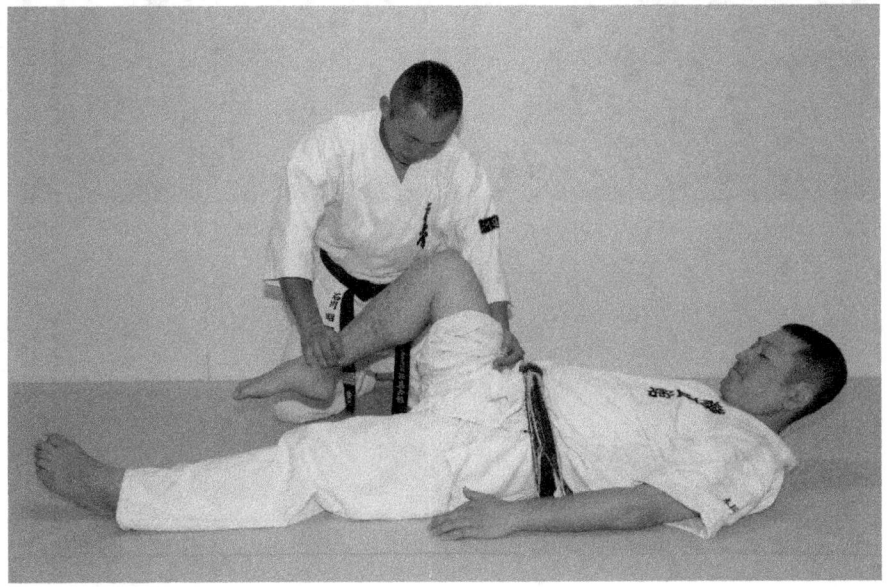

30°

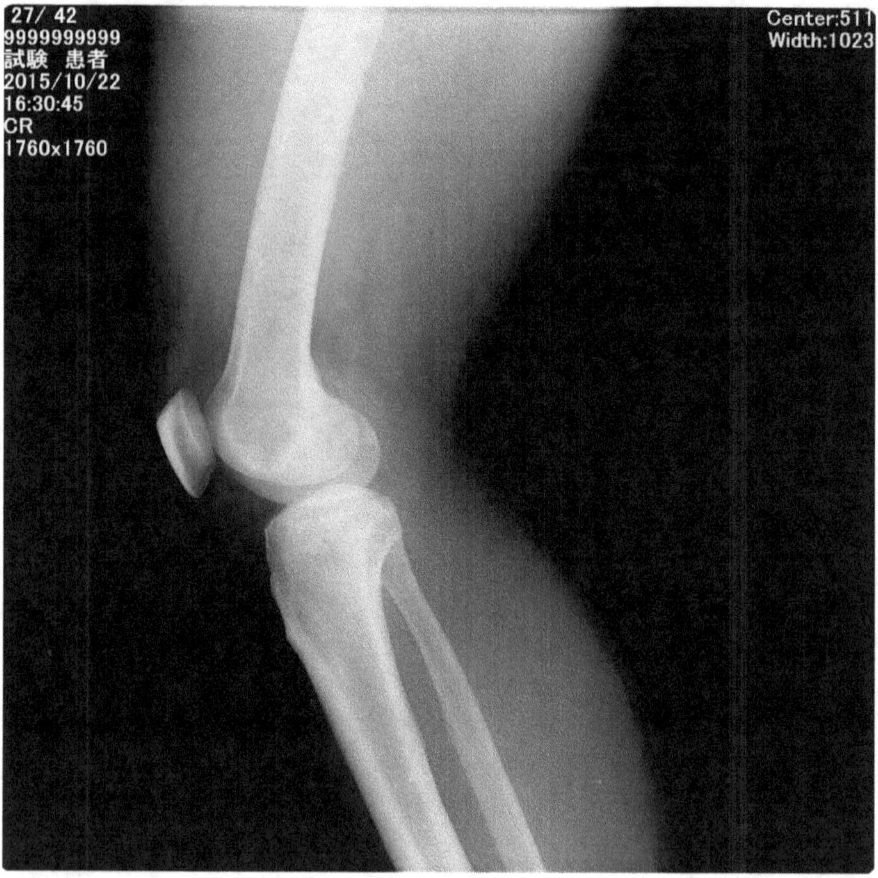
27/ 42
9999999999
試験 患者
2015/10/22
16:30:45
CR
1760x1760
Center:511
Width:1023

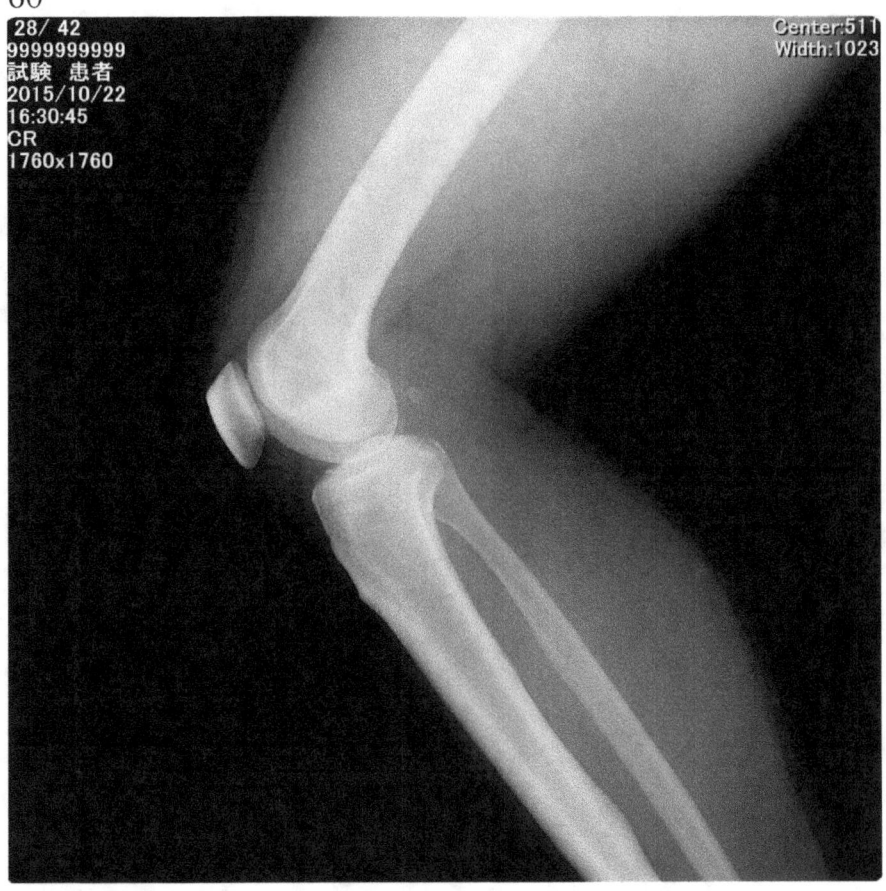

90°

29/ 42
9999999999
試験 患者
2015/10/22
16:30:45
CR
1760x1760

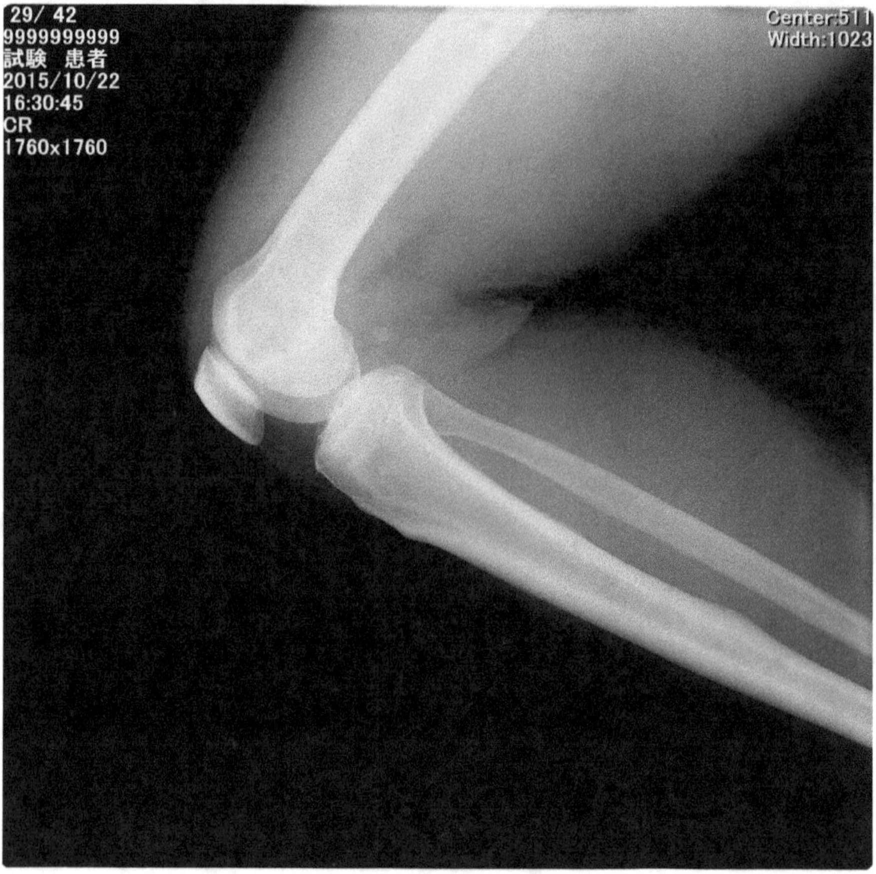

Center:511
Width:1023

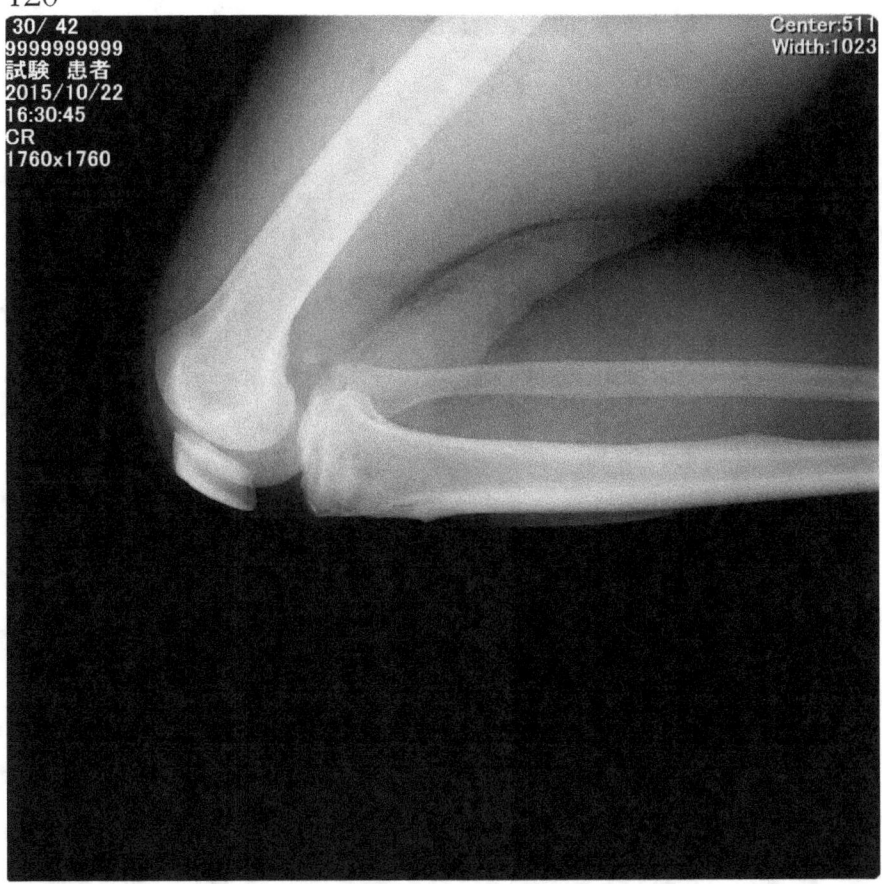

30/ 42
9999999999
試験 患者
2015/10/22
16:30:45
CR
1760x1760

60

Center:511
Width:1023

If you are a practitioner who feels that hitting a low kick but did not transmit to your opponent as a damage may be it is interesting if you try it at various angles on the angle of the knee joint when hitting the kicking leg against the opponent. This is to find "The angle where you are not really putting your power on it but it transmit to the opponent as a big damage." If the joint angle is wrong, the same output cannot be obtained without substantial muscular strength, but if the joint angle is appropriate, it becomes a large output difference. The joint angle of the knee joint will be the great help to locate the kicking form.

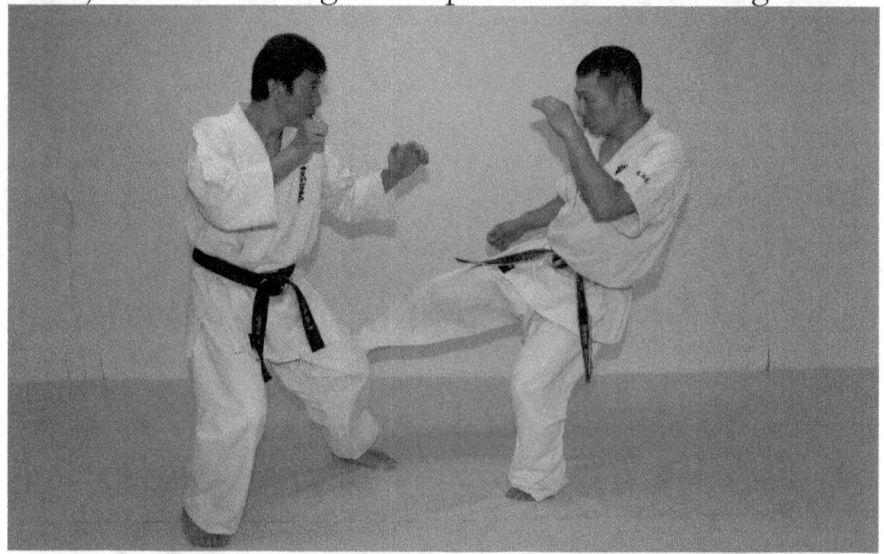

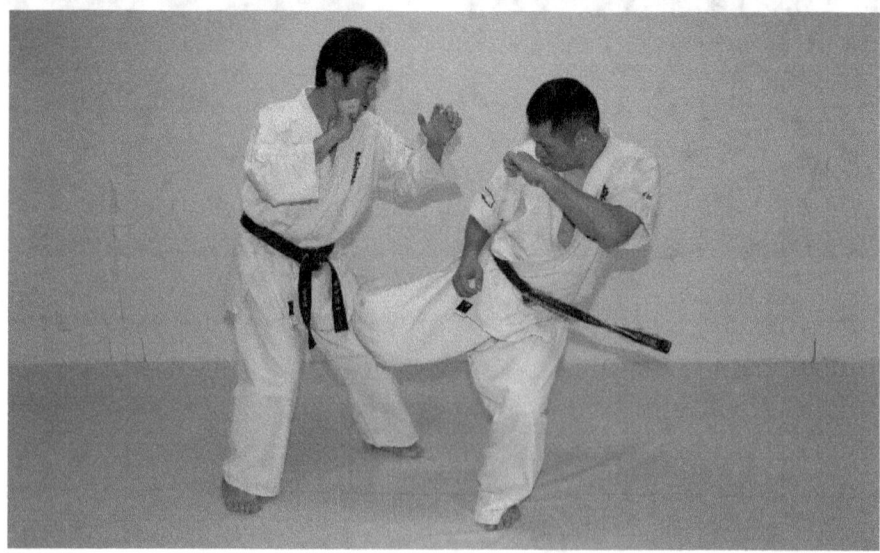

【4-6 Trunk angle when going forward】

There is a case that when you hit an opponent fighter, you are going to be held down, getting blown away. If this happens, the battle itself isn't even a battle. It is another story if it was a demonstration, but to win in the competitions, before talking about technic, you do not lose momentum of pushing each other with the opponent is a must condition. When an opponent tackles in from the front, or when you are struck on your chest etc., there is an angle of the so called "not to be pushed" trunk. That angle is 21 degrees. When setting the angle between the sacral spine from the lower back to the buttocks and the spine corresponding to the backbone to 21 degrees, it is difficult for the body to bring back to the back even if it is pushed from the front, making it harder to lose. When a Sumo wrestler tackles an opponent, when a Muaythai warrior challenges a close combat, the trunk bends slightly forward.

Make a partner and let the partner push your shoulders or chest, try to do that trunk angle at the moment his/her hands touch you, then you can obtain the strength of tackle power. At the same time, as you exhale, contraction of the abdominal transverse muscles will allow the pressure around the spine to be added to create a stronger force.

0°

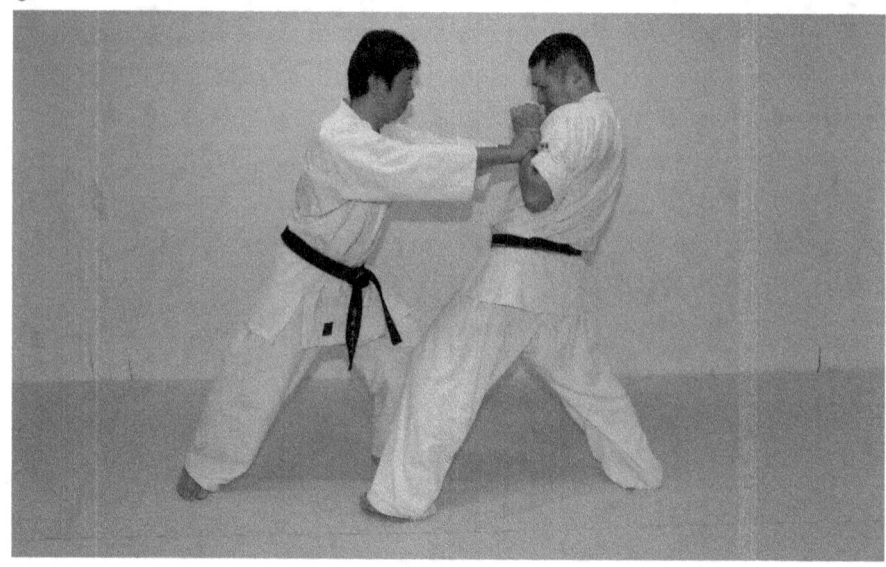

21°

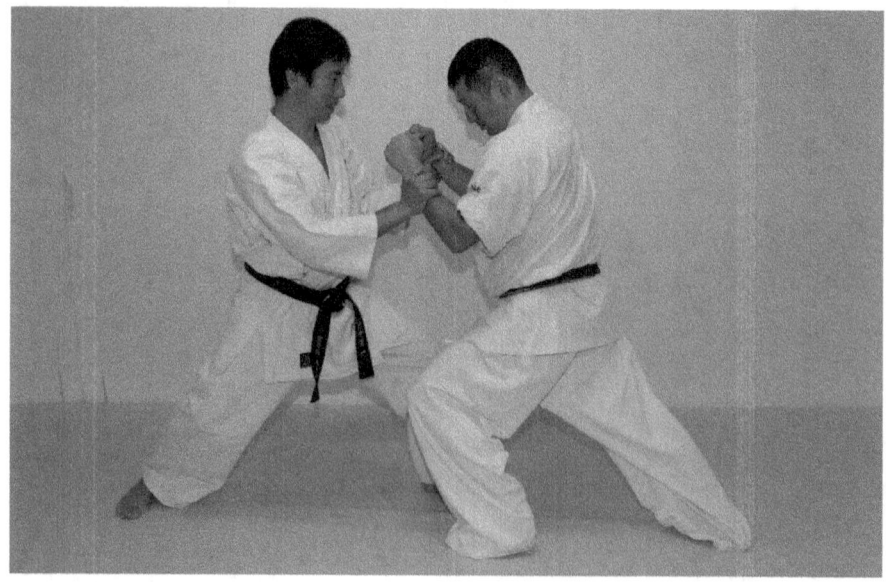

【4-7 Hip joint angle in back leg】

Let's think about the force to extend the hip joint of the back leg (bending the hip joint, that is, move the knee towards the back from the front of the body) when you make a fighting pose. The force to extend the hip joint produces the maximum output at around 30 ° flexion position. When the opponent pressures from front, bend the hip joint of the back leg slightly more than 30 degrees and move it in the extension direction to firmly receive the power of the opponent, and can withstand without pushed back.

Also, the joint angle of the back leg becomes very effective also when kicking technique with the front leg which is frequently used in Karate or kickboxing is issued. When trying to put out the front kick from the front leg or high kick from the stance of the kumite no kamae (fighting stance of Karate), the muscle group which to rise the front leg are mainly working. On the other hand, kicking from the front leg may be carried out smoothly if you move 30 degrees after hip joint of the back leg for just a moment from the stance of kumite no kamae. In Karate, the standing by bending the hip joint of the back leg is called "Koukutsu dachi", by just putting this stance into the motion for just a moment, the quality of movement will change greatly after that.

If you do not pay attention to joint angle, only practitioners whom caught the idea will improve. Therefore, while adjusting the angle of the hip joint with your partner, find the angle that will not be pushed back. By doing so, I think that you can acquire objective and reproducible strength.

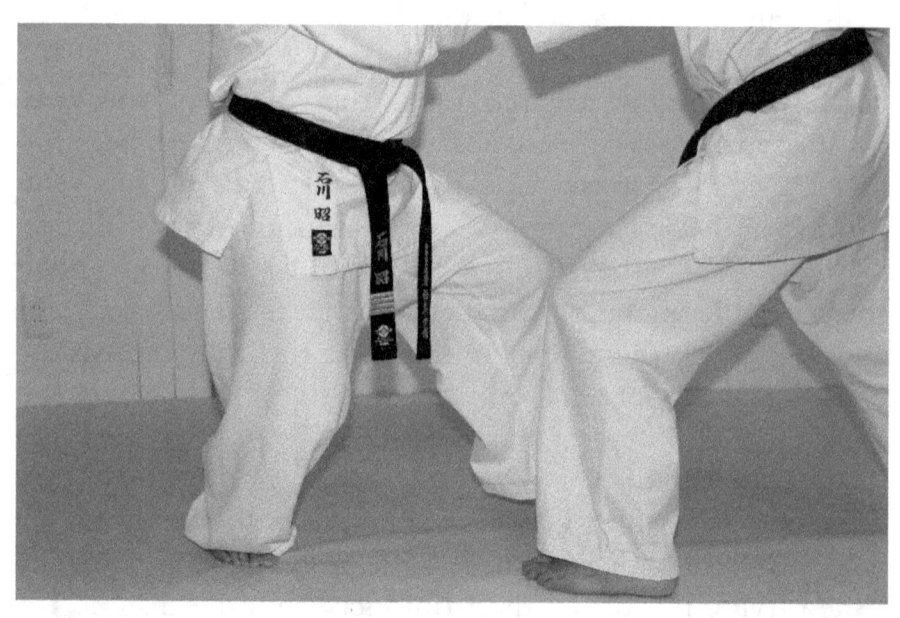

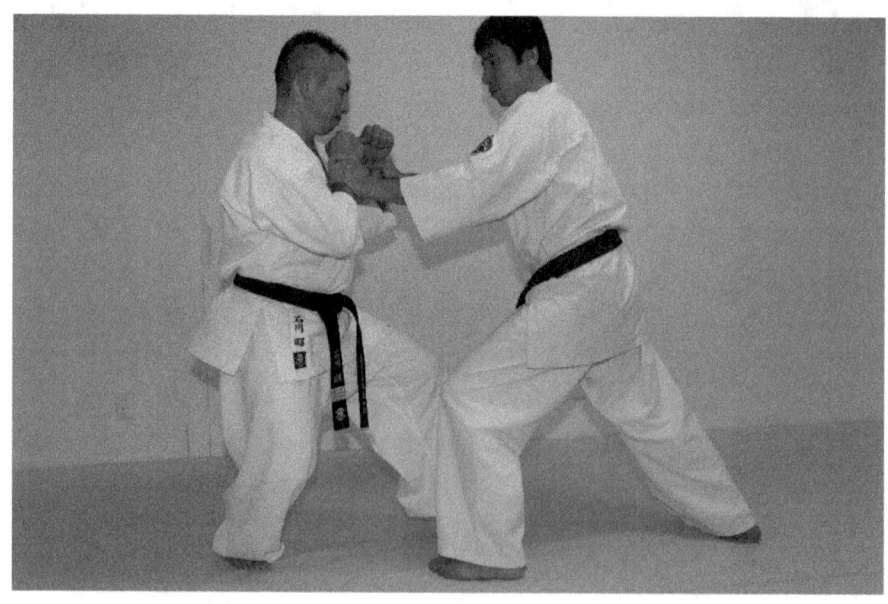

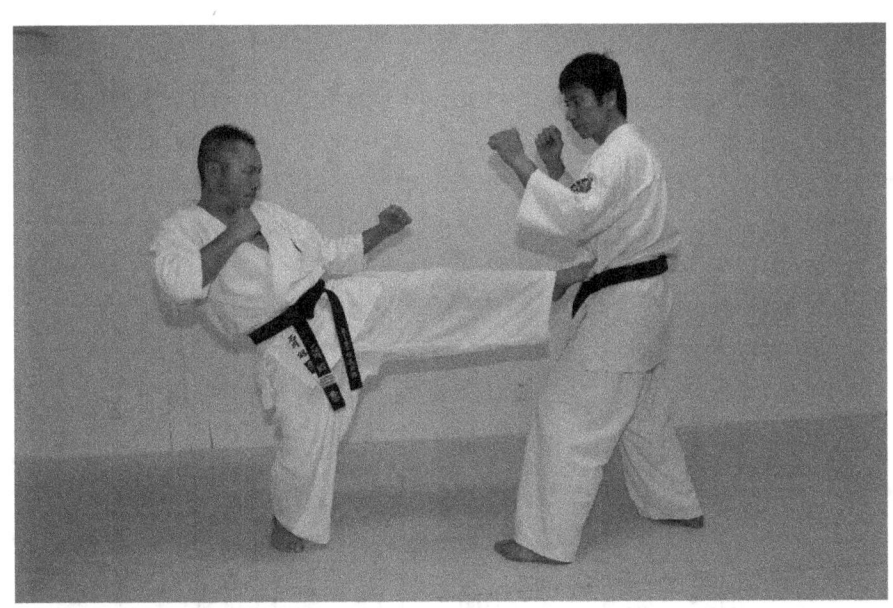

Hip joint X-ray, Koukutsu dachi

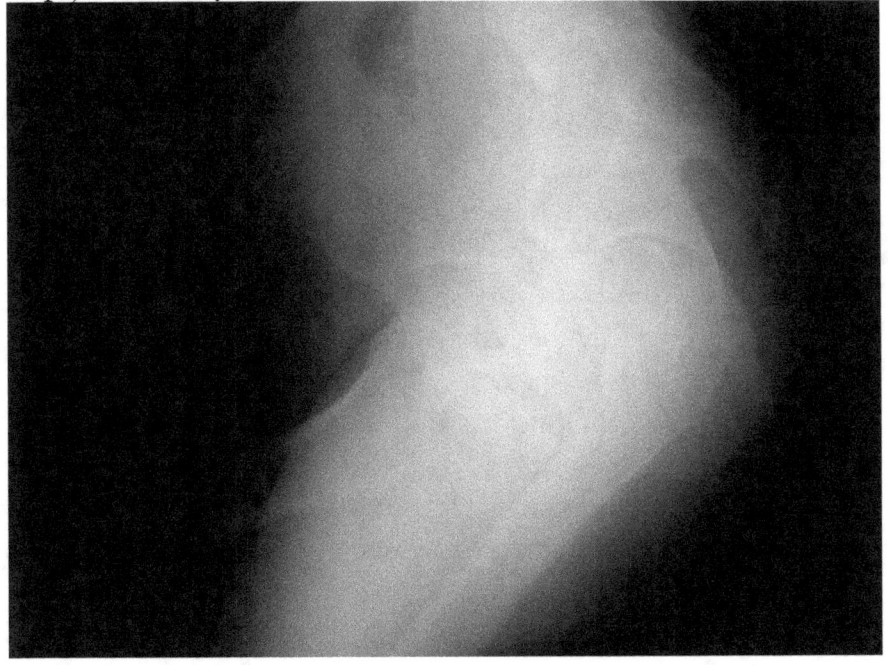

【4-8 Possibility which spreads】

In short, technique is about "How to move your body". While iterating over and over, some people get the best form, but there are a lot of people who cannot get it. One prescription for such a practitioner is a joint angle. Everyone who wants to become strong, "What is different from top fighters?" I am sure that you ask yourself a number of times. It is a waste to give up as "the talent is different", "the body structure is different", "the environment is different", "that fighter is a genius". Just by recounting the use of the body of the first-class fighter from the viewpoint of "angle of joint" as one element, we can find hints of various leaps out there.

For example, paying attention to the angle of the ankle joint of the shaft foot of the fighter who is good at high kick, when the high kick reaches the highest point, the leg joint of most of the fighters takes the bottom flexion. Bottom flexion is the direction in which the toes collapse in the direction of the sole of the foot and the calves and the Achilles tendon contract. When the leg joint of the shaft leg takes the bottom flexion position, the position of the pelvis inevitably becomes high. When the leg joint of the shaft leg takes the bottom bending position, the position of the pelvis inevitably becomes high. Stretching of the hip joint and trunk is of course important, but by itself alone the height of the kicking leg depends only on the range of motion of the hip joint and trunk. In fact, when analyzing the movements of fighters who are not good at high kicks, there is a tendency that the moment of highest point, "the ankle does not bend," or "the angle is small even if it is bending."

114

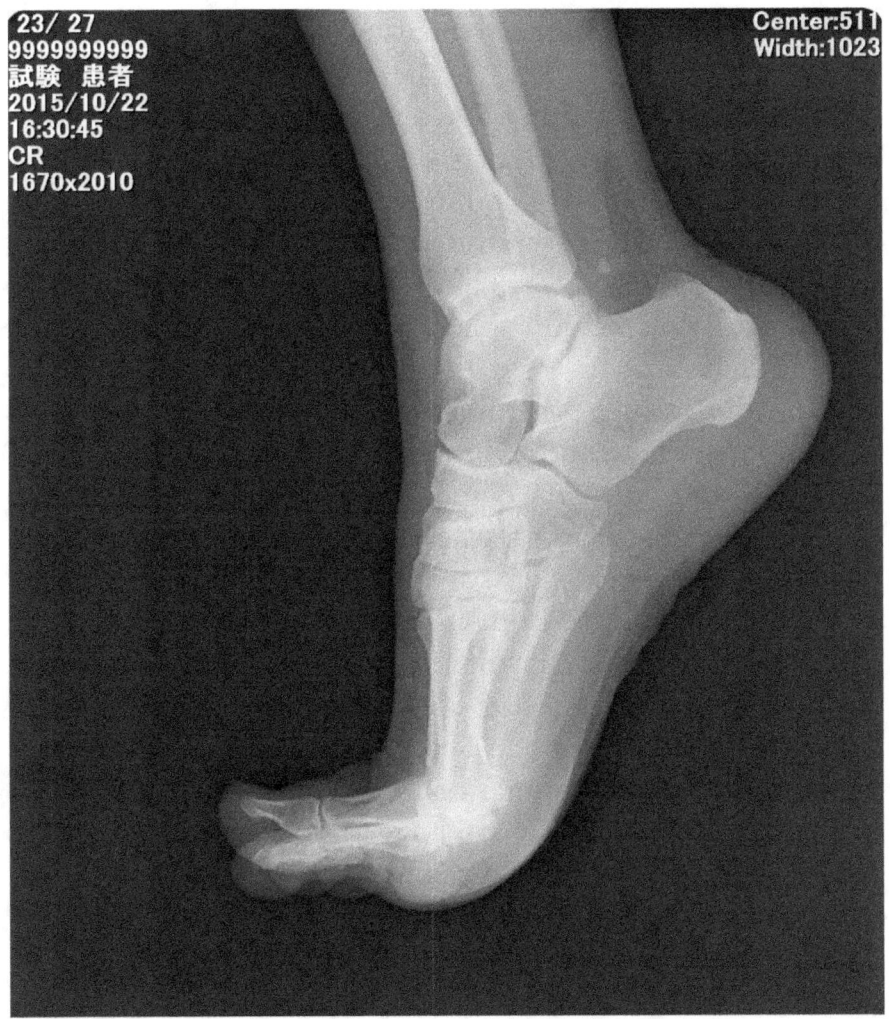

In addition, there is a tendency that there are many fighters whom good at high kicks are good at running, or like running. "Run" rather than "walk" will use the range of motion of the ankle wider. Naturally, it takes an angle of large base flexion. On the contrary, athletes who "walk" will decrease the angle of bottom flexion. I think that difference in the height of the pelvis will come out when kicking a high kick because the usual way of using the body is different.

The high kick legs also have features common to first-class fighters. It is a point where the bending of the hip joint of the kicking leg is directed to the direction of 45 degrees diagonally from the front. Some of the fighters who are not good at high kick are misdirecting the direction of hip flexion. Let's have an experiment. When knee kick is kept in front of you straight, when you first bend in the front and then go out to 45 degrees obliquely with abduction, whichever knee will rise higher? The answer is the latter. It comes from the structure of the human pelvis. Looking at the horizontal disconnection of the front of the pelvis, it is a plane with a 45 degree angle. When the hip joint is bent in the front, the thigh and the pelvis collide with each other due to the structure. There is nothing to hit and the legs are easy to rise upwards when you roll outward from the bend at an angle of 45 degrees. The result of the experiment is A (flexion only) and B (flex plus abduction) of the X ray image. Look at the line at the top of the knee at the height level of the spinal column, A is located on the lower side of the twelfth thoracic vertebra. On the other hand, if you add an abduction to B, that is, flexion, the knee line is located in the 7th thoracic vertebrae. The way of moving B is better than moving A, the highest point of the knee is increased by five thoracic vertebrae.

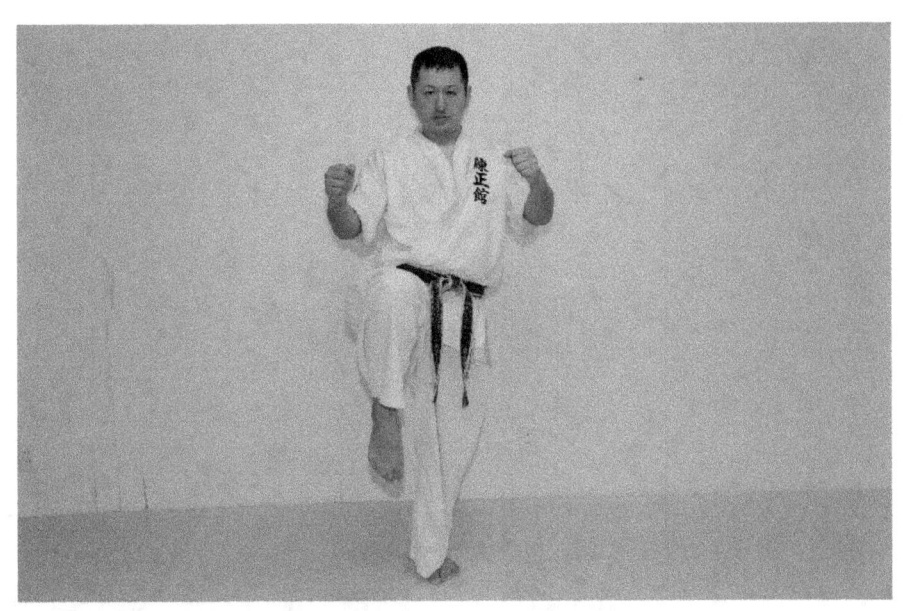

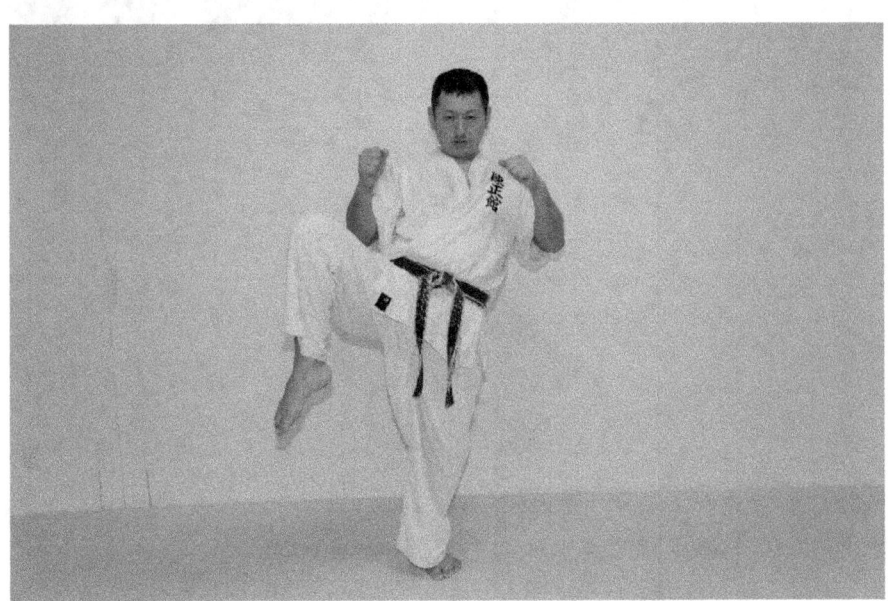

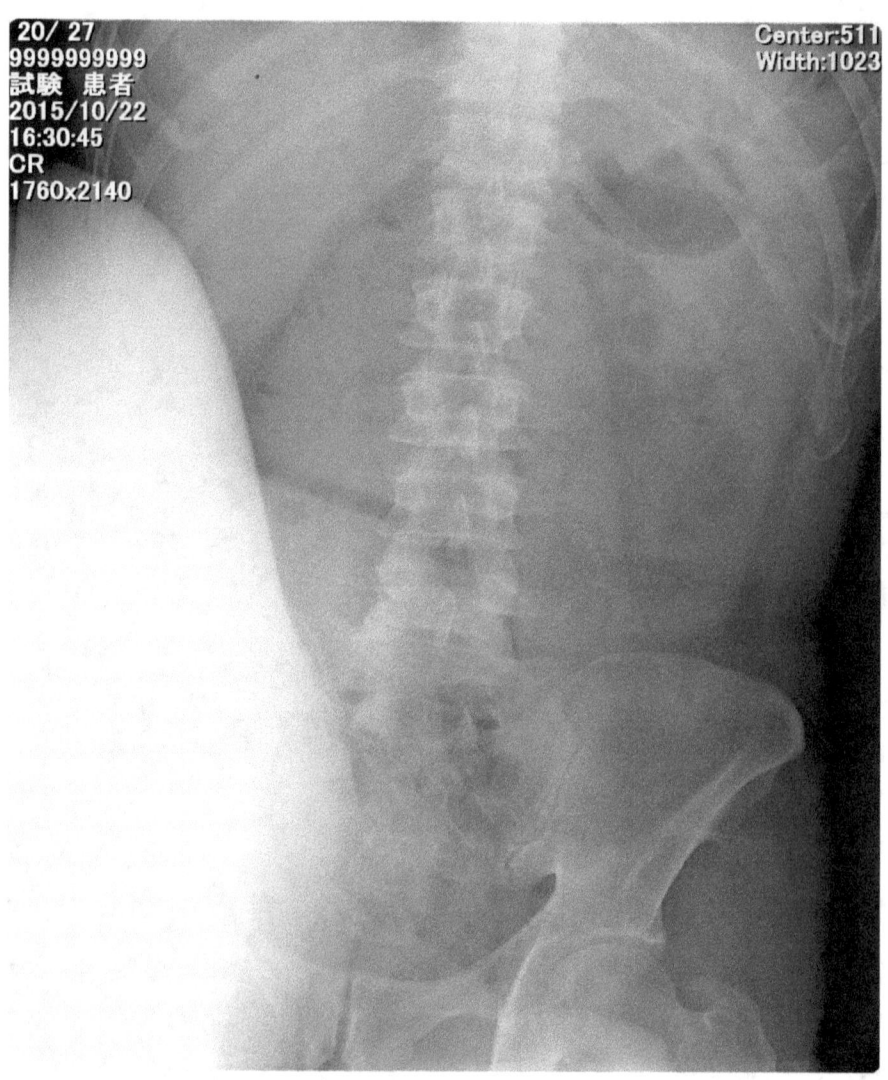

20/ 27
9999999999
試験　患者
2015/10/22
16:30:45
CR
1760x2140

Center:511
Width:1023

118

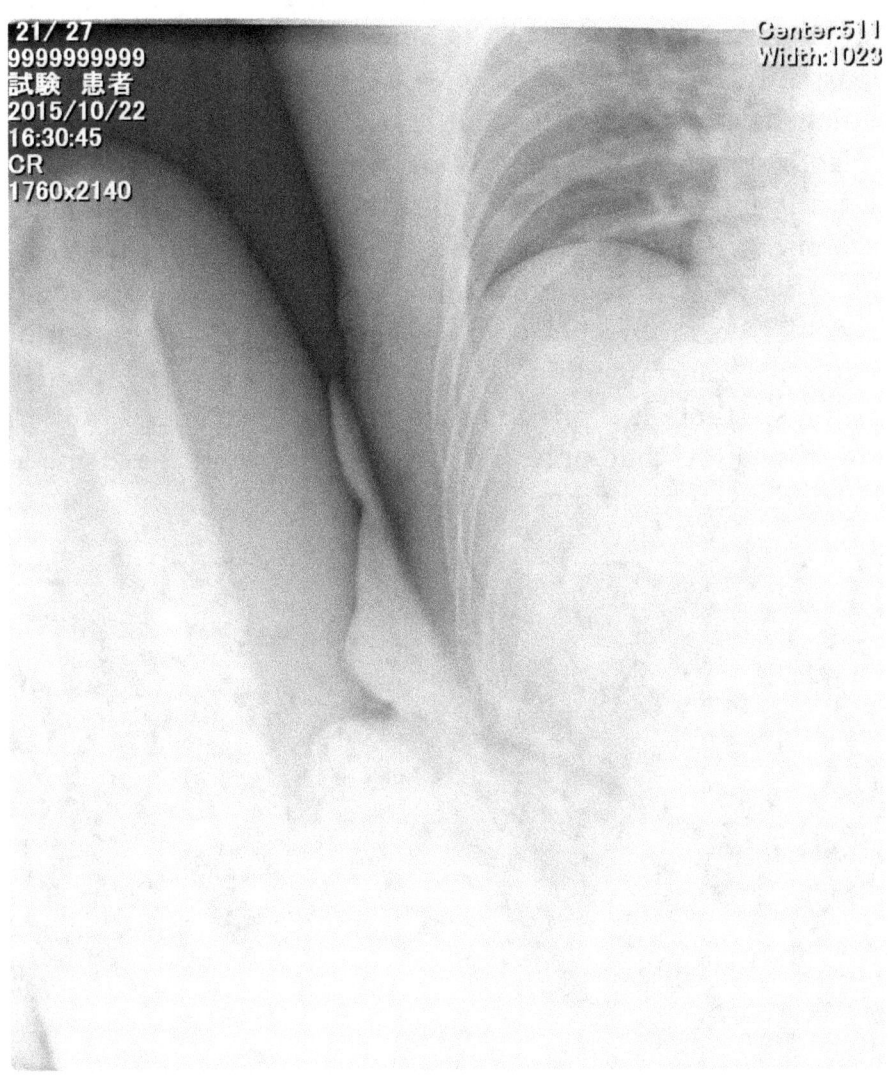

Fighters who are good at high kicks are kicking plus abducting hip joints of kicking feet in this direction. Currently, it seems that there are more fighters who are doing it subconsciously than those whom understand the relationship between such body structures and techniques. I am going to break away from the conventional thinking scheme of "Flexible joint body" → "Have talent for high kicks", "Not flexible joint body" → "Give up doing high kicks". Correctly know the joint angle and attempt numericalization within the range that it is possible. By doing so, there is a possibility to share the secret of how to use the body that only the first-class fighters have made beyond space and time.

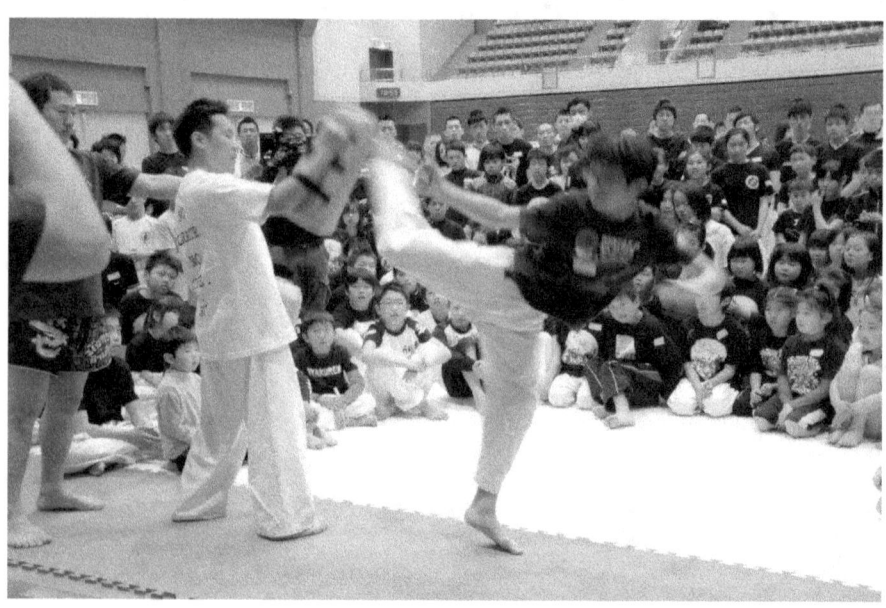

5 Stretch Reflex

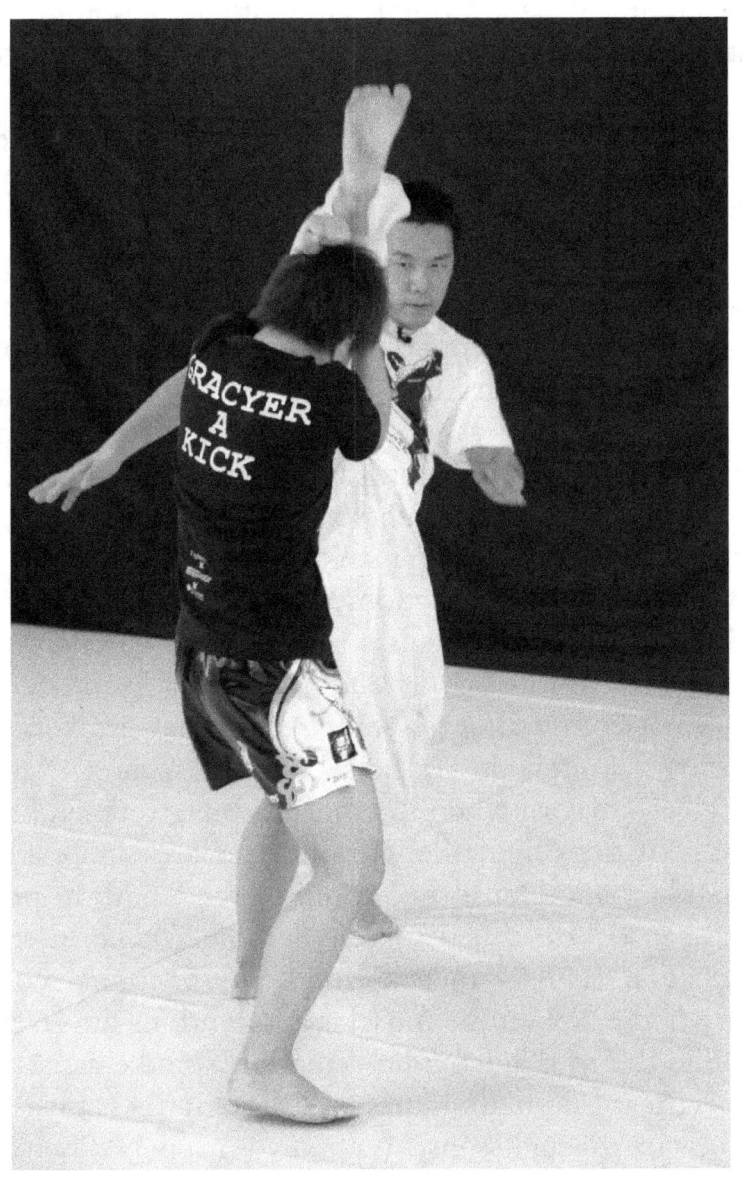

【5-1 Muscle / tendon monitoring system】

In physics, if 2 different points, for example, we say one side is point A (start point), the other is point B (end point), the shortest distance to move the fast way from A to B is a straight line which connects A and B. So that is, moving the shortest distance is the fastest to reach to the end point.

The human body is slightly different in circumstances. Let's say, for example, when hitting a punch, the position of the fist when start up is point A, and the reaching point of the fist is point B. From the point A to the point B, the punch moving the fist with the shortest straight line distance seems to be the earliest time to reach, but actually, moving the fist in the course leading to B after moving it in the opposite direction will reach sooner and the power of the punch at that time will also increase.

How does such a phenomenon occur in the human body? One of the reasons is a secret in the defense system that protects muscles and tendons. Muscles and tendons are good at contracting (shrinking), but they are very weak in being stretched. Because muscles and tendons themselves are torn when the muscles are stretched beyond the limit of the original length, muscles are equipped with high-performance sensors to monitor the length to prevent it. The sensor are called muscle spindle / tendon spindle and exist in skeletal muscle and tendon connected with sensory nerve. When the muscles and tendons are stretched suddenly, the muscle spindle / tendon spindle sense and the electrical stimulation passes through the spinal cord dorsal horn through sensory nerves (group Ia fibers), and the dorsal root, then it enters the part called dorsal horn. From there, the command of 'contraction' is transmitted to the α motor fibers through motile neurons (α cells) located in the anterior horn of the spinal cord, then the stretched muscle / tendon is contracted. This series of reactions is called stretch reflex. The system of stretch reflex always monitors "to prevent stretching of muscles and tendons beyond necessity" or even "to prevent it from being stretched and torn". This system was originally equipped for human beings, it is an automatic one that pops out without being conscious. The first-rate athlete is drawing this stretching reflection well and is leading to performance.

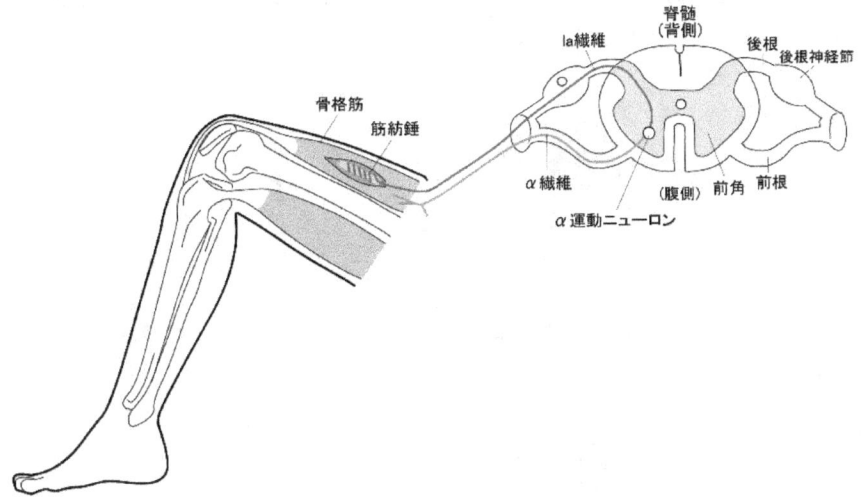

【5-2 Stretch reflex and punch】

If you punch from point A to point B, the biceps brace which corresponds to "flexed bicep" is stretched, but from the standpoint of the biceps and its tendon, if possible, it wants to avoid stretching. So, if you pull a little from A to A ', the biceps muscle contracts, so the sensor judges that "you can still extend, I can afford." Behind the flexed biceps, the triceps is stretched suddenly in the process of

123

pulling from A to A '. From the standpoint of the triceps, it is difficult to stretch suddenly, so extensional reflection will occur here. When the stretched information reaches the spinal cord, the command to activate "shrink immediately" is invoked from the spinal cord. This order does not go through the brain. The time it takes to communicate is overwhelmingly short since it issues a command of contraction with a shortcut without going through the brain. Therefore, when punching out, it triggers stretching reflection of the triceps trunk muscle group with movement of A to A ', and using stretch reflex generated there makes a fast punch.

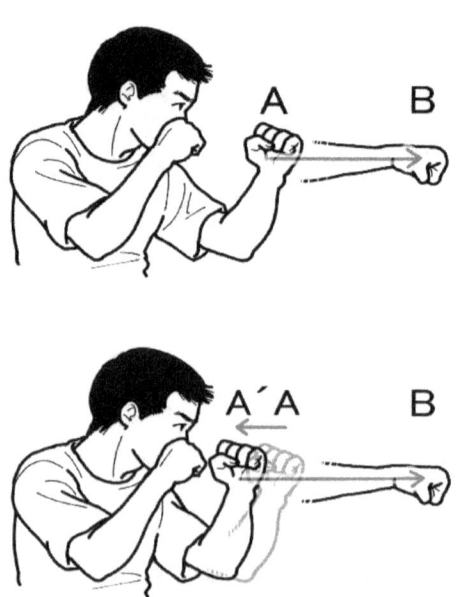

【5-3 Stretch reflex, brain image and language】

As an image in the brain, try not to think "I want to put out a punch, I want to put out a punch." or "I want to hit, I want to hit.", that's the point If you want to put out a punch or hit, reverse the motion, "pull" for a moment, make a minimal "put out a punch" issue. If you want to put it out, pull (little) and put it out. Switch suddenly with an image suddenly switching from back gear to top gear. Doing so will make stretch reflex easier and speed up. Also, at the stage of recalling the image of exercise in the brain, it may be transmitted to the opponent as soon as you have in your mind "put it out". The fighters who actually have high levels, are good at reading our images. So, changing the image and language in your brain from "put it out" to "pull then put it out" changes the movement and as a result makes it difficult for the opponent to read your movement.

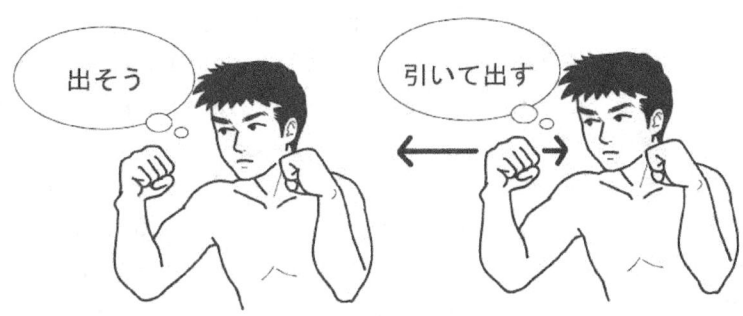

(put it out, pull then put it out)

【5-4 Stretch reflex and visual information】

Furthermore, by pulling out a fist a little, it is possible to influence the visual information which is input to the opponent. In the course of A → B, the image appearing on the retina of the opponent's eyes increases the size from small to big. The opponent approaches, the phenomenon that punches, kicks and things blow towards you, the human eye judges based on the visual information whether the image reflected on the retina becomes larger or smaller . As the image grows larger, I judge that it comes closer, so I feel a so-called oppressive feeling. It is the identity of what is called pressure in matches, the so-called pressure. In the A → B course, the opponent also reacts more easily because it gives the opponent a sense of oppression rightly. The car runs towards myself, is the image which should be close to such feeling. On the contrary, in the course of A → A '→ B, the fist moves away for a moment from the opponent. The image reflected on the retina is momentarily smaller. You are afraid if the car comes toward you, but usually there is no fear or pressure, as far as it runs away in the opposite direction. Rather, it is human being to feel relieved that the object becomes smaller. But what if this suddenly comes back suddenly the car that was running away? If it is not estimated, in the head for an instant, will it not become "blanc"? Set the inside of the opponent's brain with "???" state, create a time when he/she cannot respond, and make effective attacks. This is one of the leading fighter's techniques. Especially in boxing and kickboxing fighting which wearing gloves, KO ratio and effective hitting hit rate may increase by controlling visual information well. On purpose, some fighters use the tactics to hit the jab of A → B course, to let the opponent recognize as "easy-to-avoid blow", and to switch to the course using reflections when the chance comes.

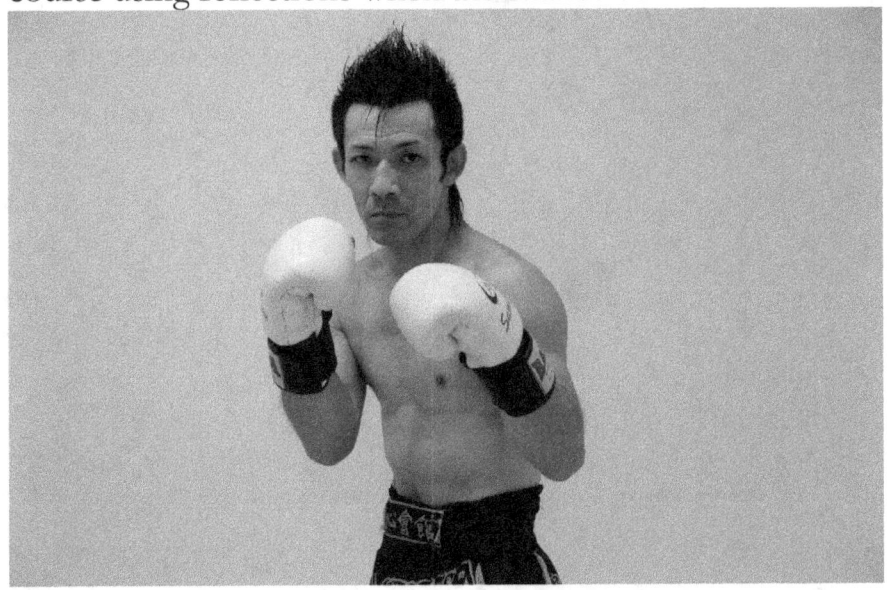

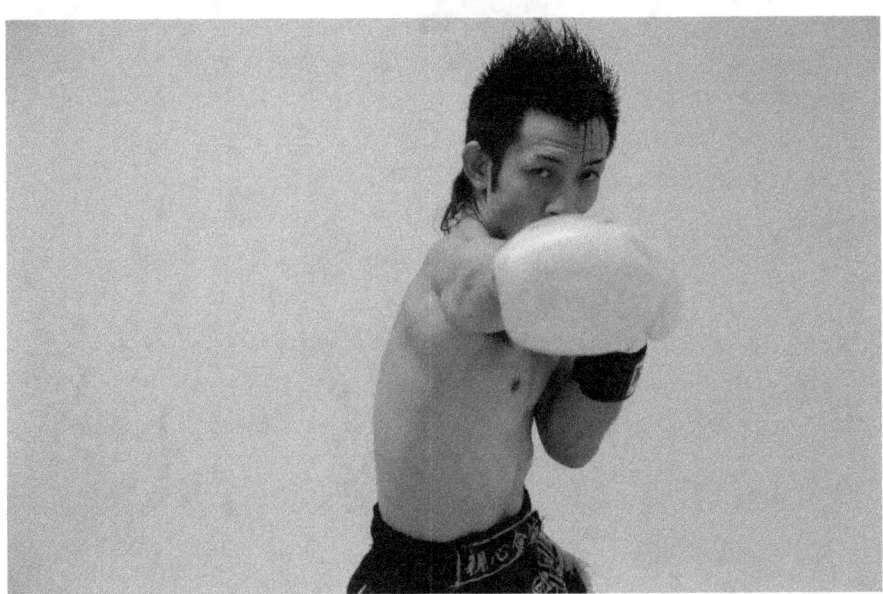

(Punch without Stretch Reflex)

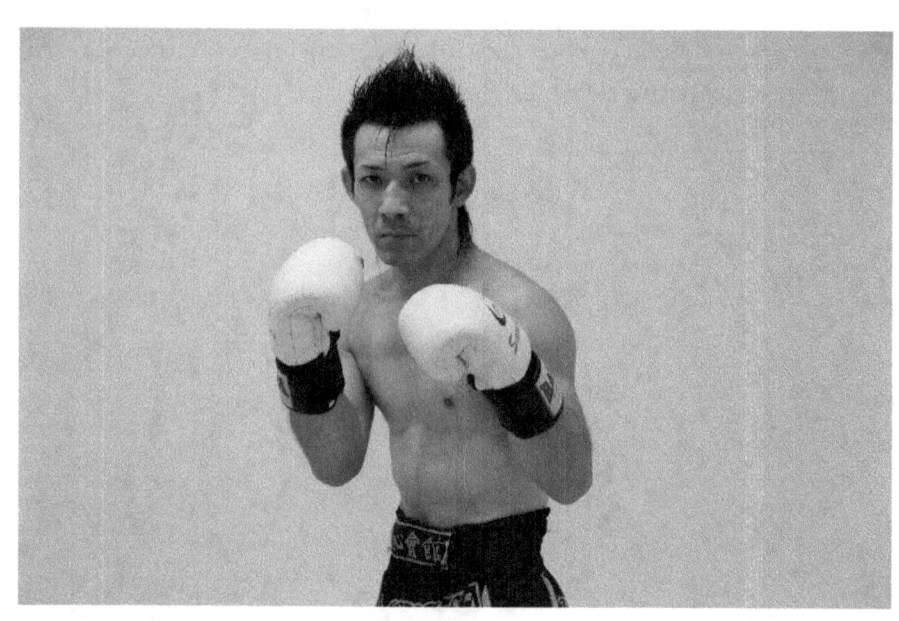

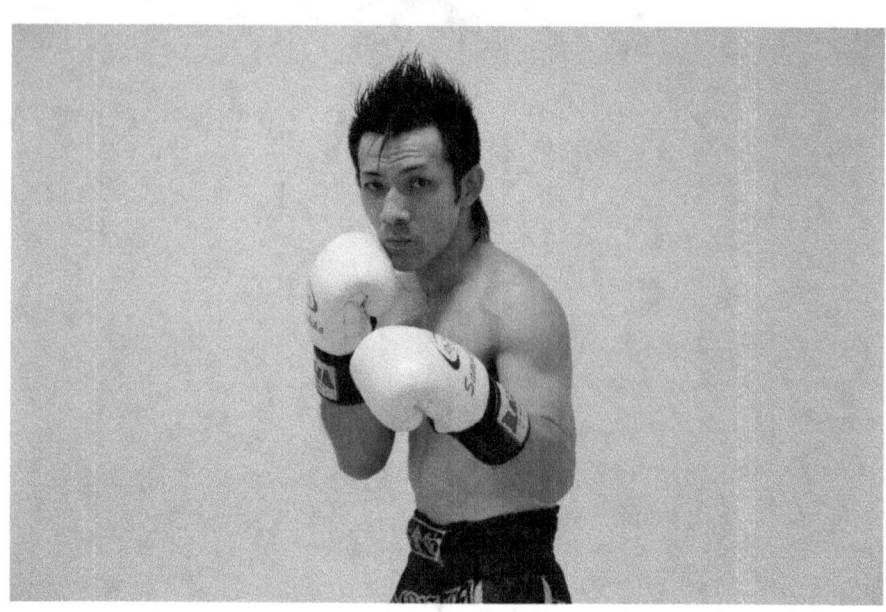

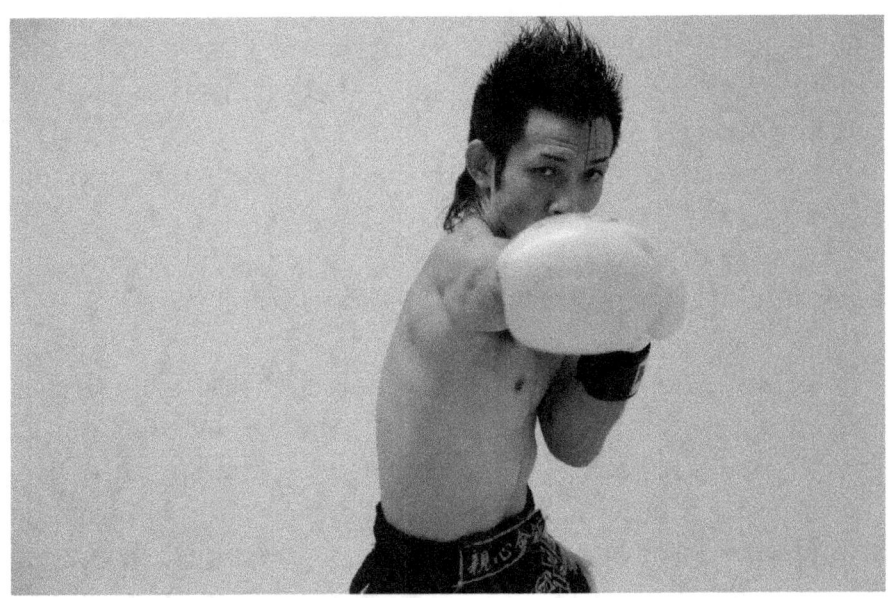

(Punch with Stretch Reflex)

To make it easy to understand, so-called "hand-hitting" - I thought about a punch that uses stretch reflex by focusing on joints and muscles of upper limbs such as a wrist joint, an elbow joint, a shoulder joint, etc. starting from a fist. Even with the same hand-held punch, I think whether there will be a difference in speed, power, easy-to-put out, etc. with a punch that utilises stretch reflex and a punch that does not utilise. Based on this, please try not only hand punching but also hit with joints and spine, such as hip joints and muscles involved in punching and striking using stretch reflex.

【5-5 Stretch reflex and kicking technique】

Next, let's think about kicking. Let's think about two types of front kick.

1) One case is kick the leg with the shortest distance course from the stance.

2) Another case, when you kick by moving the foot to the back side of the body from the position you have set.

1)'s movement of the hip joint of the kicking leg is "Flexion". One of the muscle which flexes the hip joint is, greater psoas muscle. If you kick as it is, the length of the major psoas muscle will only become even shorter from the condition you have set. We will kick legs against gravity, so movement will be slow.

2)'s case, the movement of the hip joint becomes "extension → flexion". Once the extension of the hip joint comes in, the major psoas muscle is stretched. By making good use of the stretch reflex generated at this moment and bending the hip joint, you can perform the front kick more quickly. The knee joints is the same as well. The movement of bend and stretch is used stretch reflex more than just the movement of stretching the knee joints.

(Front Kick without Stretch Reflex)

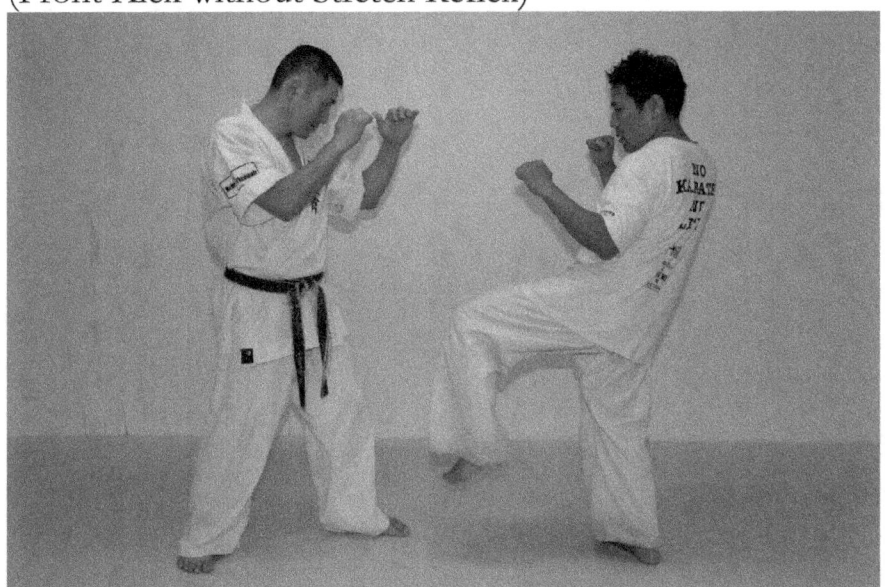

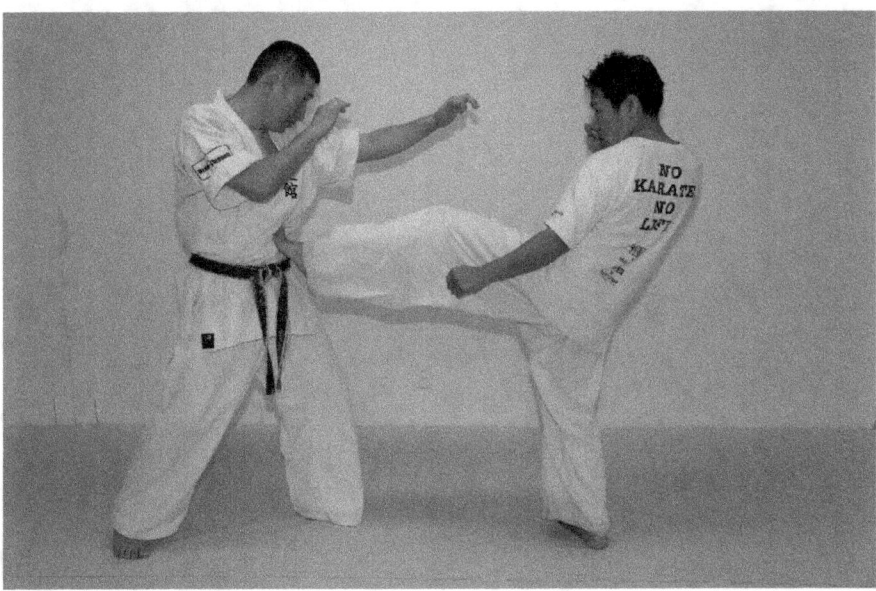

(Front Kick with Stretch Reflex)

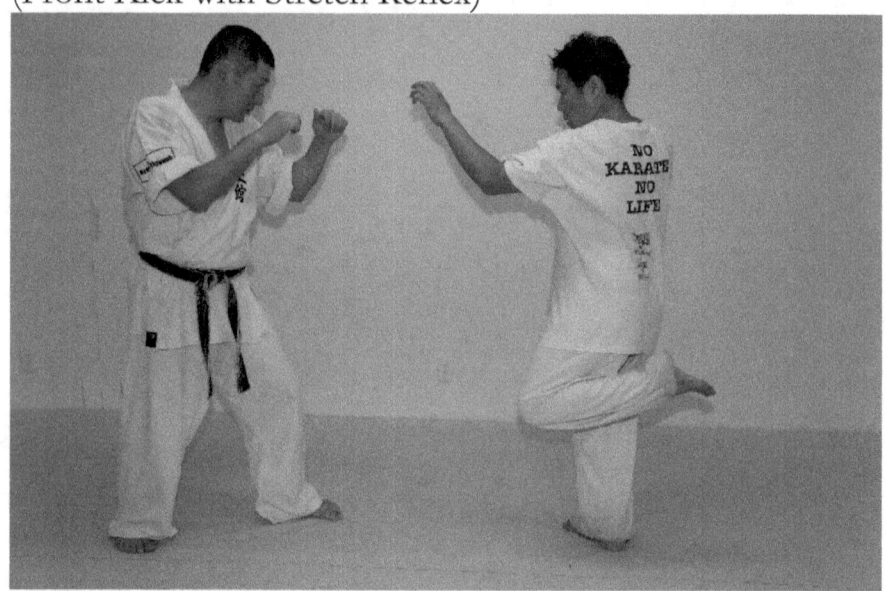

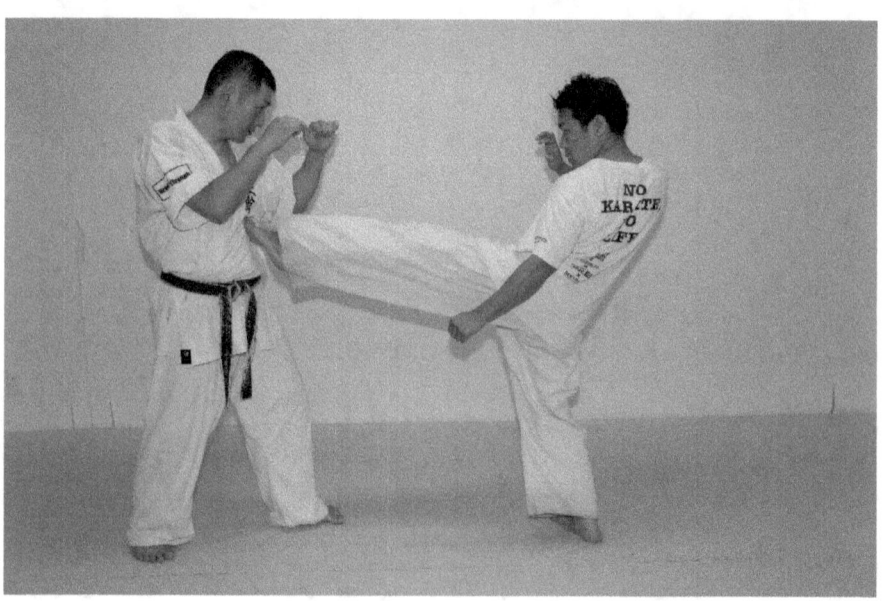

Next is about back spin kick. Back spin kick is a kicking technique that makes the opponent's face hit by a heel and the toes, but when the consciously strongly contracting the muscle group on the back of the thigh and applying it, conversely utilising the extensional reflection of the muscle group on the posterior side of the thigh There is a big difference in case of hitting. Top fighters who are good at back spin kick do not issue commands to bend the knee joints from the brain but instead extend the knee joints and the knee joint naturally bends using the stretch reflex that occurred at that time. It is fast and has power. If you want to bend the knee joint, stretch it before doing it. Even when practicing other punches and kicks, it is a very fun time to experiment, to see which part of the stretch reflex improves the power and speed.

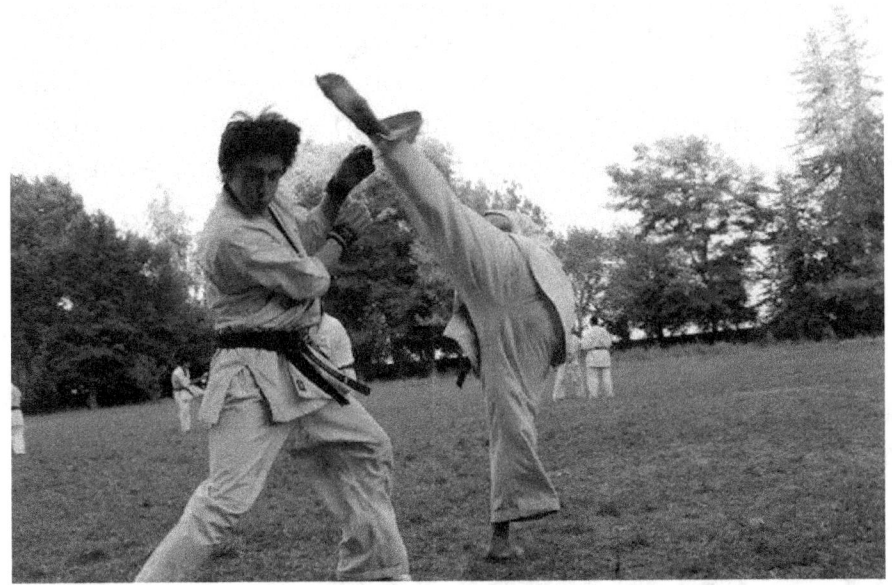

【5-6 Grappling and stretch reflex】

Even in wrestling, mixed fighting sports, jiu-jitsu and other martial arts grabbing opponents, stretch reflexes are made use of everywhere. When grasping the opponent's arms and legs, when the hand is changed from the state of Paper (of rock-paper-scissors hand) to the state of Rock (bending only), the fingers are extended in the direction of a little Paper from the state of the midpoint between Paper and Rock when comparing the case of grasping in the Stone state, I think that the latter is faster and sure to grasp.

Humans got bipedal walking and gathered the nuts and fruits at a higher position than the ground using the (foreleg) hands and have ate it since ever. "Grabbing things" can be said to be human beings are good at this movement. In that case, it is natural and reliable to move with stretch flex that you grab it after opening it wider than the width of the object once. In the grappling fighting sports, you will need a movement to grab and hold down your opponent in an instant, so you can expect a performance improvement with grappling with stretching reflection. That's why "How to open then grasp" rather than "how to grasp".

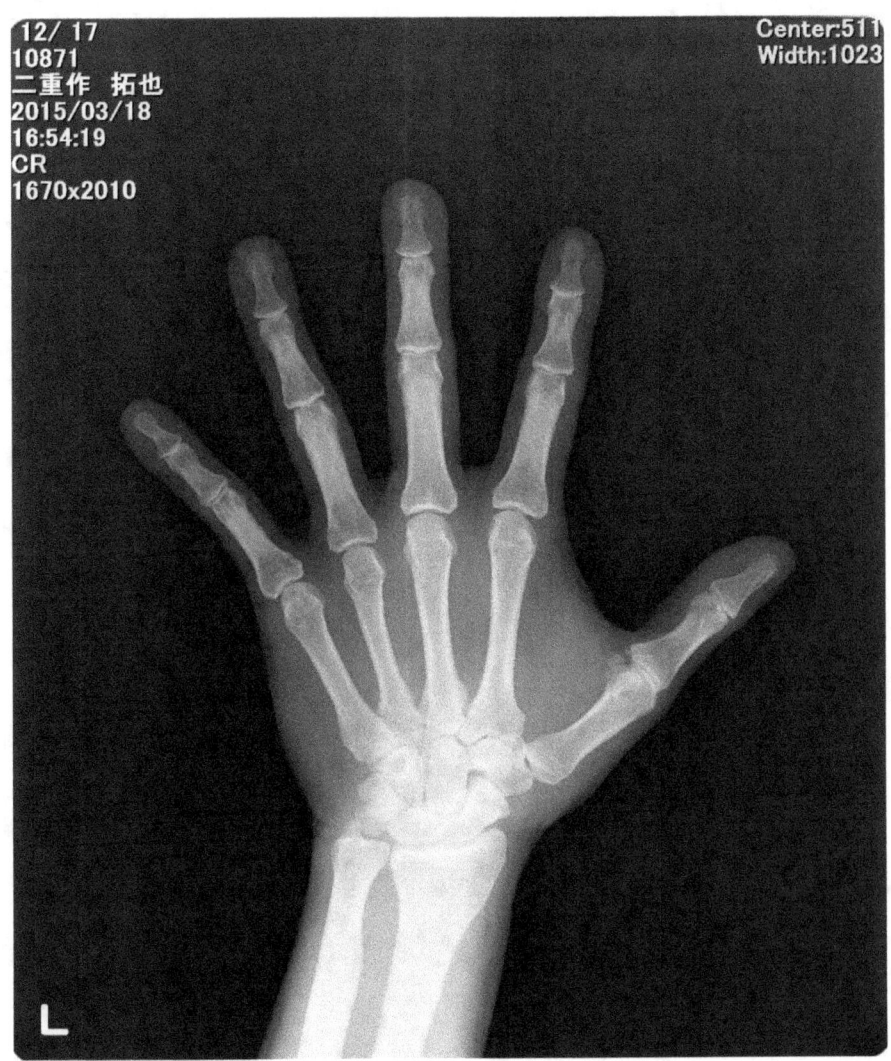

135

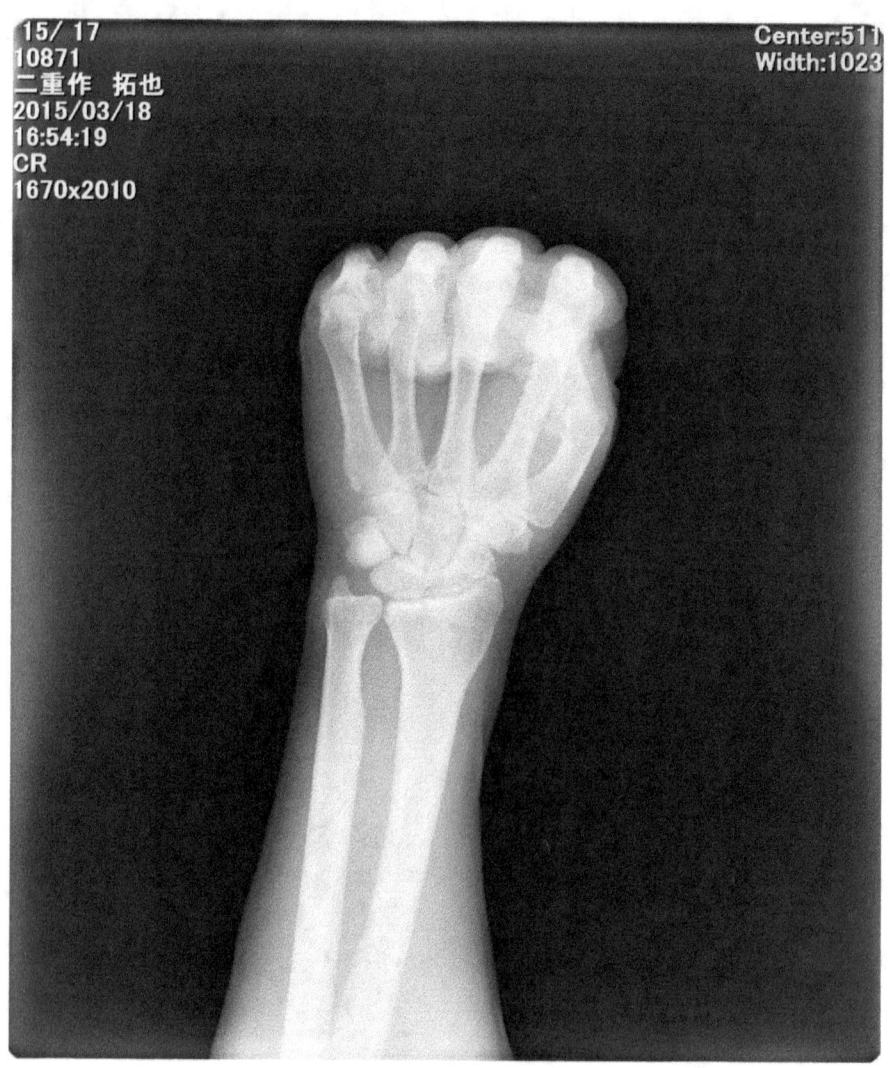

136

【5-7 Arm wrestling and the mantra of martial arts】

Let's do arm-wrestling this time. Forms and ways can be ordinary arm wrestling. How do you move your arm from the place where when it stops moving at a certain angle and enters an antagonism state? You can see frequently the muscles that demonstrate just the muscle strength and entered full-fledged competition → the one who is exhausted ahead loses.

Here is the stretch reflex. When it comes to antagonistic state, keep the state on purpose for a few seconds. Next, just 2 to 3 cm is enough, move your arm to the back of the hand. move it for a moment in the direction that you will lose. And the next moment, if you move to the side of the palm, you can win over by sweeping at once. Also, even if you cannot win, you can recover even a little. Give away to the opponent a little is a point. At that time, since the muscle group which had been contracted so far is stretched for a moment, stretch reflex occurs and it can be strongly contracted again at the next moment. Human muscles, when issuing a command to collect and withdraw, the muscular strength that can be demonstrated descending as the time elapses with the first moment contracted is the mechanism that gives the best force. At the timing when they fell each other, relax and attach stretch reflex on your side to get maximum contraction. For the opponent, although the muscular strength was demonstrated at a certain joint angle, the sudden angle changes, so the correspondence to that moment will be delayed. At first glance, compared to strength, arm wrestling that looks like, but there is a way of using the body to be advantageous.

It is possible to apply it in various scenes of arm wrestling move by utilising this stretch reflex. Even in the event of

137

sumo wrestling and wrestling, the top fighters use the technique of "giving away to the opponent then push". Even in judo and comprehension throws, using the body like "pull a little after antagonistic state if you want to push it", "pull a little after pushing in reverse if you want to draw" generates a great speed and power. Even in case of the offence side with this armlock, if you get into a antagonism state, you leave it to the power as it is and not continue pulling your opponent's arm, but if you give up only a few centimeters to the opponent for a moment, right next moment it is easy to extend the elbow joint. If you can't make it at once, just do it intermittently twice, three times, and the opponent will not know at what angle to put in force. If you do not know the mechanism of stretch reflex, the muscles performing the desired movements will only move in the direction of shrinking, so muscular strength and stamina will be exhausted unnecessarily. The result, it makes you very tired.

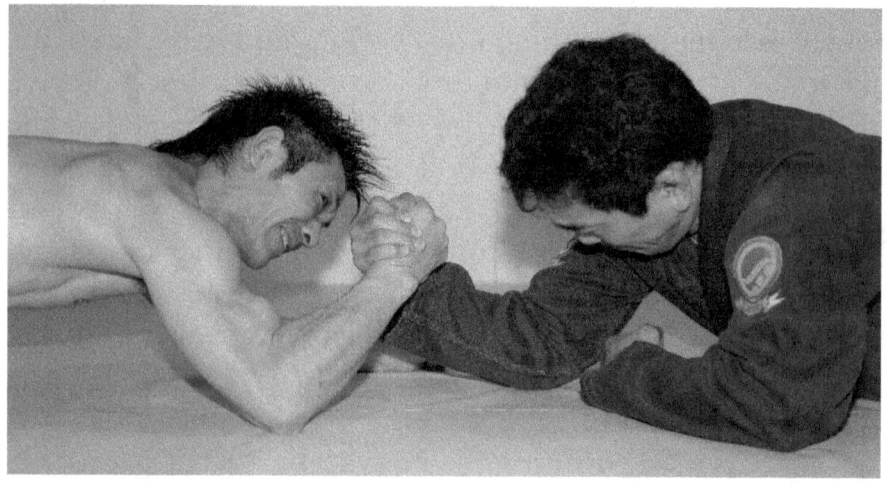

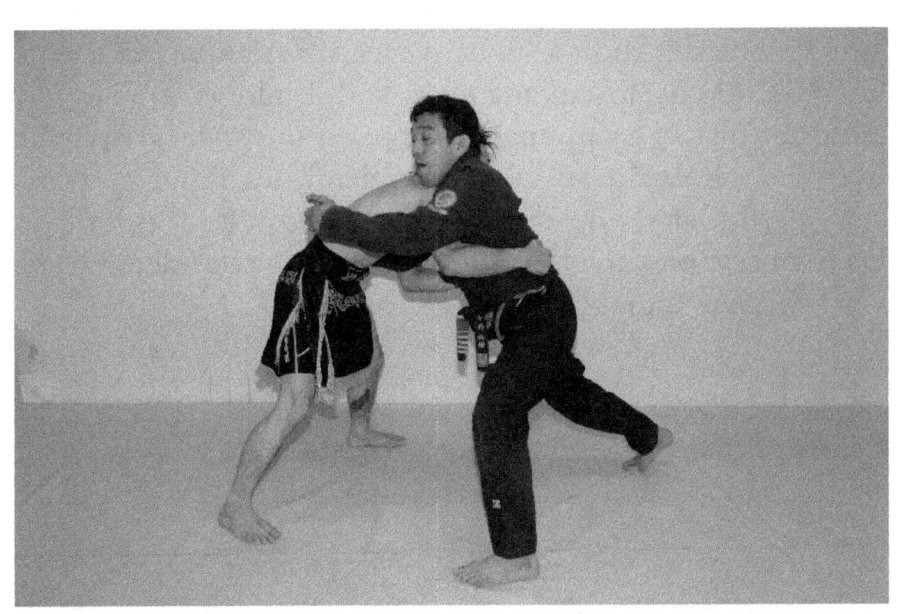

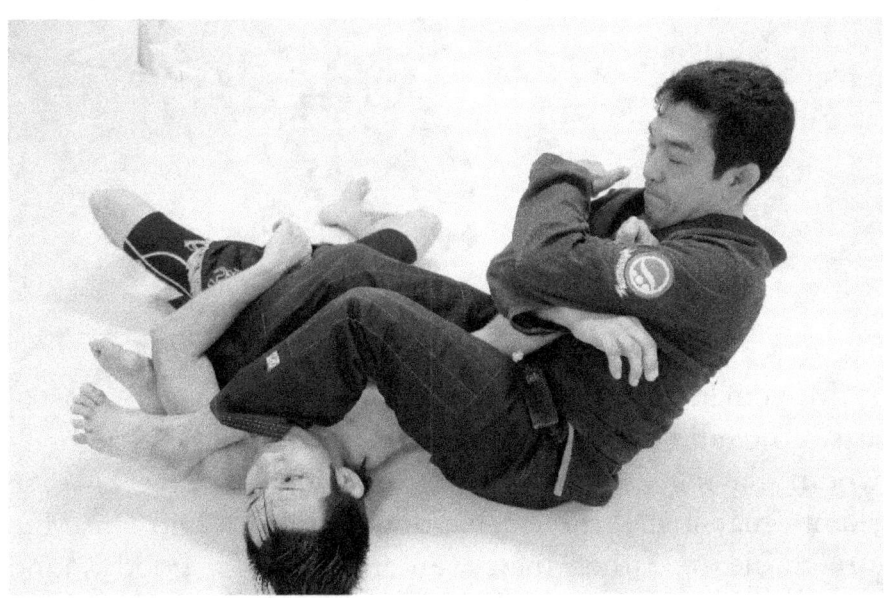

Gozo Shiota, known as a master of Aikido, leaves the word "Budo is instantaneous , and Budo is lifelong." I interpret this as a fighting medicine in the style of "pursue over the whole life to take a moment". In fighting sports and martial arts, the direction that shortens the time to keep muscle power as much as possible is considered to be very effective and makes sense.

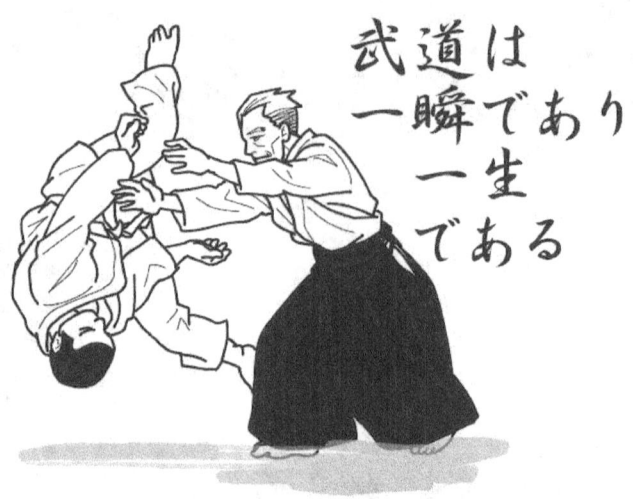

武道は
一瞬であり
一生
である

"Movement" is the deal in fighting sports and martial arts. (Including dare not move) Especially those fighters whom having trouble of improvement, fighters in the slump, may install the evaluation criteria of "Did I use the stretch flex?" rather than wether hearing a good sound whiling hitting mitts, could move smoothly or felt a good result.

6 Gravity

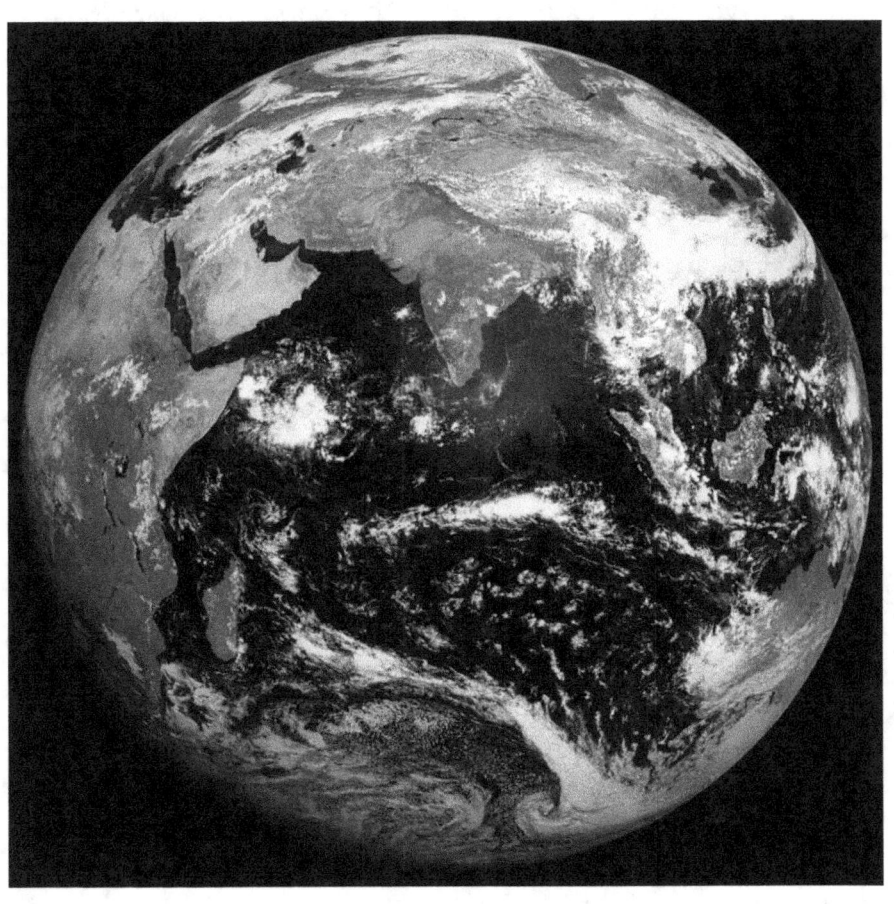

【6-1 How to use gravity?】

What if a bag containing rice weighing 10 kilograms falls from above your head? What if this was 50 kilos? What if it's 70 kilometers? What if it was 100 kilometers? Can you still remain "calm" if that right on the top of you? Gravity is given to all human beings on Earth. As you live on the earth, you will receive control of gravity proportional to your weight. So, performance in fighting sports / martial arts will change greatly with "Do you put on gravity on your side?" Or "Do you go against gravity?" Here we will examine the movement of fighting sports and martial arts from the viewpoint of gravity.

【6-2 Basic movement to ride gravity 1 ~ Drop up from the hip joint ~】

Let's first experience the gravity as a basic. Stand up with both feet shoulder width wide. From this state,

1) bending both hip joints (movement in the direction in which the knees move forward),
2) bending both knee joints (movement of the crus in the back direction),
3) dorsal flexion of the joints of both feet (movement in the direction that the toes face up),

We will do the three movements in one moment at the same time. Instead of doing it slowly, instantaneously, at the same time. Lower limb brakes are simultaneously disengaged, so that the upper part from the hip joint drops easily. When I get the timing, I think that you can get a feeling like when you fall down on a free fall of an amusement park.

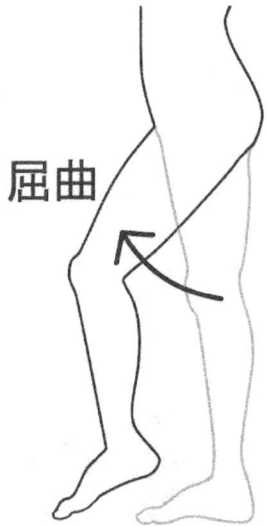

(Flexion---Hip Joint)

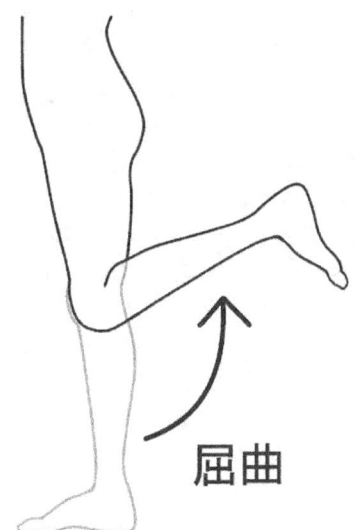

(Flexion—Knee Joint)

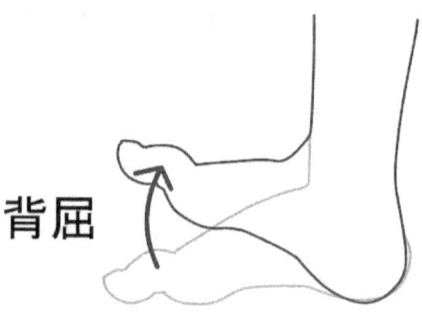

背屈

(Dorsal Flexion)

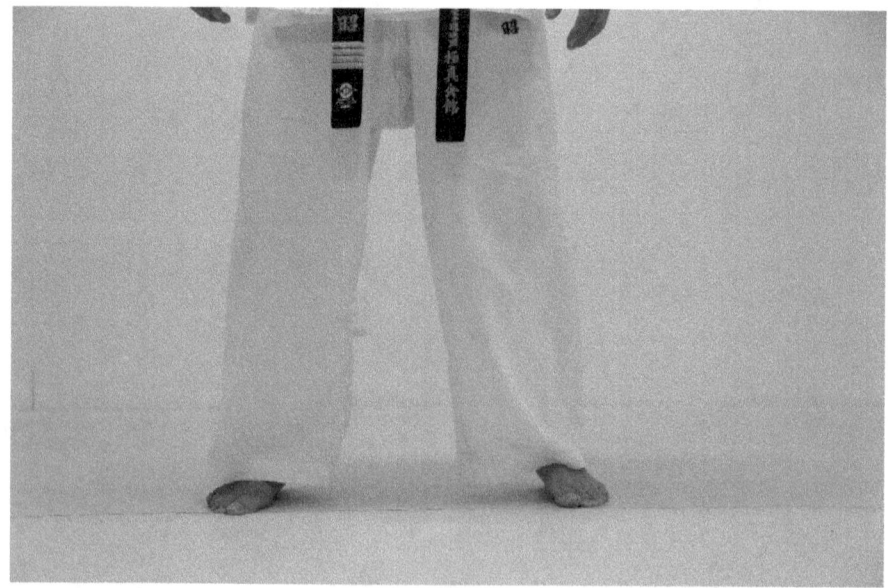

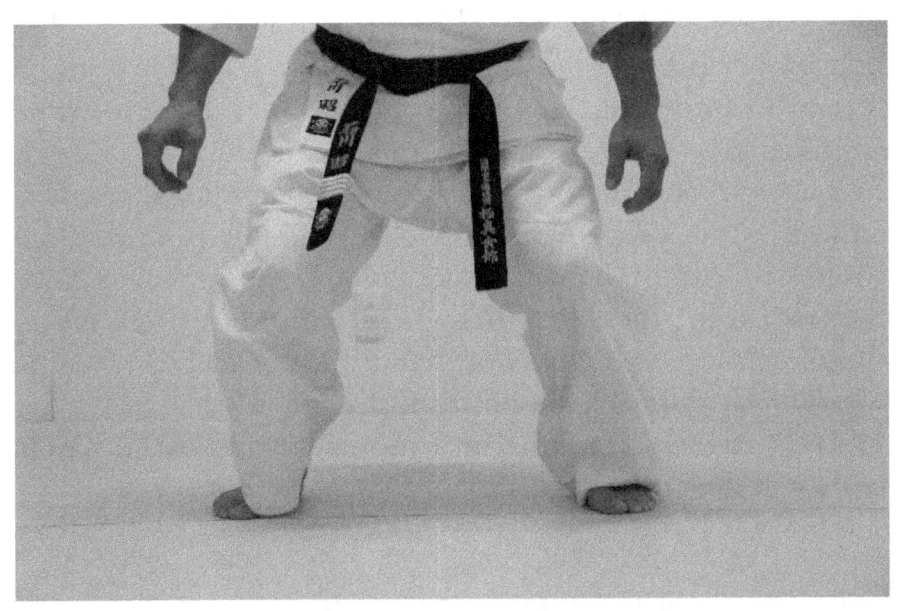

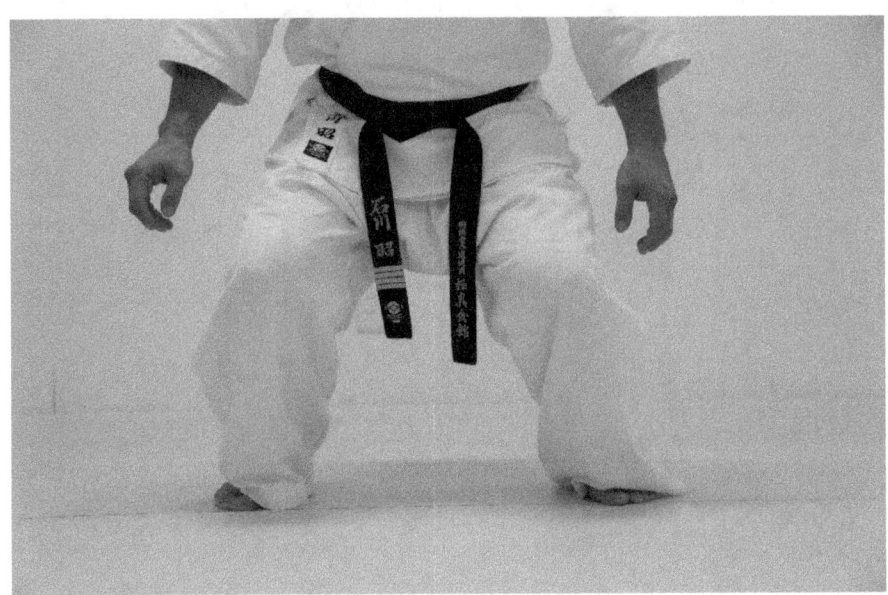

145

【6-3 Basic movement to ride gravity 2 ~ Suspend the bottom of both feet ~】

If you can do this, 4) Let's run 1) 2) 3) at the same time so that a gap of several centimeters can be formed on both feet bottom and the ground. From the standing state, it is an image that uses lower limbs "as suddenly both feet are shortened". If both hands suddenly disappear 5 cm from the bottom of the sole, "bang" the entire body will fall in the direction of gravity. Try practicing the feeling that the whole body falls as a chunk from the sole of the feet, doing 1) 2) 3) at the same time in a moment so that the whole body will float in the air while it falls.

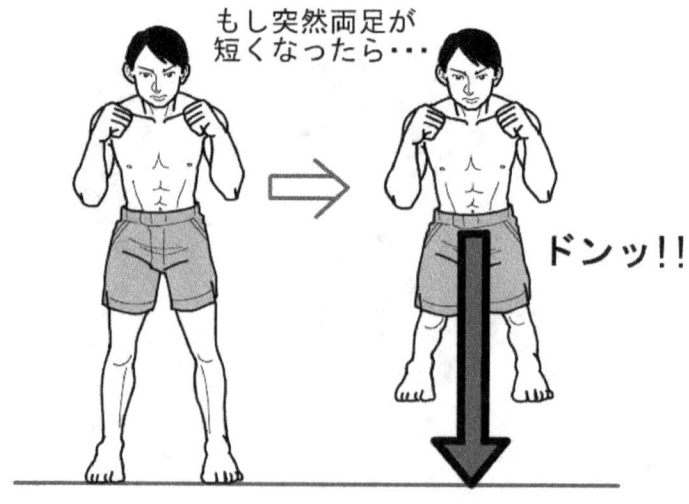

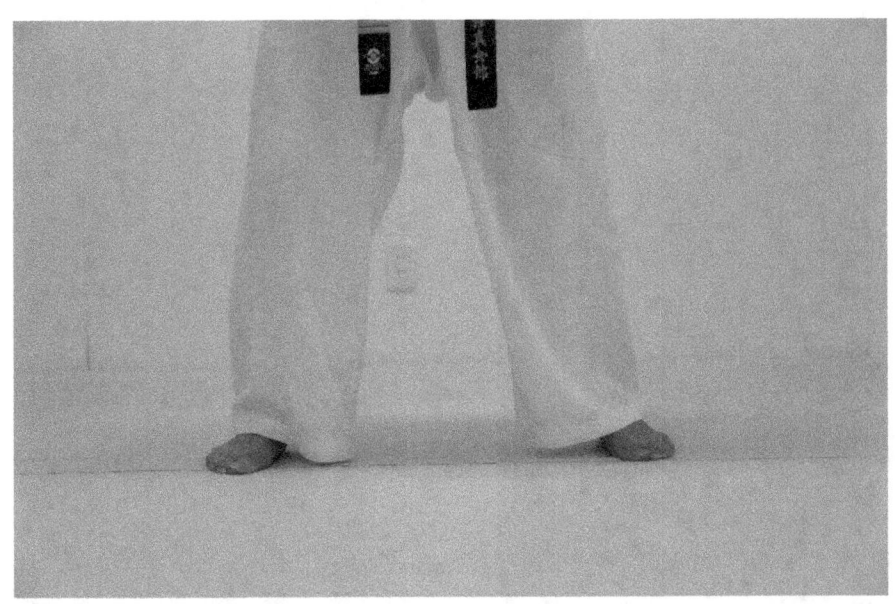

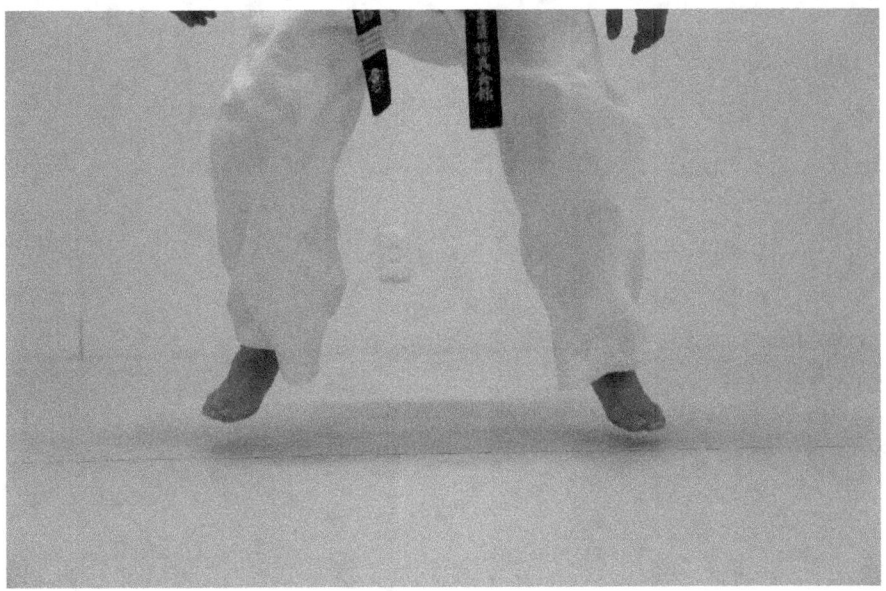

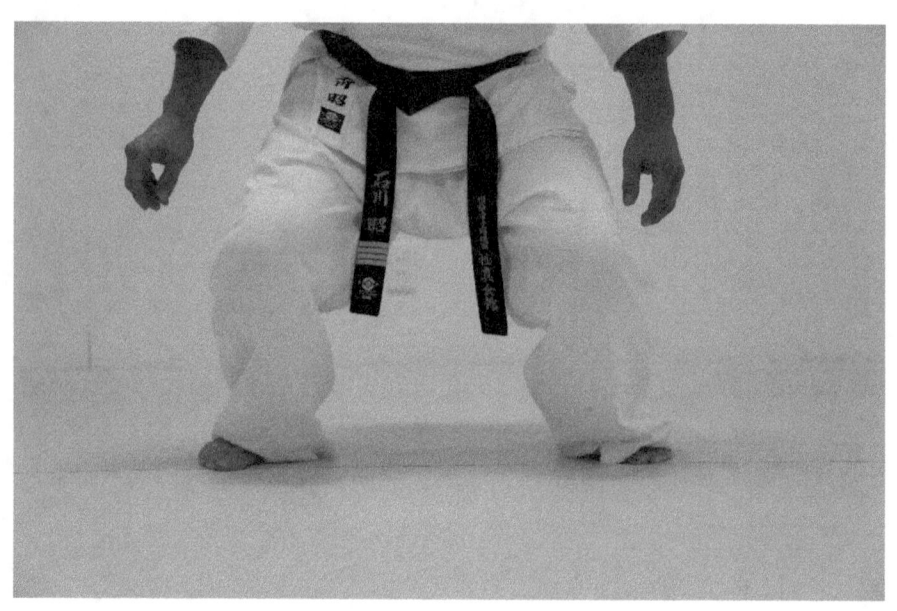

【6-4 Basic movement 3 riding on gravity to float one foot bottom】

Let's do basic movement 2 with one foot. Something like, having only the left leg or only the right leg. If you can do it with spreading your feet with a shoulder width, with so-called fighting style (in the set state), make it fall to the front foot (if the orthodox style with the left foot front, is on the left foot, southpaw on the right foot). Also, it falls to the back leg (if the orthodox style with the left foot front, is on the right foot, southpaw on the left foot) from the standing state. Like the movement of tap dance, please imagine and move as "one leg suddenly got shorter".

Front

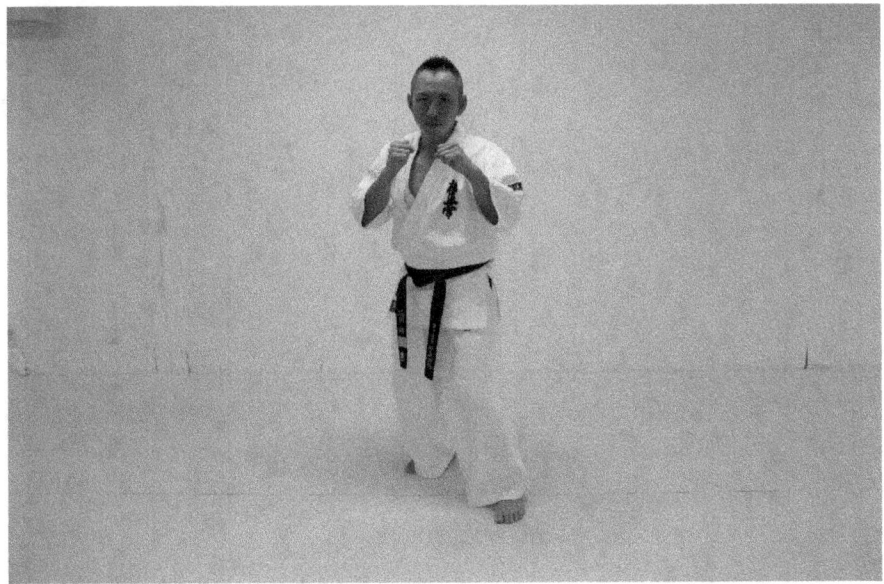

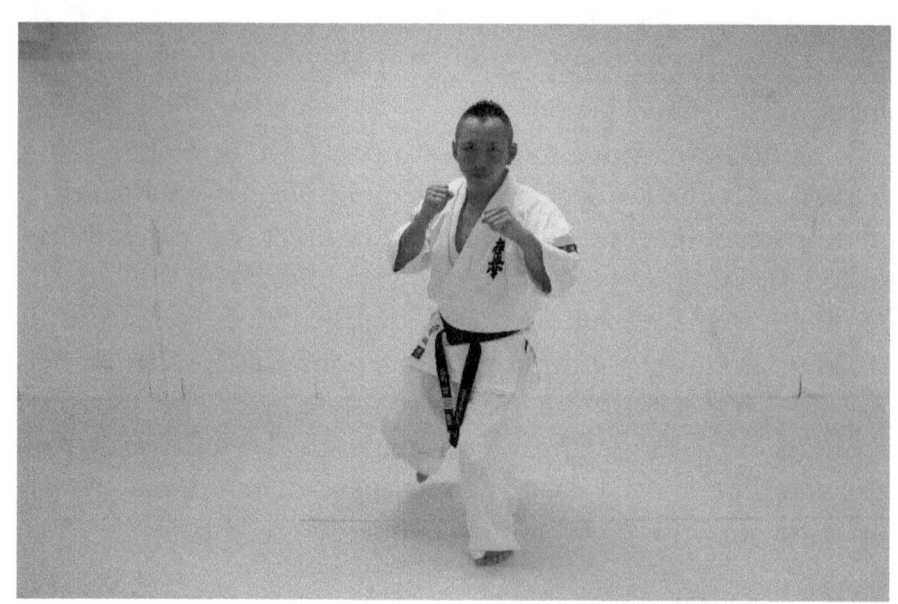

Back

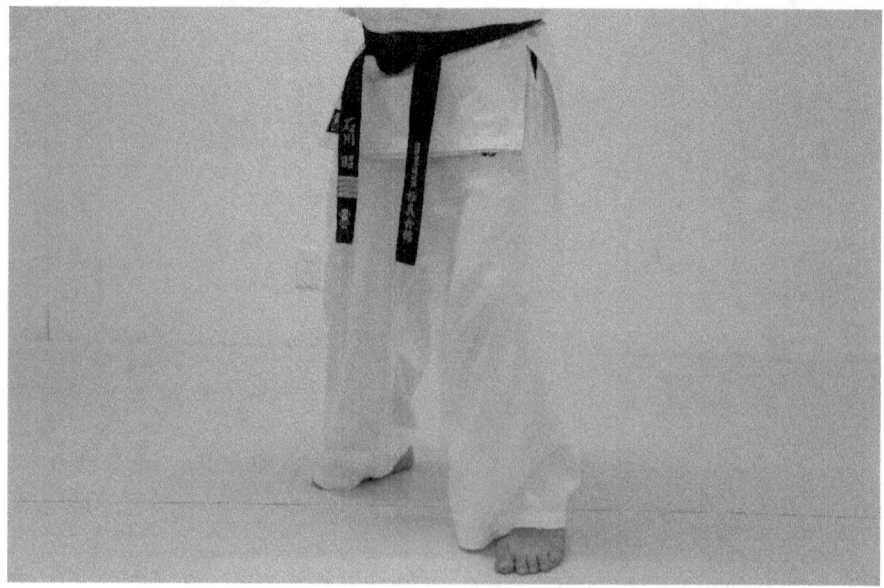

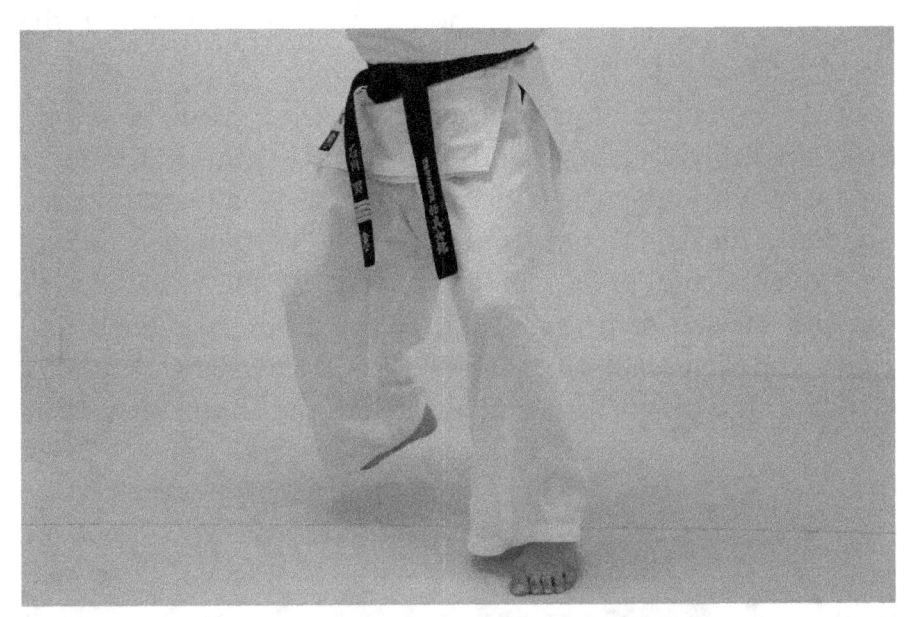

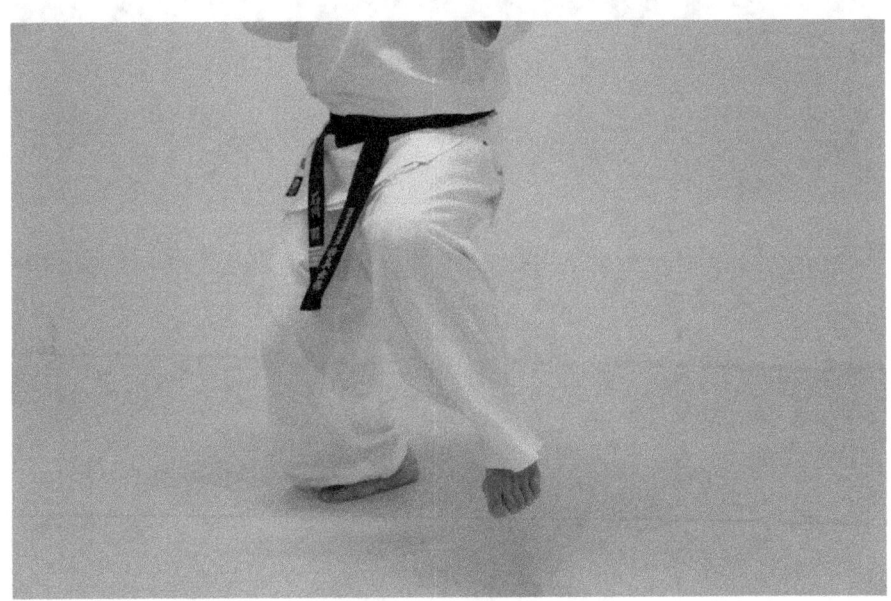

【6-5 Basic movement to ride gravity 4 ～ Expand the width of feet ～】

Stand by spreading your feet about the shoulder width, and spread your feet to the left and right at the next moment with a snap. If the initial width is 50 centimeters, suddenly make it 70 centimeters or 80 centimeters. Then, as a result, the pelvis and head fall in the direction of gravity. In the same way, please try both feet back and forth and diagonally in various directions. Also please try with the initiating width narrower than the shoulder width.

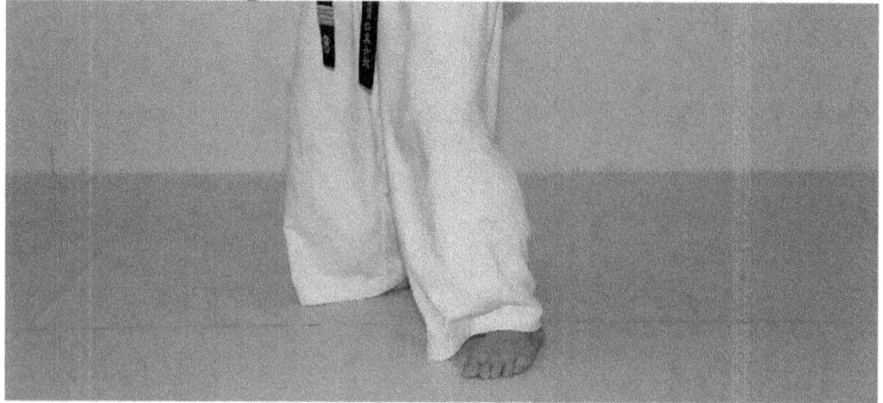

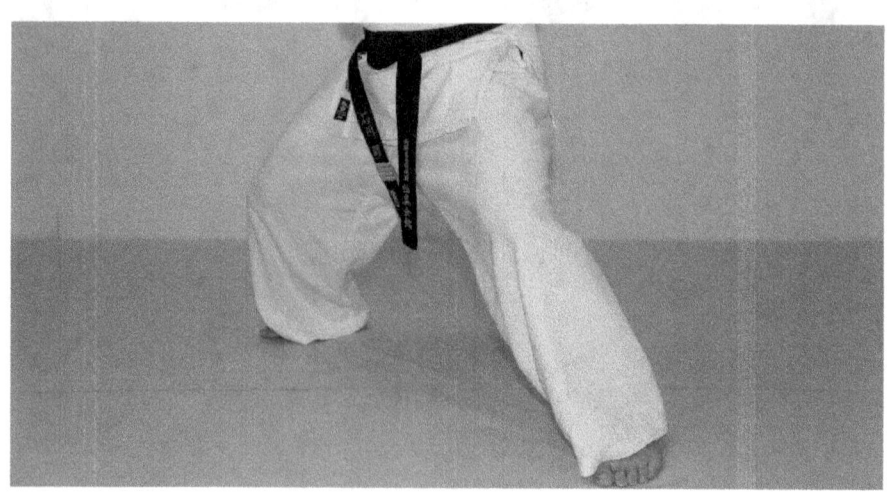

【6-6 Movement using reaction of gravity】

This time, let's try using the reaction of gravity. As the basic movement 2 riding on gravity is easy to understand, I will explain this as an example. When falling to the lowest point, a large counteraction will be added to the bottom of the sole, so let's just use that reaction and jump up. If expressed by words, it is a movement of "falling → going up". In the case of "falling", it takes the gravity and goes up using the reaction (the force that the ground pushes back the foot) generated at the sole at the lowest point. This is a movement similar to dropping basketball on the floor. If you drop the ball, it bounces off the floor and moves up. Instead of using only the muscular strength you are going to rise, you use the falling reaction to jump. At the lowest point which fell on gravity, the thigh involved in extension of the gluteus muscle and knee joint (movement in the direction of extending the knee) related to extension of the hip joint (movement of the hip joint when the knee moves from front to back), the musclus triceps surae group related to the planter flexion of the ankle (movement of the toe from the top to the bottom) has been contracted and stretched. In this way, "a state in which the muscle length contracts while it contracts" is called "eccentric contraction", but the eccentric contraction is shorter than the concentric contraction which contracts while the muscle length is shortened , there is a report that fast muscle fiber are frequently used.

Fast muscle fiber is a muscle fiber excellent for instantaneously demonstrating a large force in addition to quick muscle contraction speed, also called white muscle fiber. White flesh fish such as sea breams, flounders and anglers are not good at swimming long distances, but the instantaneous speed of taking food is extremely fast. In contrast, red flesh fish such as bonitos and tunas are good at swimming at a steady speed for long distances. Humans have both of these muscle fibers and can be used properly. The fact that fast muscle fibers are easy to use means that speedy and instantaneous movements are easy to achieve. Because stretching reflection also occurs in this, it can be moved faster than "going down" rather than "going up from below". If you could catch the feeling with this, try to use the reaction of gravity even with other basic movements! The principle of utilizing the reaction of gravity is common, just by using different muscle groups and joint angles.

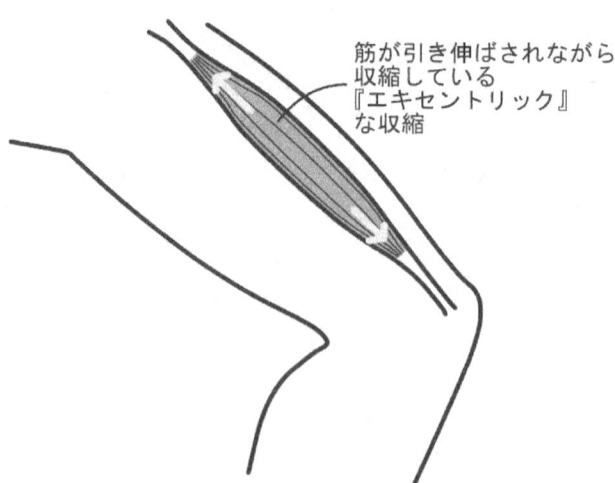

筋が引き伸ばされながら
収縮している
『エキセントリック』
な収縮

(eccentric contraction)

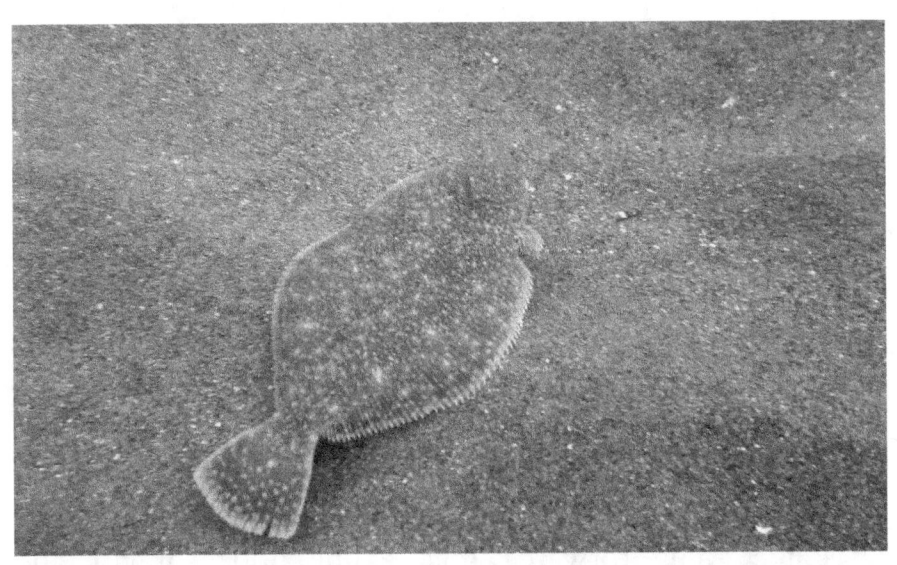

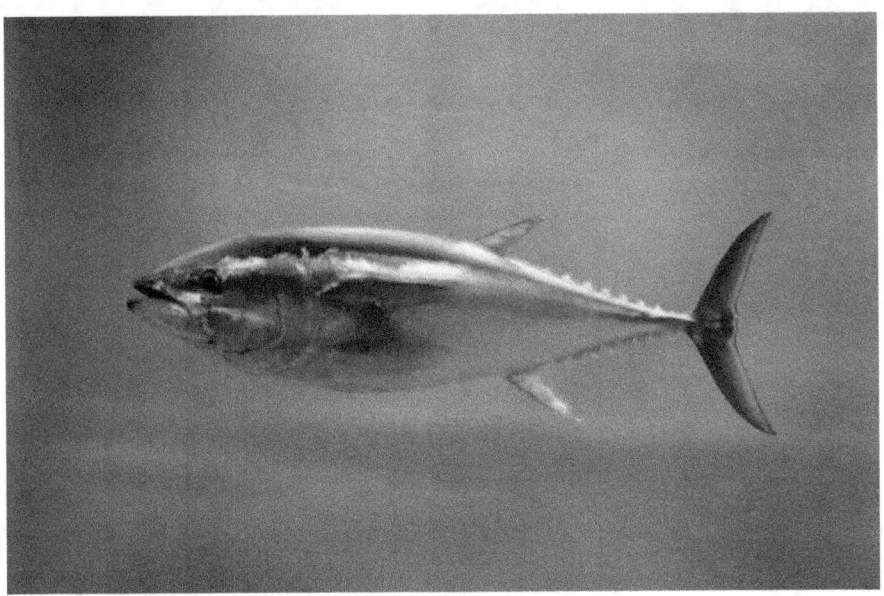

【6-7 Relationship between Ichiro's batting and walking】

I was watching the slow motion movie of batting practice of Ichiro, a major extraordinary major leaguer from Japan, and I noticed certain features. When swinging his bat from the back to the front, his head and the pelvis traced the trajectory of falling in the direction of gravity once, then going up again from the lowest point. Because it was a movie I happened to find on the internet, it may be only that time, but when I saw the movement, I was convinced that "This is it!"

If Ichiro 's movement was seen from the side as alphabet, it was moving in V letter or U letter shape. Venture to say, it is like going forward while falling under gravity and sending the ball out with the body using the reaction of gravity from the lowest point. Rather than striking with Ichiro's own muscle output alone, not going against gravity, rather riding gravity and getting the resultant reaction. It was a beautiful batting form like flowing without stagnation.

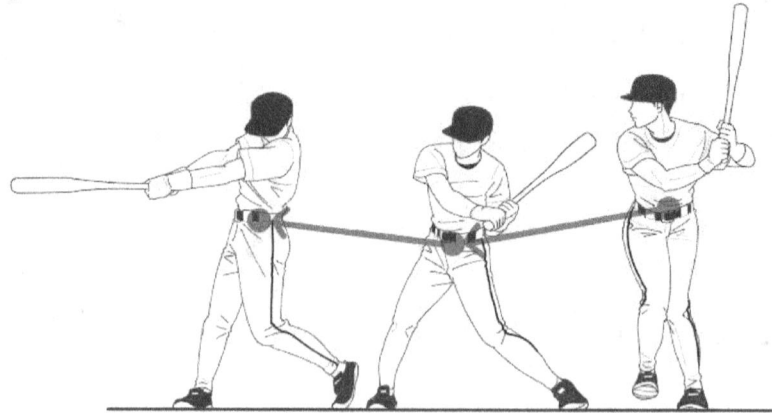

The normal walking of a human being is also a moment when the head and pelvis fall to the lowest point in the direction of gravity when the leg is opened (when the right foot and the left foot are most separated), the moment when the back legs overtake the front leg (when the right foot and the left foot come closest) The head and pelvis return to their original heights. It is hard to be conscious of walking with narrow stride, but I think that you can see your head and pelvis will go down as you walk with a little wider steps. Ichiro's batting and our daily walking movement. What is common to these is that the movement to move forward involves more or less vertical movement.

【6-8 Punch and gravity】

Let's take the movement of fighting sports / martial arts actually based on these. First of all, I will try the punch of the front hand from the state of the fighting stance. Please try out the course of the fist, in parallel to the ground or slightly downward. At this time, I will try the movement of the basic movement 2 riding on gravity with only the front leg. If you are standing at orthodox (left hand at front), hit the left punch while instantaneously performing hip joint flexion, knee joint flexion, ankle dorsiflexion at the same time so as to create a gap between the left sole and the floor, the body blow that combines the force to fall to the left front and the force to bring the arm forward. (It is an application of the basic movement 3 riding on gravity 3 ～ floating one foot bottom side ～ It is a feeling that putting the falling body by gravity as is, on the punch. Should it be expressed as left punch on gravity? This way of hitting is a method which fits when you hit a place that is equal to or lower than the shoulder, such as the chest or body, or when the opponent is shorter than yourself.

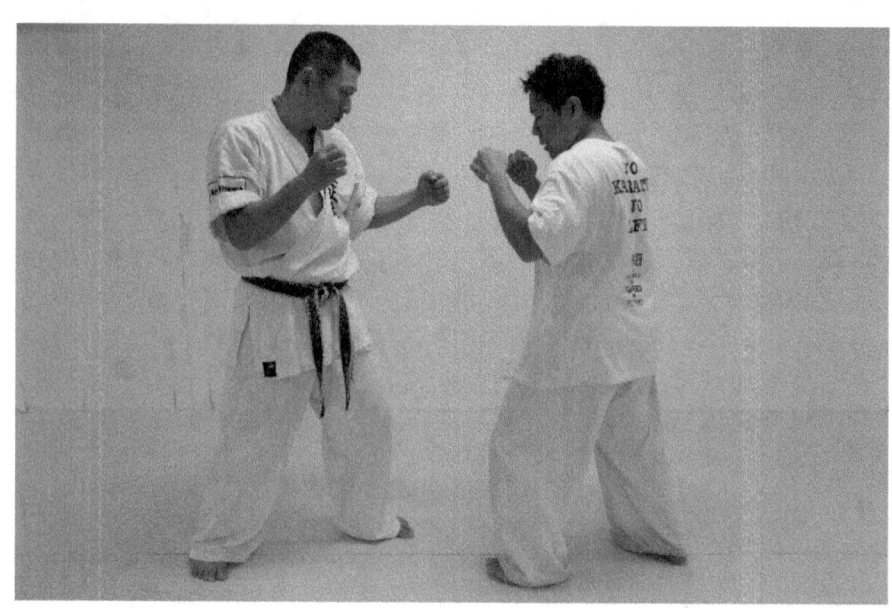

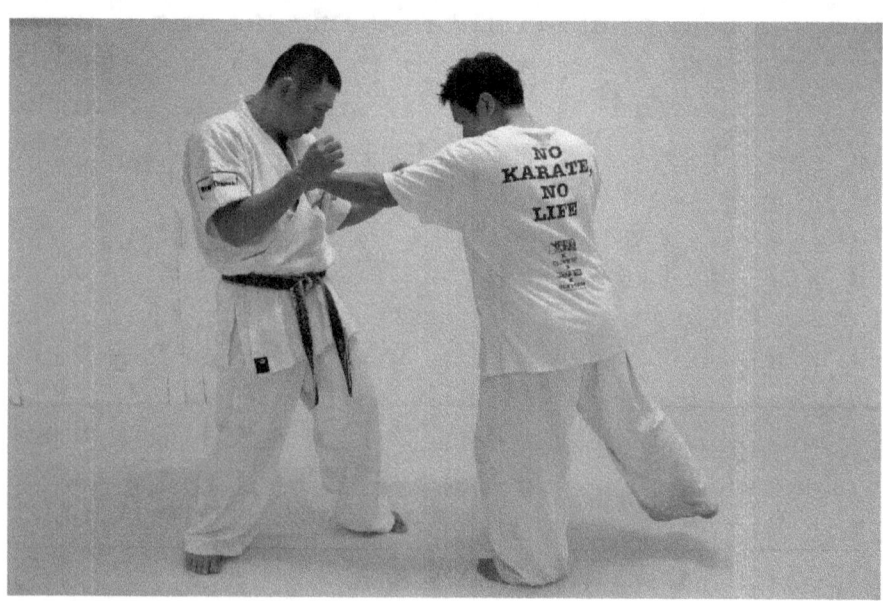

If you strike above the shoulder, you want to use the reaction of gravity. From the fighting stance, create a gap between the bottom of the left foot and the floor and fall onto it. If you hit the left punch while raising using that reaction, it will be a left punch using the reaction of gravity. Since it is a punch to be put out when it "falls then rises", it will behave like two movements.

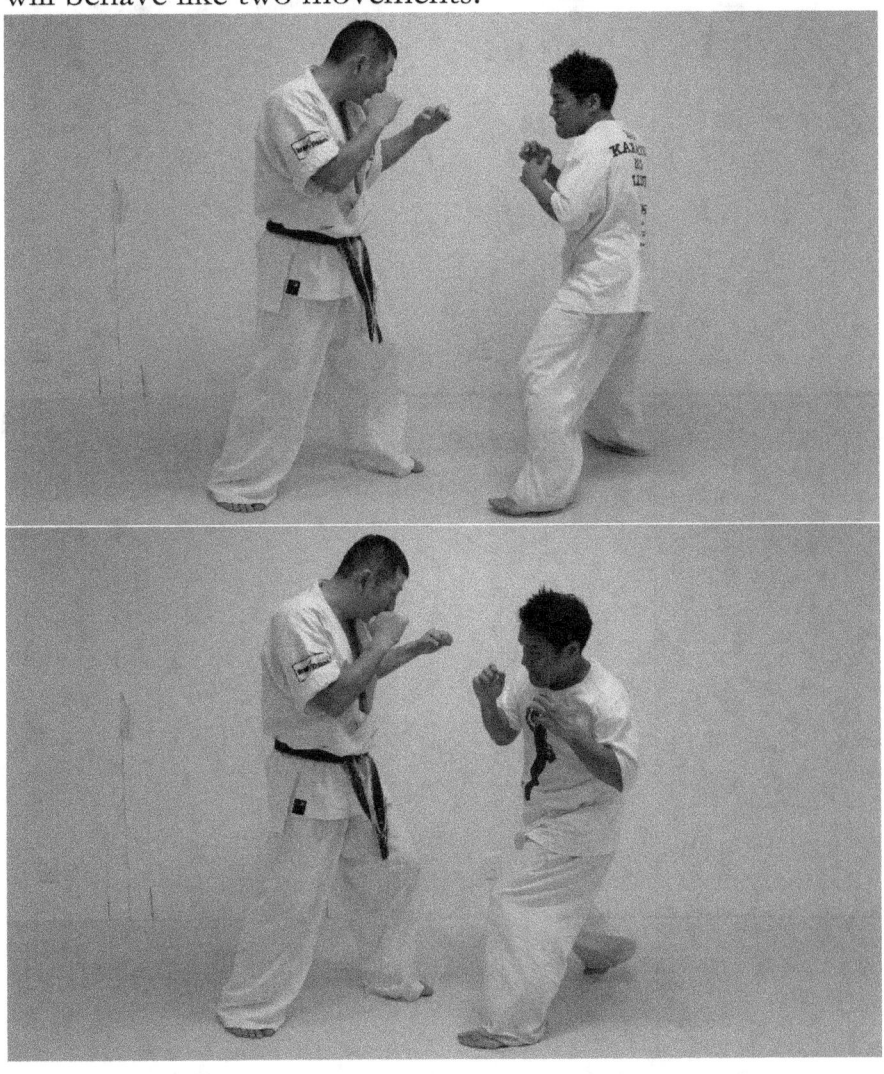

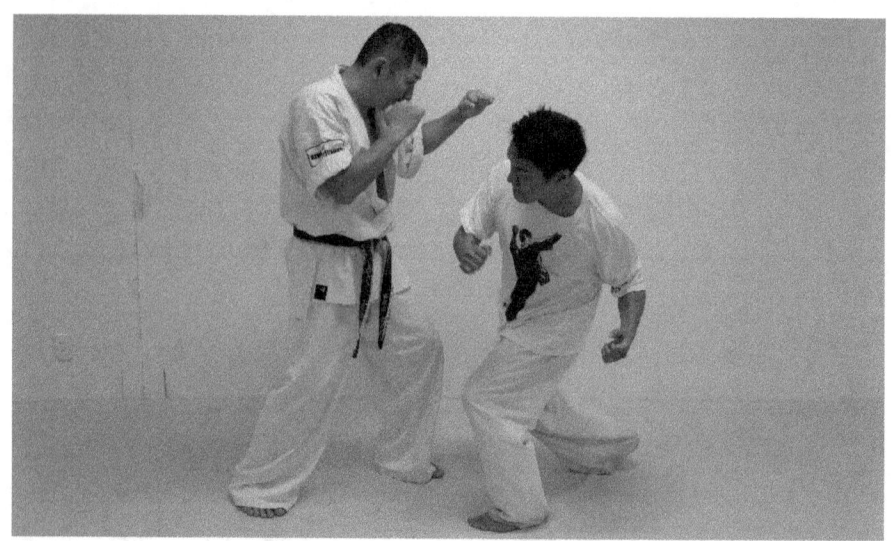

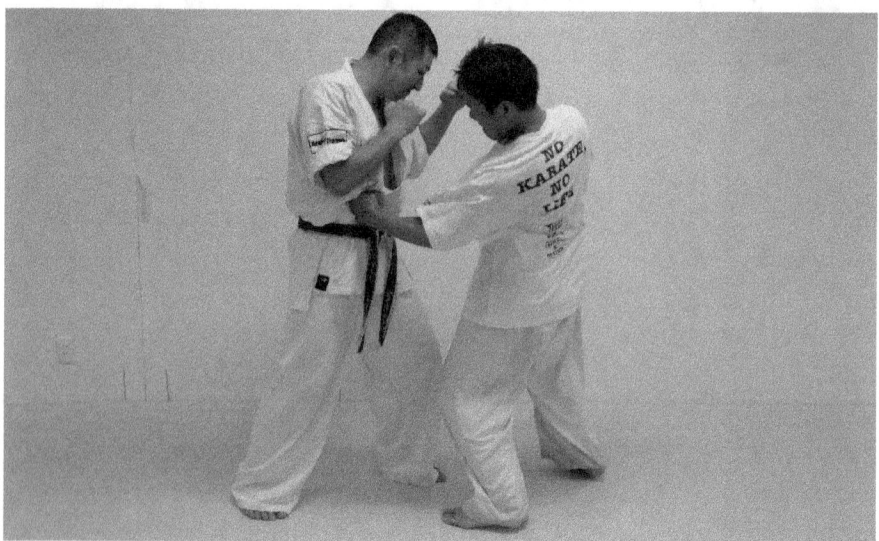

Like this, even with the same left punch, there are two kinds of movement depending on how gravity is used. (The body falls down to hit high, the body rises to hit low, the vectors of force conflict with each other.) The reason why we introduced two kinds of front hand punches is, to let you understand there are 2 ways, using the body that the movements of fighting sports / martial arts use gravity as it is, or use gravity reaction. This is to make gravity easier to use.

【6-9 Technique is】

Even the world champion of fighting sports or martial arts does not fight all the people all over the world. If in an individual match, to every single opponent. If in tournament matches, win with reliability to the fighter whom won through the tournament. That's a champion. Simply put, it's a one-on-one correspondence accumulation. A legendary martial artist, Royce Gracie, who made the name of the Gracie clan all over the world left the word "techniques are drawers". We use techniques that match the opponent and modalities, the relationships that are mutually exclusive, not using them conversely, sometimes add up, or assemble by subtraction. I interpret Royce's word as "withdrawal of drawer itself is technique". If you have advantage on your reach or your height, the dropping jab is very effective. Just dropping from the top slightly, the probability that you will hit your opponent at a hard-to-reach distance will also rise. On the contrary, if the opponent has that advantage, you have to shorten the distance, so it will be hard to hit the dropping jabs. Even only talk about a jab, it will change depending on the person's body and the relative relationship with the opponent. If there is a method weak in your skills, it may be resolved by reviewing gravity and how to use the body. Left jab, but the way is not one.

【6-10 Knee kick and gravity】

This time, it's knee kick. Suppose you are kicking the right knee kick with your orthodox stance. From the stance, you bend the right hip joint, the knee joint also bends, and when the ankle does planter flexion, it becomes a knee kick shape. However, since this is a movement of "raising the right leg against gravity", the right leg is heavy, it does not produce power, before all, you get tired soon, so if the match is prolonged, your stamina will be exhausted, then knee kick will be difficult to put out. The knee kick using the reaction of gravity is placed in front of the left foot and puts in motion to widen the foot width. (Basic movement to ride gravity 4) Then the pelvis will fall in the direction of the floor. This is the first half movement of V shape. At the timing when the pelvis reaches the lowest point, the right hip joint is extended, the knee joint is also extended, and the ankle is dorsiflexed (the movement with the toes facing upward). Extended reflex is generated in the muscle group of the right lower limb extended at that time, it becomes a kicking leg of hip flexion, knee joint flexion, ankle base flexion, and the hip joint of the left foot which is the axis foot is bent at the lowest point, The next moment it becomes easier to extend. From the lowest point until the knee kick hits, it will be the second half movement of V shape. It is the difference between "Raise the right knee" and "Mix in the movement of easy to raise the right knee in the movement of fall then rise". Introducing this way of using the body may change from "raising the leg" to "the leg and the whole body are rising." Because the number of muscle groups participating in kicking also increases, the power also rises.

Knee kick with raining left leg against gravity

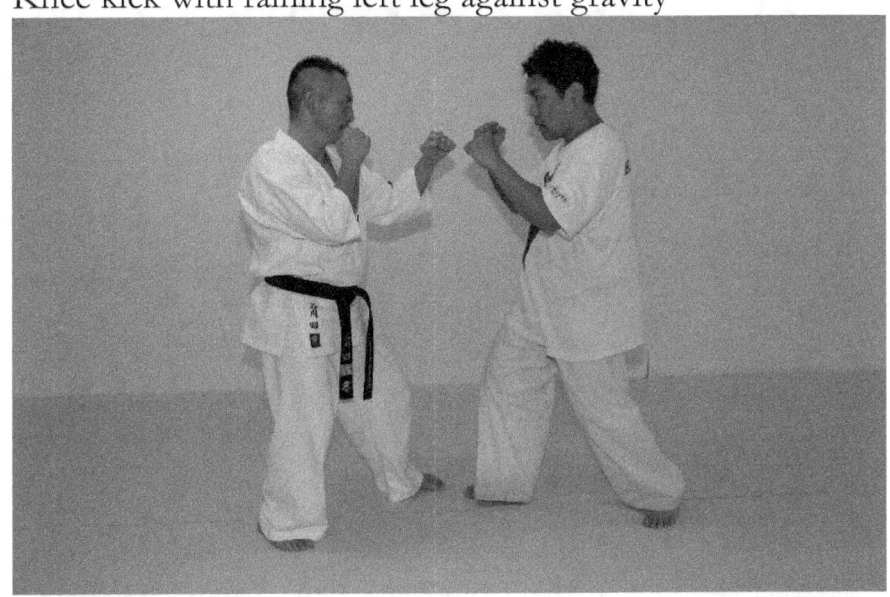

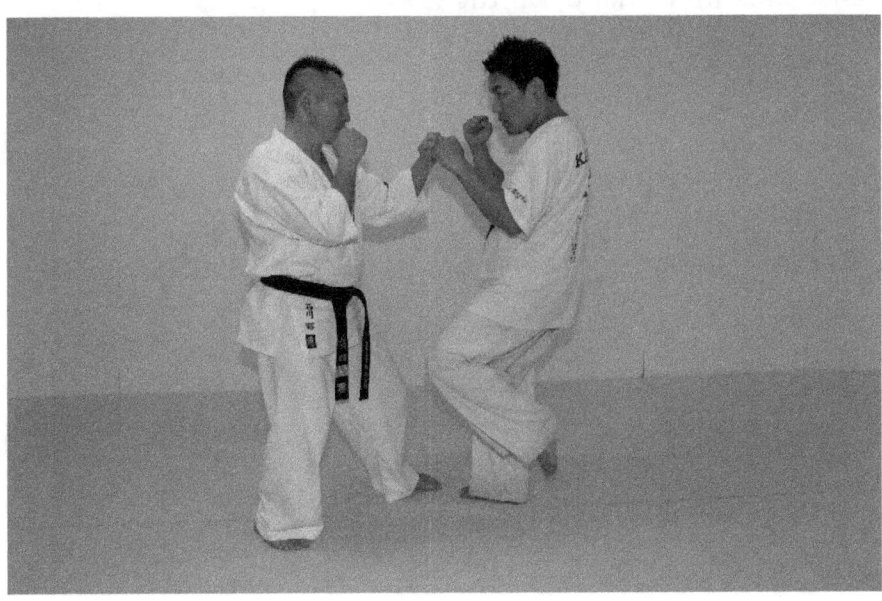

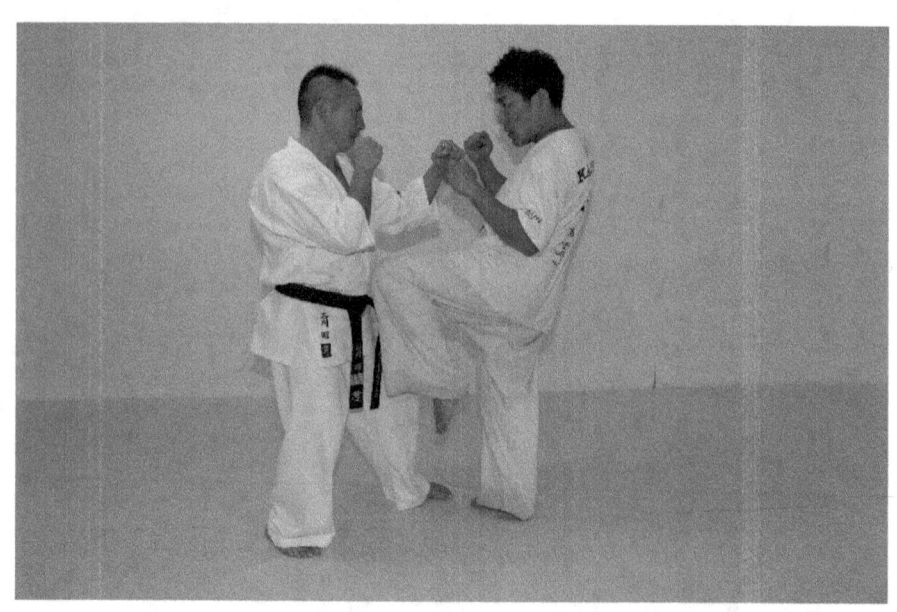

Knee kick in V shape, on the gravity

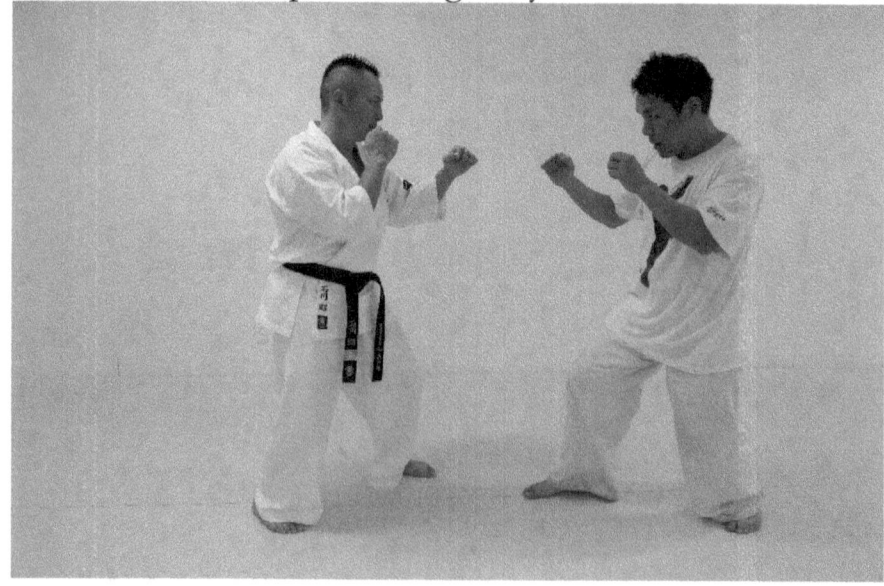

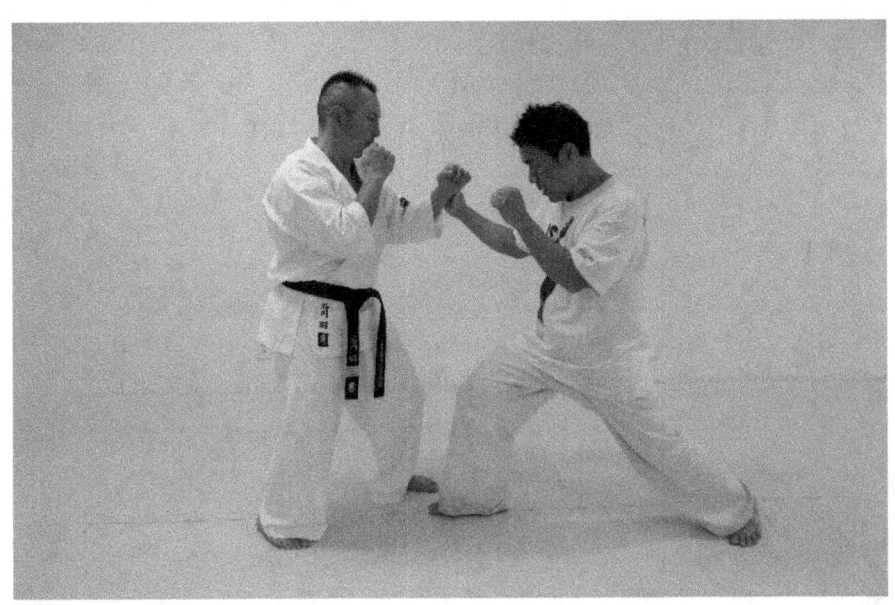

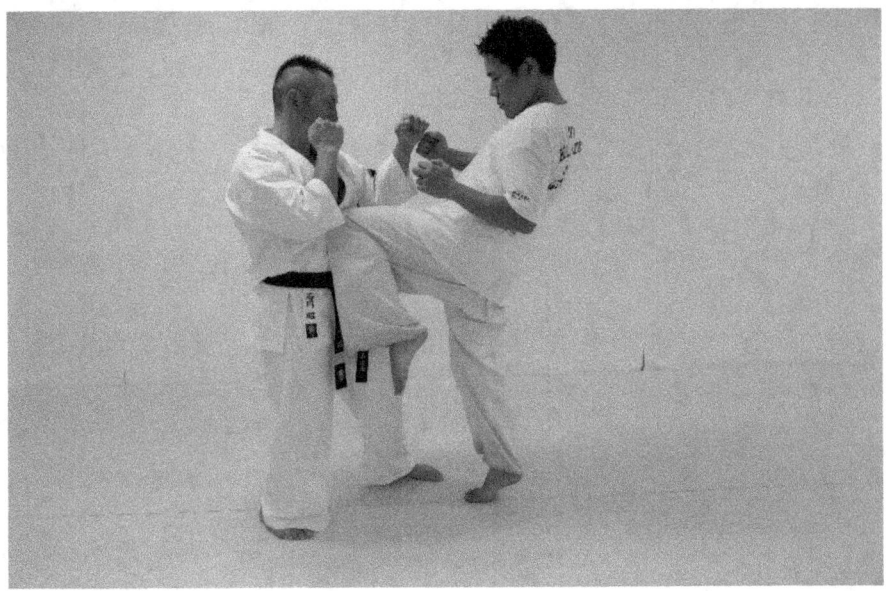

Of course, there is also a method of knee kick without widening the width of the foot. Fall above the left foot using the movement of "Basic motion 3 riding gravity, float one foot bottom ~", and use that reaction to connect to the right knee kick. If you put your weight on the right foot before the movement falling on the left foot, the load moves with the right foot → the left foot, so the right knee will be easier to move forward.

【6-11 Objective verbalizing of movement】
   As described above, when practicing skills, which weight is on which leg is now on which foot? It is necessary to have ability to monitor. So when I practice with the players, I try to quantify and verbalize it as much as possible.
"Now we are standing with both feet 50% load on both side"
"Front leg zero percent, back leg 100% as head gets on back leg by raising the front leg"
"I felt the reaction on the toe side"
"In the current step the body moved freely as stretch reflex worked."
   Like this, I make the fighters easier to also understand their movements themselves and loads objectively. "Movement" is unsettled and does not stop, so it is quite elusive. It is difficult to make it unless you consciously and objectively observe it. In competitions where figure skating and rhythmic gymnastics compete for sophistication of movement, there is always a coach to observe the movement. It is not easy to match the feeling that you are moving and the feeling you see from the outside when competing for sophistication of movement. Therefore, in order to make it easy to catch even invisible movements, we introduced numericalization and verbalization. As a result, athletes grasp their movements themselves and

repeat trial & error. Until then, the fighter who rely on feeling and intuition also understand "where and how it should be improved" if you are in a bad condition and know "what is collapsing" correctly. So, I started to explore while making conversations with the body and the ground.

It is the same as stomachache , whether it is painful due to excessive eating, whether it hurts due to stress, food poisoning or gastritis, if the cause is clear, possibility of improvements gets high. I believe that the medical point of view will be positive for practice that makes you stronger.

【6-12 Low kick and gravity】
Let's see the relationship between low kick (gedan mawashigeri) and gravity. It is a case of kicking the low kick to the opponent's front leg (left leg) with the right leg from the orthodox stance. From the stance, first let the left leg, which is a shaft leg, float once, and perform a preliminary operation so that a 100% load is applied to the right leg. At the next moment, while forwarding the left foot a couple of centimeters, landing on the ground from the left foot while simultaneous hip joint flexion, knee joint flexion, ankle dorsiflexion of the left lower limb. At this time, move as the whole body weight 100% goes onto the left foot. "Basic movement 3 riding on gravity to float one foot sole ~" "Basic movement to ride gravity 4 - Expanding foot width ~" This is these two types of movements combined.

From the stance → 100% load on the back leg → 100% loading as it drops on the front leg slightly spreading the feelings of the front leg and back leg. Like this chain movement, it becomes possible to create the condition of dropping the mass of a person of 50 kg is 50 kg, 90 kg for

90 kg. By combining this with the movement of the low kick of the right leg, we can add power in the direction of gravity to the point where the kick is hit. A normal low kick practices a low kick form as one form, but if you do not understand the principle of movement, you might possibly go to the direction of "How to hit the kicking leg, how to swing the kicking leg swiftly". It is a very interesting work to create a movement using gravity, while interacting with the body, "Become an iron ball for your own weight and drop on the front leg".

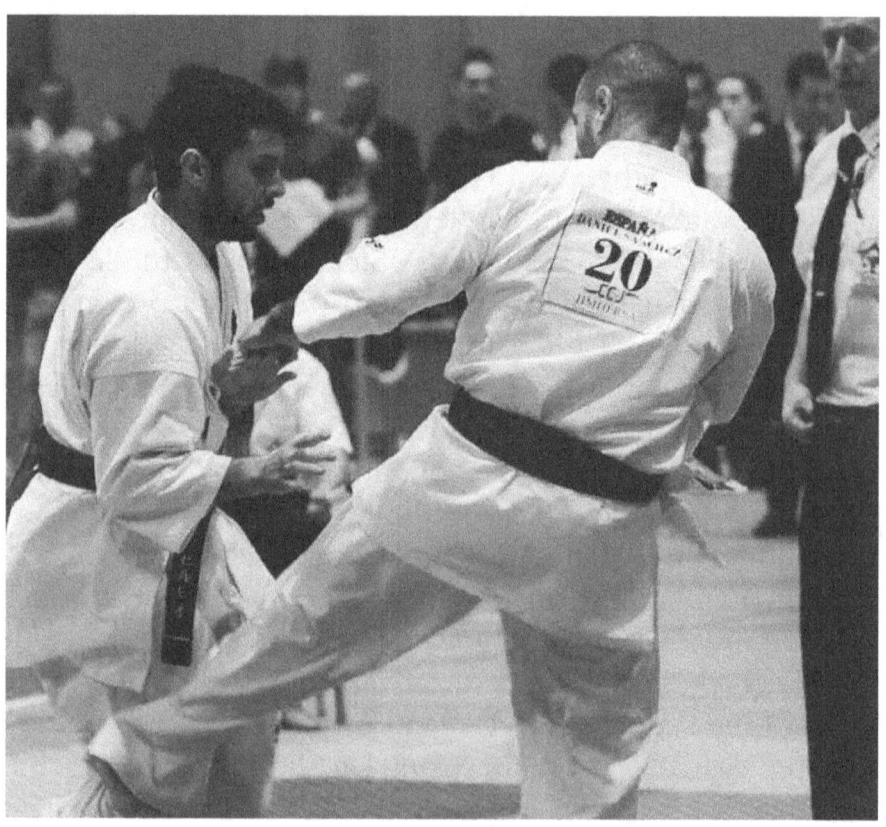

【6-13 Inside low kick and gravity】

Lower kick to inner thigh, inside low kick is easy to kick with the reaction of gravity, the damage transmitted to the opponent also increases. If you kick the inside of the thigh of your opponent's back leg (right leg) with your right leg, you will move against the gravity as you raise your right leg and kick it while bending the right hip joint. However, the top fighters kick the inside low kick using the reaction of gravity.

Movement at the low kick, from the stance → 100% load on the back leg → While slightly expanding the feeling of the front leg and back leg → 100% load so as to fall on the front leg, while using the reaction feeling to the front leg that fell at this next moment Please try kicking the right inside low kick while moving the flexed hip joint in the direction of extension. The hip joint of the shaft leg will tend to stretch and reflex generated by the bending of the dropping motion and the kicking leg, right hip joint will have the movement of extension when moving forward the left leg, so the muscle group related to the hip flexion gets extended, the the flexion becomes smooth. When seeing the motion of this inside low kick from the side, the pelvis falls and goes up. It becomes the trajectory of V shape.

Raising right leg

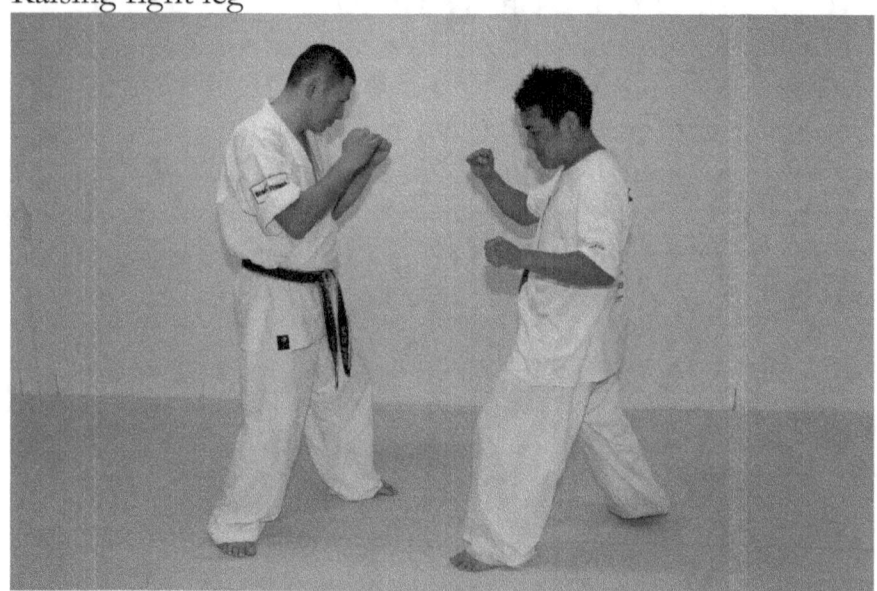

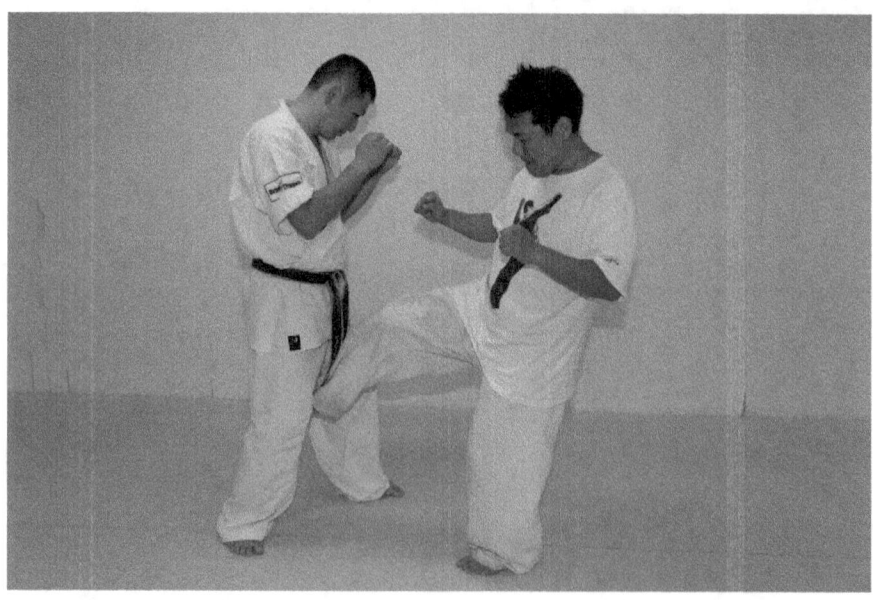

V shape

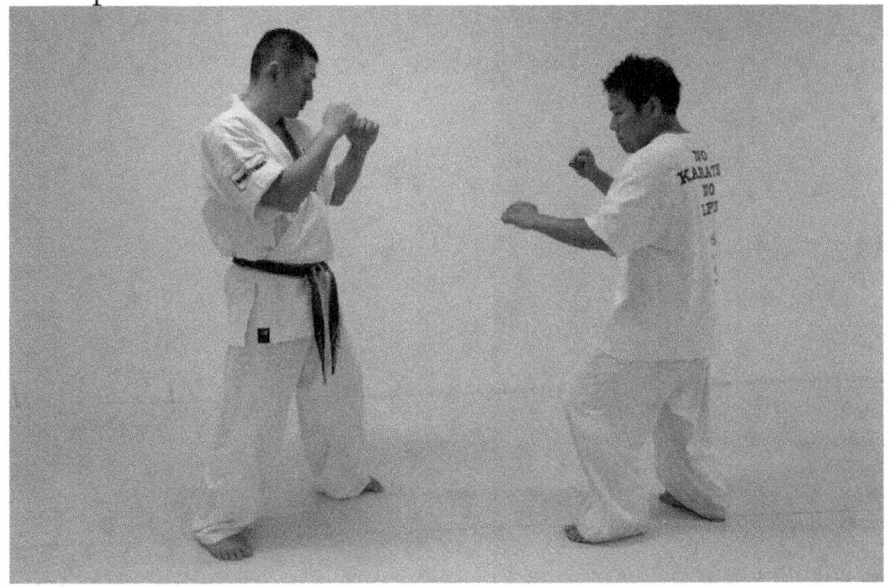

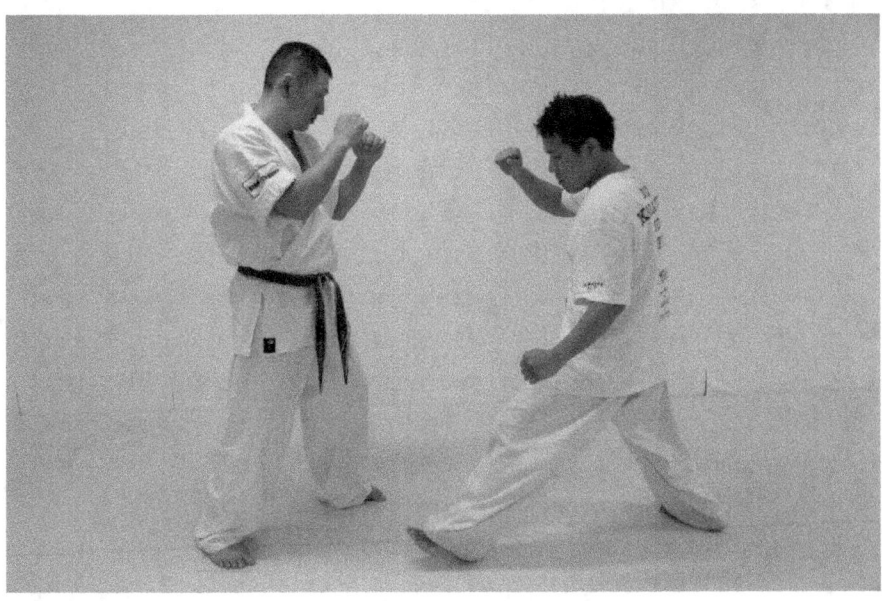

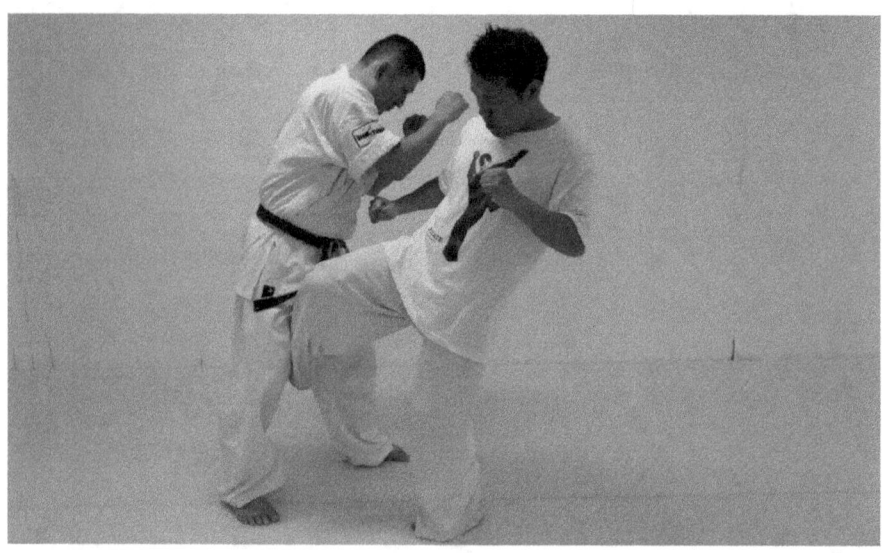

【6-14 High kick and gravity】

High kick, though there are a variety of kicking methods, here I would like to analyze the movement of the high roundhouse kick with the back leg. From the orthodox stance, put the front leg, which is the left leg one step before the half step. (The distance between the left foot and the right foot at that time, pick the width which you feel comfortable with.) At this time, the front leg and the back leg separate so the pelvis heads to the ground. It is the first half of the V letter movement of the scene of Ichiro's motion explanation. When falling to the lowest point, reaction of gravity is generated. Taking the reaction of gravity, the whole body rises upward, but what is important at this time is the angle of the ankle joint of the shaft leg (in this case it becomes the left leg, the front leg). The greater the angle of the backbone (the movement of the toe in the direction of the back side of the foot), the higher the position of the pelvis, and when the angle of the bottom flexion is small, the position of the pelvis is low, making it difficult to make a high kick. When observing the movements of high kick master fighters, there are many cases where their ankles take the bottom bending moment when the kicking feet are at the highest position. As the height of the pelvis is as high as possible, the pelvis is lowered in the direction of gravity with the previous movement, and the pelvis rises up by the reaction at the next moment. Instead of "ordering the muscles to get the planter flexion at the ankle", instead of "moving the dorsiflexion of the ankle to the bottom flexion of the ankle while using extensional reflexes" and "lifting the pelvis up", make it as "the pelvis is rising". This corresponds to the second half part of letter V. Also, when the front leg comes forward, the right hip joint is stretched. I will bend the extended hip joint with the next movement, but here let's be aware of the course of the hip joint which we explained at the joint angle. Just bending the hip will lock the joint with the femur (the thigh bone) and the front of the pelvis, so in order to prevent it, to prevent bending movements and abduction movements) are added. When base on the standing posture with the toes closed, the movement of the hip joint in the direction in which the entire right leg draws a circle in the right direction with the pelvis facing the front while centering on the right hip joint, the right toe is outside The movement of the hip joint in the direction facing it is called outward rotation, but if you take a course with slight bending and outgoing direction while bending, it is easy to obtain the highest value of the knee height as a result. Search for a course that is comfortable to rise the leg with the reaction of gravity High kick is not going to be a burden.

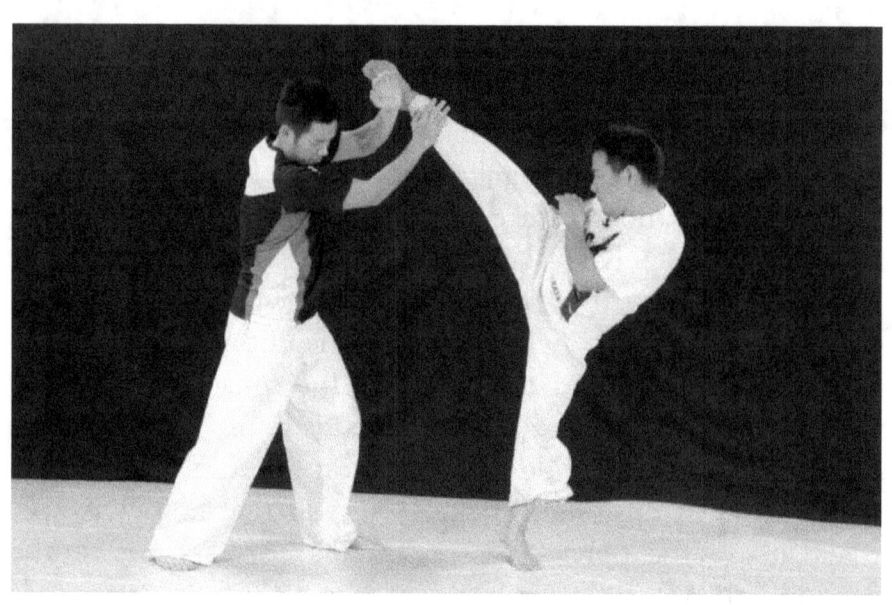

【6-15 From "Raising my leg" to "My leg rises up"】

Sports doctor of specialized in fighting sports. Doing such a rare job, I receive a lot of questions like "Will you check my movement? Because I can't high kick well" I often hear it at the dojo and at the gym, "Raise higher your leg !!!", I do not think it's right in kinematically thinking. (Now, yes. It was completely wrong in the past.

When you are told that you have to raise your legs, humans try to get out of the brain a command to contract the muscles to raise their leg, which is transmitted to the target muscles. As a result, there are quite a lot of people trying to raise kick legs against gravity. You get tired if you go against gravity. If you get tired, you cannot win against those who are not tired. If you brought it to exhaustion warfare yourself, I feel a waste if you are unconscious of the exhausted movement.

High kick, good athletes probably do not just issue 'directive to raise their feet'. First of all, using the whole body in the direction of gravity, while using the reaction (professionally called floor reaction force) generated at the floor and the sole of the foot well, it generates the stretch reflection of the muscle group necessary to raise the foot, It seems to be connecting to the high kick on that movement. So the high kicks of the top fighters do not make you feel like "purposely kicking". There are even things that "kicks are sucked into the other's head". It means not to "raise your feet" but "to pursue how to move your body as the foot will rise (as a result) the next moment before the foot rises up".

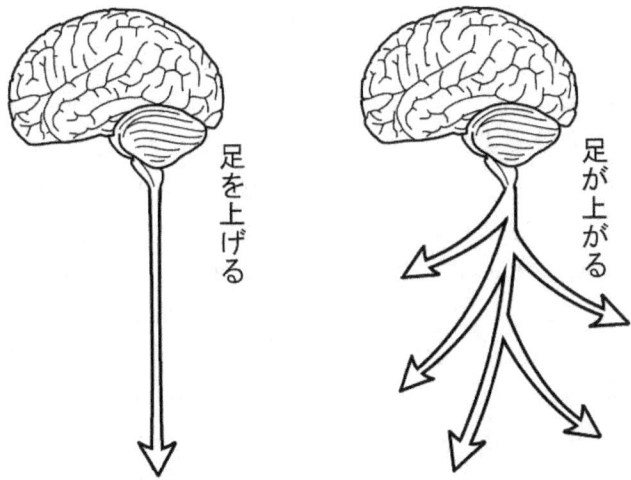

(When you issue a command to raise your leg from the brain, an order comes out to the muscle group that raises your foot, and when you give an order to the muscle group whose legs rise from the brain, then the leg will rise)

【6-16 Kicking technique of front leg】

If the person does not have experience of martial arts or martial arts at all, if you ask him/her for punch or kick, most will use back hands and legs as punches and kicks. I think that those whom are experienced substantially control the front jab and the high kick from the front leg. Using the front arm and front leg as weapons requires a certain degree of training, and many fighters and practitioners are longing for kicking accurately with the front leg.

By using the front leg kicking technique (front kick, high roundhouse kick, inward roundhouse kick, axe kick, side kick, etc.) from the fighting stance, using the basic movement 3 riding on gravity ~ floating one foot bottom side ~ It is easier to understand and makes it easier to move. While kicking with a touch to the floor with the front leg (left leg) from the orthodox stance, bending the hip joint and the knee joint of the back leg (right foot), ankle dorsiflexion, these are performed at the same time, and create a space within a moment between the sole of the back foot and the floor. In the next instance, the weight of the whole body falls on the back leg, so it will move forward using the reaction of gravity that occurred at that moment. While using the force generated by kicking the floor with the front leg and the force generated with the back leg, advance forward and kick with the forefoot. With this method, since the propulsive force using gravity is accompanied, it becomes an intense kick because the power by the propulsion is added to the power by the kick when the opponent hits the kick, and this also makes our side hardly pulls back.

Let's experiment with the middle height front kick against the partner with the mitt.

A) When kicking with the front leg led from the stance, ① front flexion of the hip joint, ② knee joint extension, ③ bottom flexion of the ankle becomes the main, so if your partner is heavy or comes out forward front, it becomes "pull back with the reaction from kick". On the other hand,

B) When you kick with gravity and its reaction from the stance, the whole body moves forward, so it will be difficult for heavy weight opponent or powerful opponent, or even against the opponent who comes forward, not easy to be pushed backward.

A-1

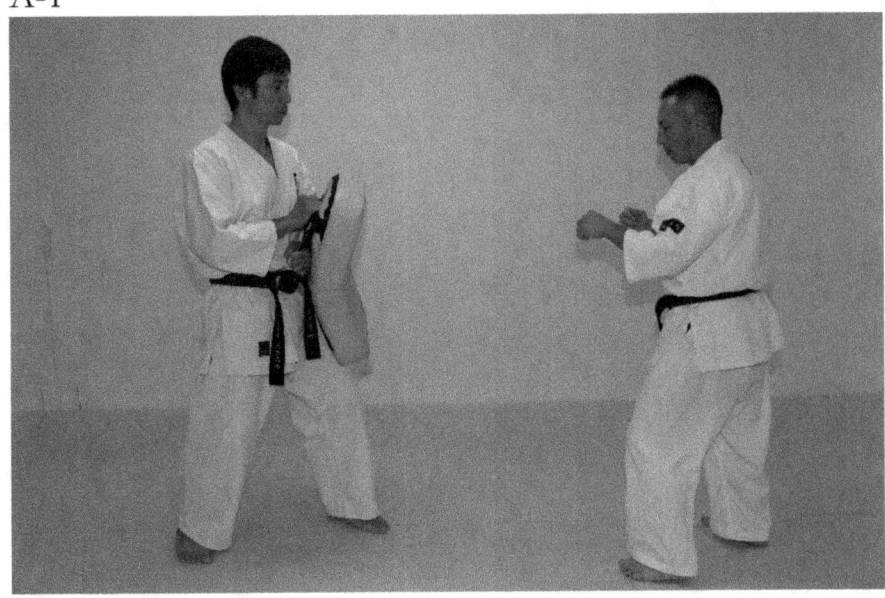

A-2

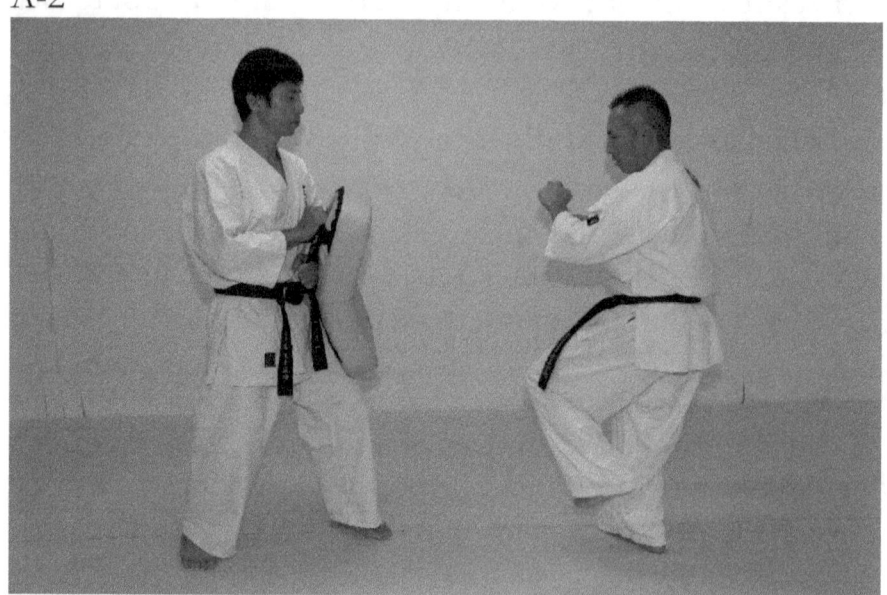

A-3

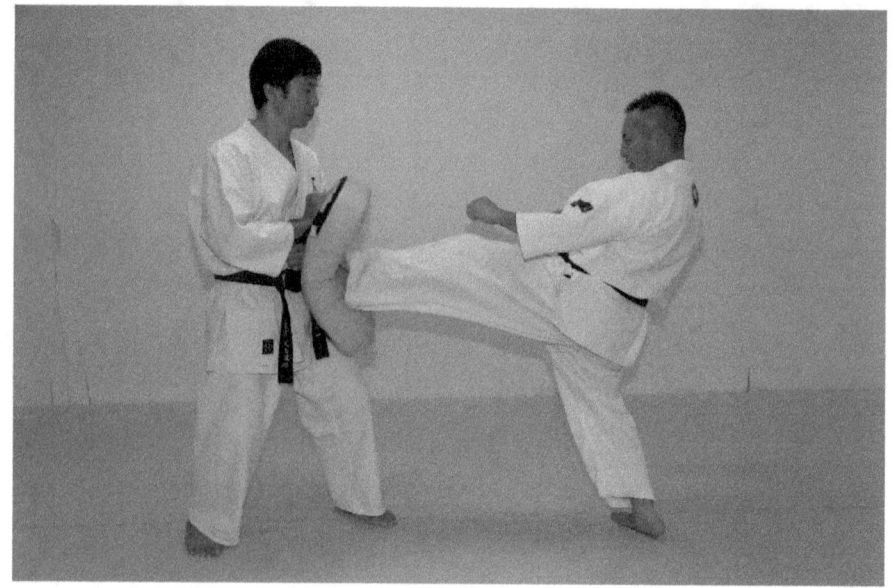

A-4

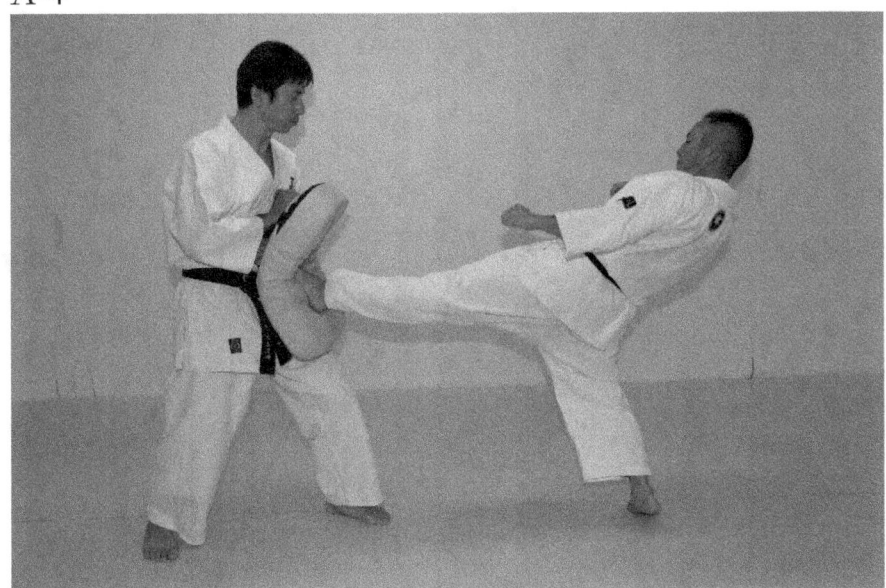

B-1

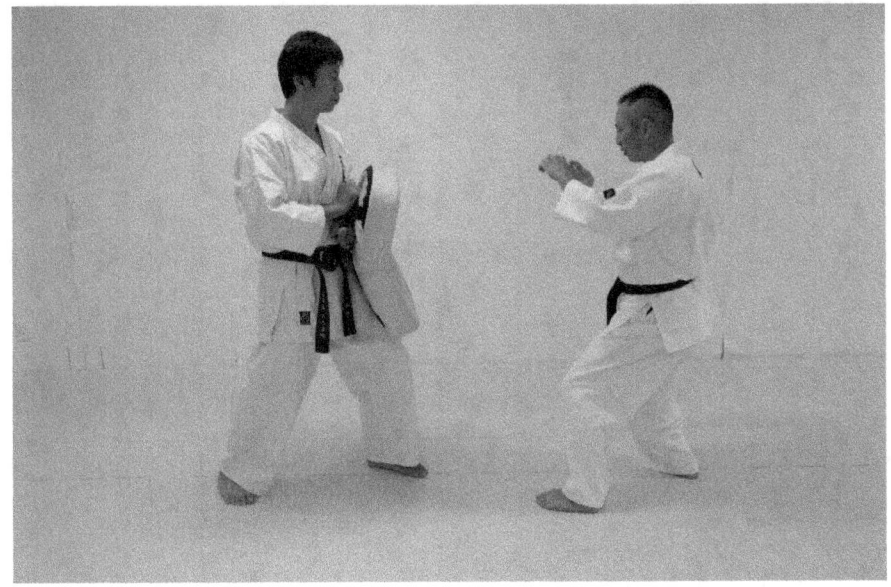

179

B-2

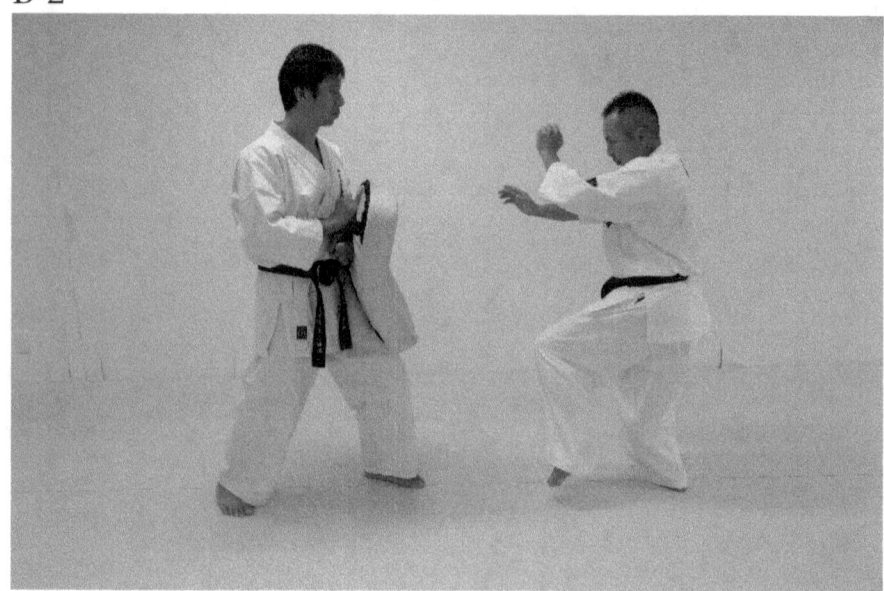

B-3

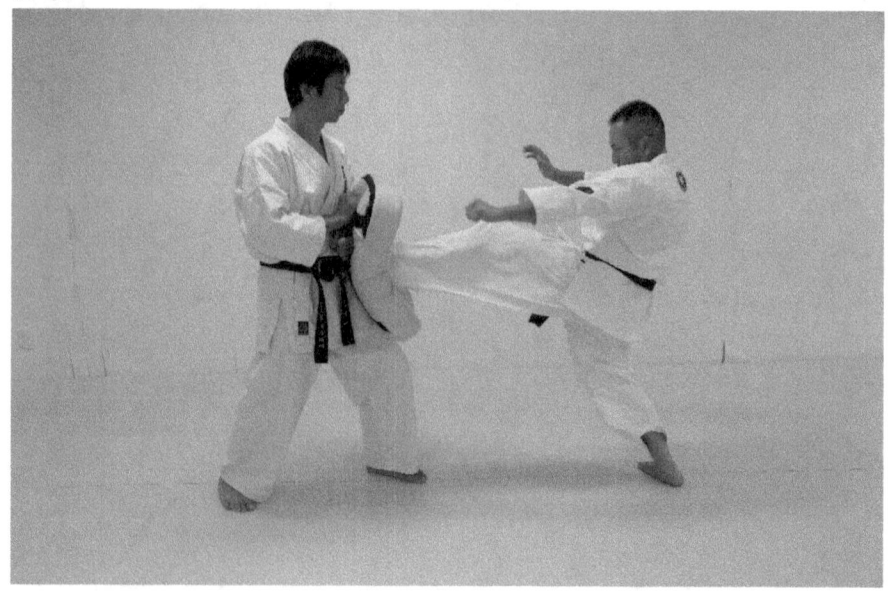

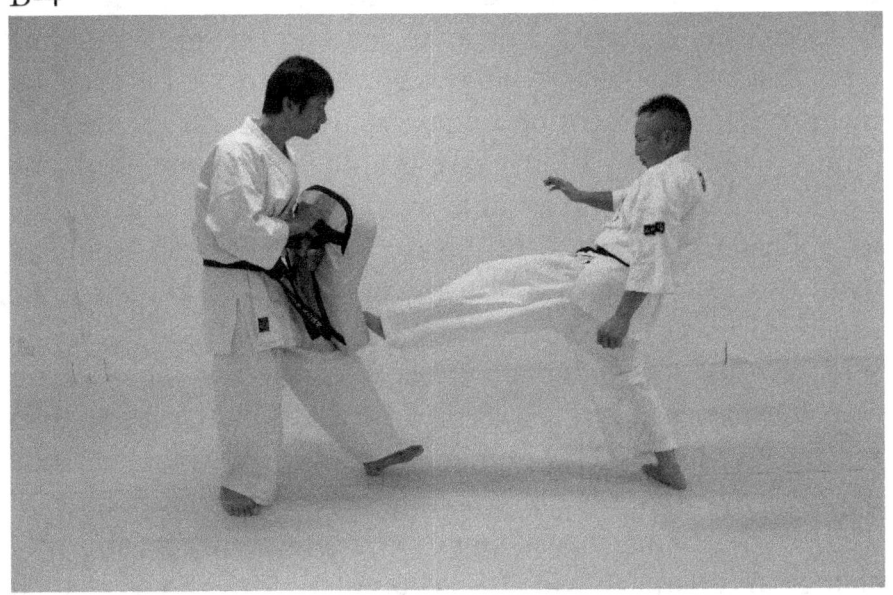

【6-17 Know why that movement can be done】

If you see the movements of players who are suffering from "weak in the ability to go forward" or " lose because pulling back during the match", the tendency that the person himself/herself has declined unaware themselves, the tendency of punching and kicking out. The tendency that the body itself is left in its original position, another way to say, I can observe the tendency to try to let the opponent backward with "the power of technique". If you follow the "law of conservation of energy" which we learn in science and physics, if you want to let your opponent pull back, your weight must move forward. Punches and kicks also function as "medium" or "bridge" to convey your weight shift to your opponent.

Through this experiment, I think that it is important to understand the difference between A) and B) from the head and the body. Of course, some fighters are able to do B) from the beginning, but there are a lot of fighters of that type that cannot do A) in reverse. A) cannot be done, it means that you cannot be aware of any differences or points from A) to B). By being able to dig into both, be able to understand A, be able to understand B, and be able to understand B from the vision of A, and understand A from the vision of B. Knowing two leads to knowing the square of two.

If you do not understand this to some extent why you can do that, you will have difficulty rebuilding when you fall into a slump. The human brain and the body change day by day. Metabolism and digestive function change as well. If the living environment changes, body weight will change and damage will also accumulate for exercisers such as muscles and joints, by accumulating the exercise practice and career. It is a common story that "I have become impossible to move like I used to do", "I am moving like a different person at my golden age". By moving while searching for differences in movement between A) and B), you should find several checkpoints such as "If you move this like that way it will be like this" and "Such an image will be like this". In the era of information overload, various hints are overflowing, but I think that the real answer to strengthen yourself is in the trial and error to be repeated over and over.

【6-18 How to use gravity, of Mike Tyson】

Up to this point, we have mainly mentioned striking and gravity, but the important thing is to review the movement from the viewpoint of "gravity". Even now as a world champion of boxing, Mike Tyson boasts a tremendous popularity and influence. Before he releases his left hook, he gets his legs as if they were sinking into the ring when turning from the right leg load to the left leg load. While bending it will make the whole body smaller. At the next moment, Mike Tyson, who was taking a small posture, suddenly jumps big and feeds the left hook with the jumping flow. From the gravitational movements, it seemed to be producing a deadly KO punch with the reaction of gravity. Actually, when I look at the image of the training menu of Mike Tyson at that time, he was doing a menu called "Change jump height while jumping rope". While jumping at normal height suddenly shorten both legs (bending the hip joint and knee joint, dorsiflexing the ankle joint), jumping rope with the pelvic falling height, and returning to the original height. That was the training about. As the fighter with overwhelming muscle strength, speed and weight moved with gravity and its reaction, it should be strong already. Tyson was "keeping the earth on his side".

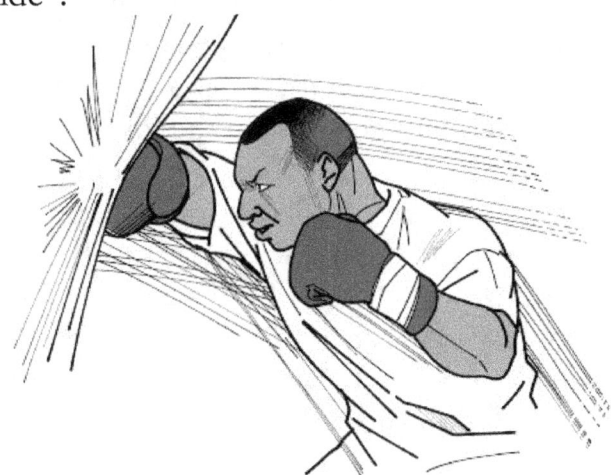

To everyone, not only hooks, uppercuts, body blows, front kicks, axe kicks, back kicks, back spin kicks, side

183

kicks, inward roundhouse kick, ..., no matter what kind of skill, use the "gravity" as I would like you to try and use it while feeling that you are using or using "gravity" and "reaction of gravity" in combination. Practice of dropping punches leaves as it is also becomes practicing dropping low kicks. I think that in many brains of fighters, memorize and recognize which are called "punch and low kick are different techniques" are processed, but by moving by feeling gravity, punch and low kick would link each other. When linked, the neural circuits which were separate in the brain are super strongly tied! If it is a complex separate folders, it is hard to take them out, but if you make them simple, it will be possible to retrieve them instantaneously. This is also one of invisible strength.

【6-19 Pushing each other】

Let's face each other in pairs and try to push each other. Let's try both the pattern moving the pelvis and the head in parallel to the ground and the pattern falling in the direction of gravity and going ahead in its reaction. The pattern which tends to fall during pressing is a movement which you stop yourself and get stiff on the lower limb, and push with the arm. If it is this, it becomes dependent on your muscle power, and it will be disadvantageously steadily because muscular strength decreases with the passage of time.

When you grapple with each other, drop the pelvis and head in the direction of gravity while advancing the front leg and go forward to go up from the lowest point. "Drop then rise" of the trajectory of V shape, it is. If you incorporate this movement when you interfere, you can enter between the opponent and the earth. By becoming the shorter one of the Japanese character "入", you can push your opponent from diagonally while making the earth as your ally. If the opponent is powerful, if you scale down the V shape and attack it several times lightly, it will be easier to let the opponent go backwards.

Drop in the direction of gravity by opening the legs or making it short, when the opponent seems to be pushing. And go forward at the next moment. If you try to go forward without moving in the direction of gravity, "opponent's pushing force" + "you pushing back force" will overlap and may fall back to the contrary.

Pushing Horizontally

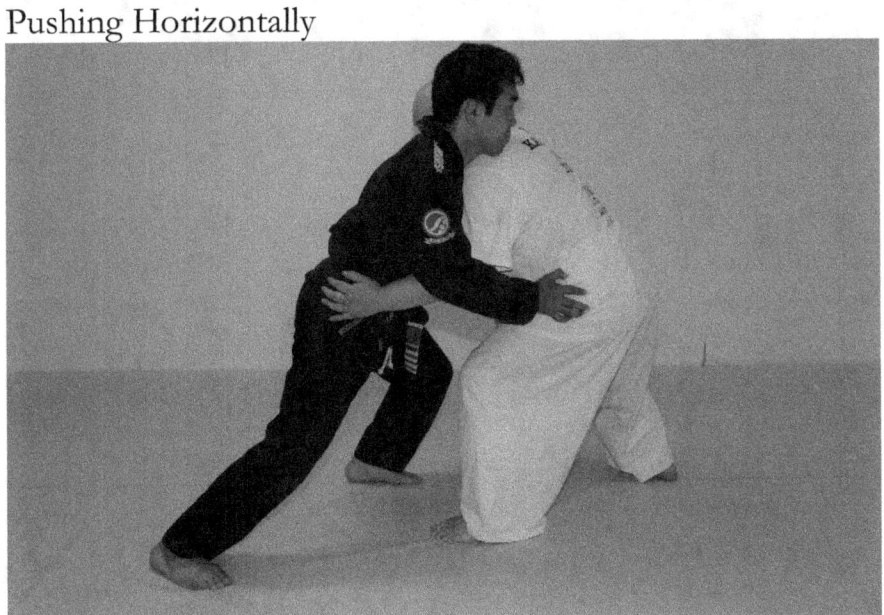

V shape

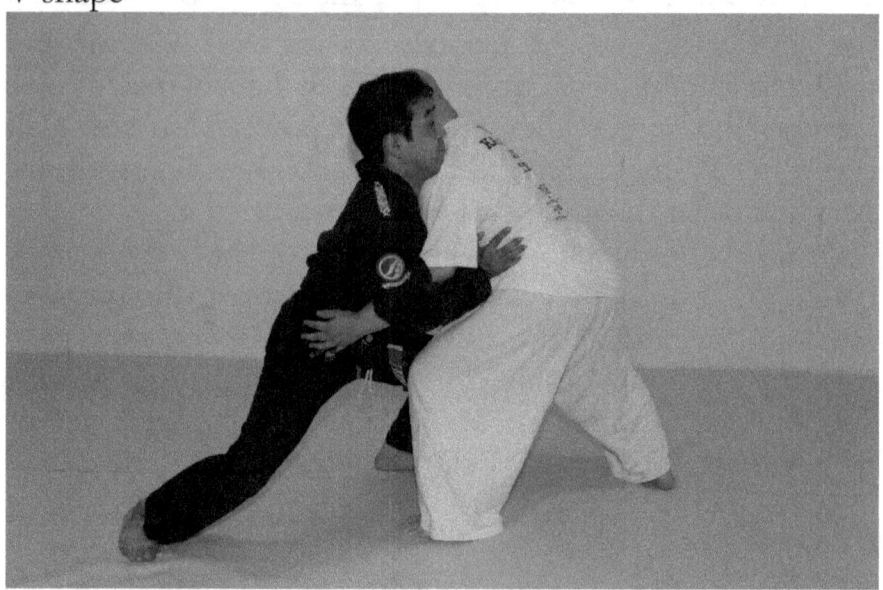

【6-20 Lifting, & Throwing】

Let's compare the movement of throwing with arms around your opponent's body. "Stop at crouch once and lift by grabbing your opponent's torso." This will be a movement against the gravity. Fall in the direction of gravity by himself using the basic movement 2 riding gravity with floating the bottom of the feet itself, grappling the opponent at the lowest point and moving the opponent in response to gravity reaction, it will possible to lift up the opponent in an instant with feeling less weight. And the lifted one would also feel like the body floats with a fluffy, please try it by a pair.

Mr. Toshihiko Koga, a genius judoka, "Sanshiro in Heisei era", including the winner of the Barcelona Olympic Games. That high level technique has influenced beyond times and genres. As Fighting Medicine, Mr. Koga's footage is full of discovery and awareness as research subjects, but his one-arm back throw was a "shock" in particular.

Mr. Koga himself is also floating in the air the next moment when he thought that he wandered under his opponent in a moment after separating the bottom of the sole and the floor. even while throwing, he doesn't stop nor stand firmly. There is no pause at all. As we are constantly moving weight, at the moment when his opponent is lifted, Mr. Koga is no longer under him. So his opponent eventually has to fall. Until then, I myself thought that 'lifting, throwing' are to firmly step with the lower body and stabilized, demonstrating muscular strength, but Mr. Koga's one-arm back throw is "Drop with an instant → Himself rise with the opponent "is a perfect expression for this movement.

There is no "I am stopped and move opponents." The essence of the movement "the energy that you move is transmitted to your opponent". Even though it looks alike, I noticed what is important to the world's best technique.

【6-21 Mount position】

Mount position frequently used in mixed martial-arts and jiu-jitsu. It's an important skill that sitting astride the opponent with his face up, then continue to joint locks. The opponent who is under you, will somehow try to escape from the mount, turn over, or conversely use the mount to attack from the bottom. Those who are taking mounts cannot make an advantage unless you control the person under you, but there are also cases where this will work well if you take advantage of the reaction of gravity and gravity well. When you get on the top, you can move a few centimeters and move the pelvis up and down. Continue gravity → reaction → gravity, as if the ball repeats a small bouncings. Doing so will make it difficult for your opponent to recover from being mounted. Regardless of how much the opponent moves, gravity is applied instantaneously and intermittently from the top to the bottom, with acceleration in response to that phase and aspect, which makes it easier to control your opponent.

If you continue stabbing like stabbing insects with pins for insect specimens, keep on stabbing like that, your weight will take on your opponent multiple times and your opponent will be hard to respond to it. If you are stopped while mounting from above, it will be easier to turn over as the opponent only needs to move the other person who stopped.

The Jiu-jitsu family, the Gracie family who created the current mixed martial arts and jiu-jitsu wave has introduced 'horseback riding' as one of essential training. Speaking of which is stronger, horses and humans, is a horse, not to mention. The horse's weight ranges from 400 kg to over 550 kg. Even an opponent of fighting sports, there will be no opponent of 400 kg before all.

"Movement" is important to control a horse when a human rides a horse. Because communication by language doesn't work, they say that you cannot control horses unless you can express the difference between "Will you stop?" "Stop." "Stop already!!!" by movement. You cannot be looked down or ignored, but you should not be regarded as an enemy either. The fighting sports competition also holds the aspect that you control yourself, control your opponent, and control the relationship between you and your opponent in a certain kind of trust that rules and conditions are mutually protected. Among the loads of "Can you control the horse?" Or "You get shaken down by the horse?", In addition to the neural circuit of fighting sports typified by the mount position, I suppose you are training the ability to control yourself and your opponent in a more general idea.

Training of the Gracie family, is putting the great weight on how to manage themselves in "nature", such as running in the mountains or moving the body in the torrent of the sea or river, as a feature. It is considered conscious of how they feedback to the scene of interpersonal competition. While also mentioning the strength on the ring, there are also places to link the themes that are likely to be perceived as seemingly different, "horseback riding" and "fighting sport", is the magnitude of the Gracie family who carves in the history of the world of fighting sports.

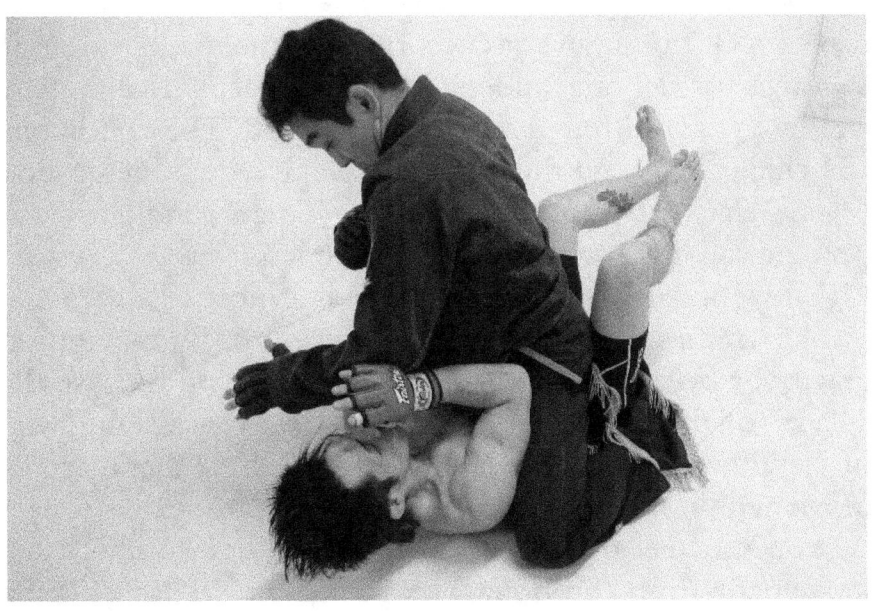

【6-22 Utility of Gravity】
Gravity cannot be ignored if you live on the planet earth. You cannot escape from gravity. By daring against gravity, you can create a strong body and you can create movement by putting gravity as your ally. Punches, kicks, throws, mounts, tackles, clinch, footwork, defense, etc. Do these movements of martial arts under the awareness of "only my muscle strength" or "consciousness of myself plus the earth". This difference is very big.

Although we cannot usually be conscious, the skills of fighting sports and martial arts are bound to the "place". The top of the ring, the tatami mat, and the top of the mat are made of a flat surface. It is a premises that there is a flat face for all of the skills like a bone cracking intense middle kick, a knocking out punch with a single blow, and a thrilling throwing skill. Even with the same kick, it will change on the top of the mat and on the ring, and the hardness of the ring varies according to the organization. If it comes to fighting underwater, the effective technology will be greatly different from that on land. The conditions will change even on the mountain slope where the ground is not flat. How to make use of that condition also becomes an important element of strength.

The technology that you are building now is also based on the premise of the "place" on the earth. By moving on gravity or by using the reaction of gravity, you can use the "place" of the earth as a friend. This is a very useful point of view for objective movement of ourselves, the image of movement in the brain will be bigger and stronger as well.

As you can feel the gravity, you will be able to check the movement from the point view of gravity. That is, some conversations like "Oh, the punch just now could use gravity", "I just raised my feet against gravity" "I pushed my opponent with the reaction of gravity" are generated, and could do a self-evaluation. It also makes it easier to understand the structure of techniques that you could not do so far. For example, when mastering the technique of "axe kick", the difference is "to raise and lower the kicking feet" and "drop the body in the direction of gravity and raise the kicking leg with each other by the reaction and move in the direction of gravity" will be clearly felt eventually.

Furthermore, becoming able to make a large part common to movement is also a big advantage to install gravity. The number of folders in the brain will increase rapidly as you place practice punching is in the practice punching folder, memorizing in sumo wrestling practice is in the sumo wrestling folder in the brain. The movement of the punch using the V shape and the sumo wrestling using the V shape are "common" movements from the viewpoint of using gravity and taking reaction of gravity. If you can find out the common terms, if practiced you can practice sumo wrestling can be a practice of punching and kicking. I also get to say that the movement standing while straddling a little bouncing without being trapped by the strap in the train links to the practice of control at the mount position, and the fighter who practiced knee kicks and front kicks separately. However, when you notice that it does not change much except how to move the kicking leg, you will be able to distinguish according to the distance.

"While making the thickest common part of the movement even thicker, create individual skills" " Make the thick part even thicker while practicing various techniques and movements" "The practice of a certain technique could be a practice as well." "Easier to be able to understand the movement of the other sports." Gravity also gives a lot of hints for leaping, such as "It will also be practicing skills" "Movement of other sports becomes easy to understand".

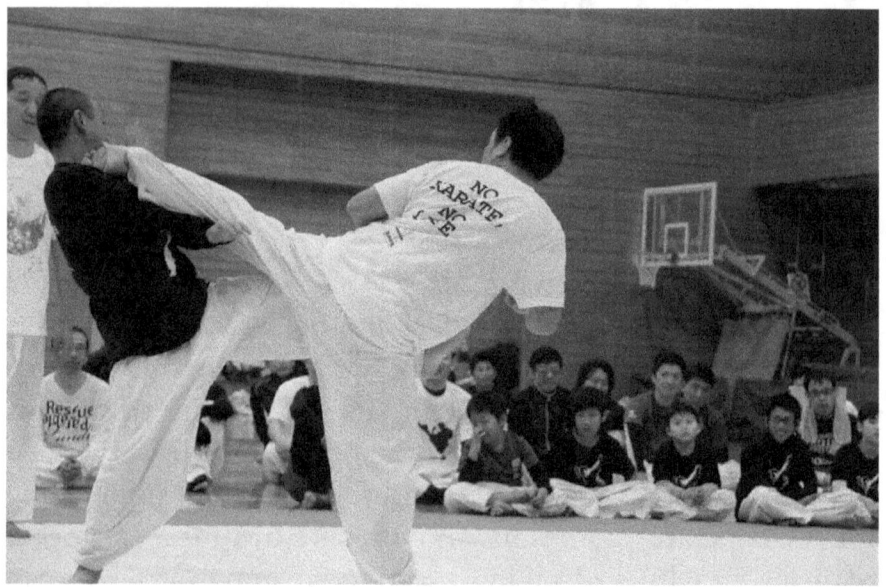

7 Motor Unit and Impulse

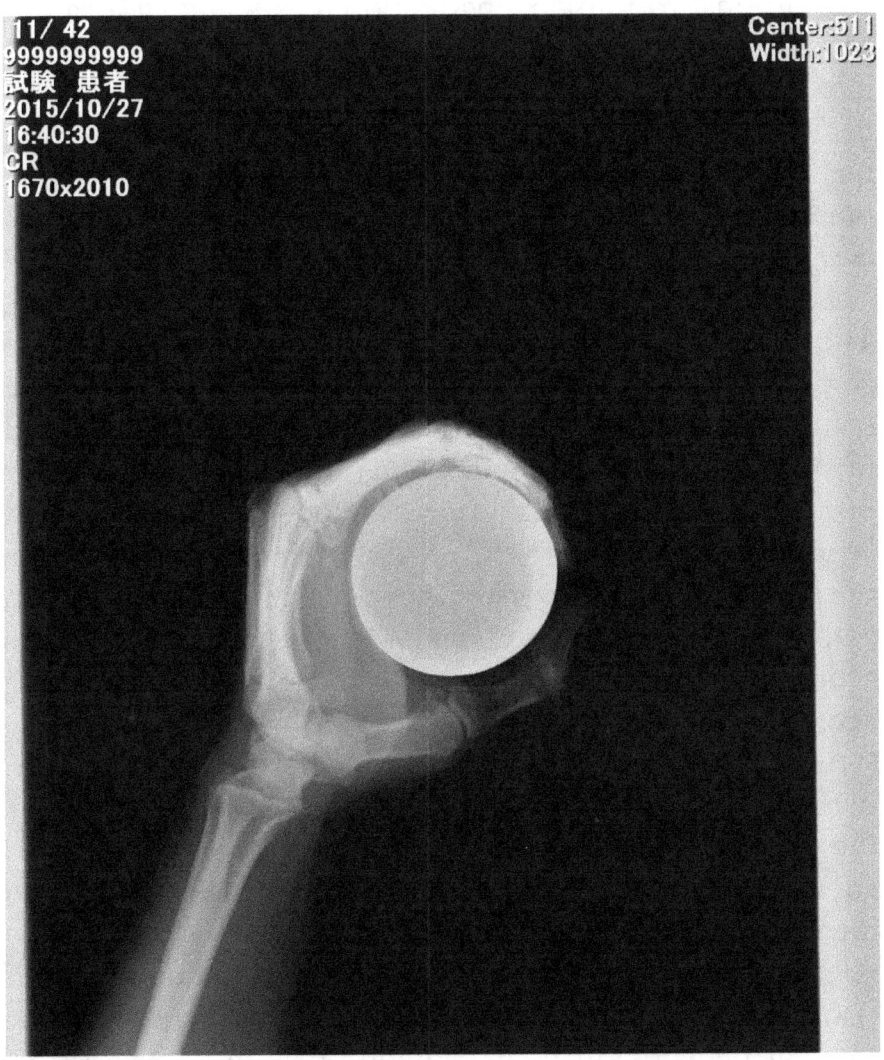

【7-1 If you are thick, does that mean you are strong?】

There is an experimental result that "muscular strength is proportional to muscle length and cross-sectional area". If it is the same length, the larger the cross sectional area of the muscles, the greater the muscle strength can be demonstrated. If you strengthen the muscles and increase the cross sectional area, you will be able to feel that the muscular strength you can exercise will increase if you have ever trained your body.

Let's step on to a micro world one more step from here. The muscle fibers that constitutes the muscles are composed of myofibrils and sarcoplasm. Myofibrils are composed mainly of actin filaments and proteins called myosin filaments in bundles. And myosin has many protrusions called cross bridges. When the command of "contraction" reaches the muscle through the nerve, calcium is released from the sarcoplasmic reticulum, actin and myosin are activated, and the cross bridge sticks to actin. It is a system that contracts in the form of attracting actin towards the center of myosin.

As myofibrils increase, the more the actin and myosin overlap, the greater the contraction force of the muscles. If the myofibrils increase and become thick, the muscular strength increases. On the other hand, the sarcoplasm also increases. However, it is said that sarcoplasm is not directly related to the demonstration of force. That shows, even if you say that your muscles are thick, or the muscles became thick, it depends on their contents. It is said that load of high weight and low number of times is effective to increase myofibrils, and load of low weight and high number of loads is effective to increase sarcoplasm. (Of course there are also overlapping parts.)

Both sides are necessary for fighting sports and martial arts. A momentary overwhelming power is also necessary, and there are also cases where it is advantageous to have the size of the muscle itself in terms of struck strength and robustness. Depending on the type of competitor and the tactics depending on the rule of the competition being practiced, the appropriate proportion will change according to age even for the same player.

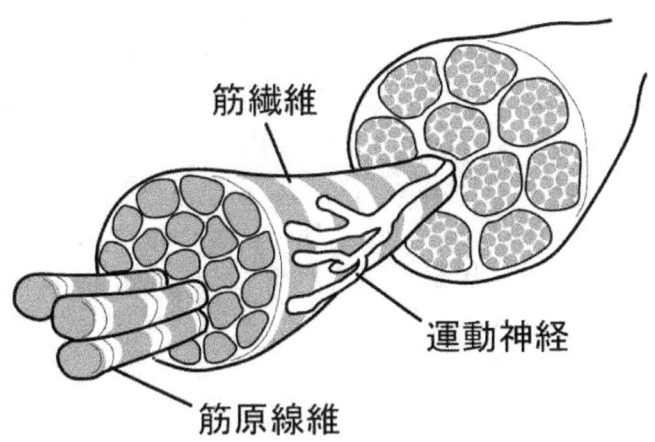

運動神経 motor nerves
筋繊維 muscle fiber
筋原線維 myofibrils

【7-2 Motor Unit】
There are motor nerve cells in the motor cortex of the cerebral cortex and the anterior horn of the spinal cord. From one motor nerve cell, the motor nerve branches off and is connected to the muscle fiber, receives the command of contraction, and transmits it to the muscle fiber. The number differs from several to several thousand,

195

and one motor cell and the number of muscle fibers it controls are collectively called a motor unit (movement unit). Motor nerve cells range from small to large, small motor nerve cells for thin motor nerves, large motor nerve cells for thick motor nerves.

A motor unit with a small size is rich in endurance, but the speed at which it can demonstrate is slow, and the power is weak. A motor unit with a large size is poor in endurance, but its speed is fast, it is characterized by strong ability to demonstrate. There are seven kinds of muscle fibers, I, Ic, Ic, IIac, IIa, IIax, and IIx. Type I is classified as a slow muscle and type II is classified as a fast muscle. The more right, more the size gets bigger, I will be the first muscle fiber of the motor unit to be mobilized first, II x the most difficult to mobilize, but once mobilized, we can it's the motor unit that demonstrates explosive speed and power

【7-3 Principle of size】

Not all motor units are used when exercising. When demonstrating power, there is "order of appearance" in the motor unit to be mobilized. At the beginning, the smallest motor unit I appears, if it cannot be handled, it will move onto bigger one with the next size and next size. "Big man appears at the end!" Phenomena common in human society is also occurring in nerves and muscles. Small motor units are mobilized soon, but big ones are hard to be mobilized. "Ultra large one" does not even appear easily.

The fact that the order of motor units to be mobilized according to the magnitude of the force to demonstrate in this way is determined corresponding to the size is called "principle of size". At first, a small light footwork soldier takes the field and big one appears only when it's necessary.

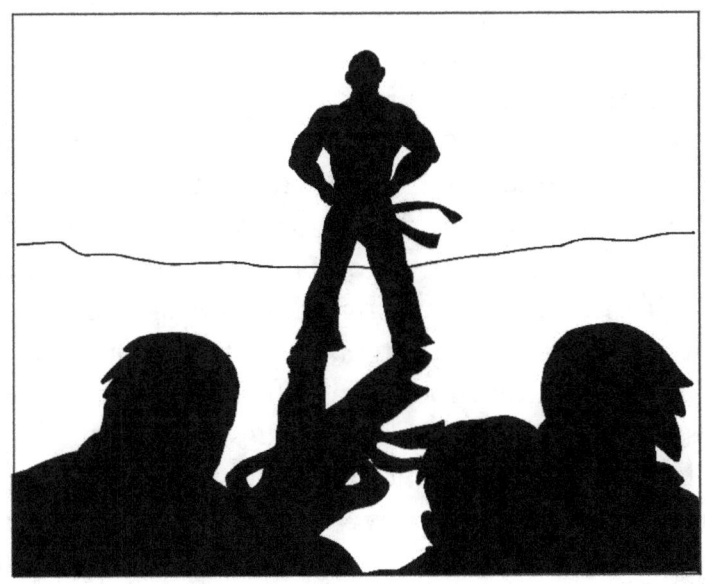

【7-4 Exception of the principle of size】
However, in a recent study I realized that there seems to be "exception" in the principle of size. It is suggested that there is a possibility that a motor unit including II x may be used right at first.

(1)Danger avoidance in protecting the body
In highly urgent situations, you must demonstrate great power quickly and instantly.
"I helped someone who was about to run over by a car with incredible speed"
"In the case of a fire, the elderly person exercised the muscular strength that we cannot believe normally and carried the baggage out"

I think you have heard of the episodes like that. It is the so-called "adrenaline rush". In such a special psychological state, there is a possibility that the brake will be released so that we can use a motor unit that is not usually used much. Even in practice and training of fighting sports and martial arts, here is the essence of meaning to practice with "opponents that are overwhelmingly stronger than yourself" or "who you do not know what to do with". It's easy to put a trick or demonstrate to the opponent you know from the beginning that he/she does not do anything, but it is hard to get down to the opponent whom is already in battle mode. Therefore, even in practice, it is necessary to positively create the situation of "What will you do to someone who you do not know what to do with?" "How can you move to an unknown opponent?" I hear "I cannot move in the match although I can move in practice" frequently. I was one of them. There was a period of time, I was thinking "If the movement of practice gets out in the match ... I can win." After that, it was the method of condition setting that learned from the fighters who gave results in the matches. From the stage of practice and training, "If I cannot take the counter attack within the first 5 seconds, I lose myself at that point" "Be sure to use back spin kick more than 10 times during 2 minutes of sparring" "Always update the 50 meter dash record" "Always make a high kick hit within 20 seconds"

It is the distinctive point that they set up their own criteria, and applying great pressure to themselves. The fighters who get results at the match is creating a situation where "practice is harder, matches are much easier". Do not practice for practice. Practice is more troublesome than a match. In a match I can move freely. I feel that how to hold consciousness around here is the characteristic of the fighters and leaders who produce results.

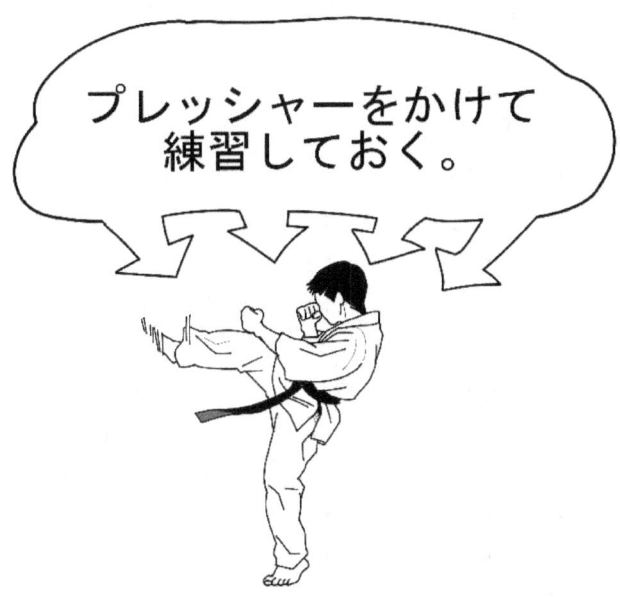

(training under pressure)

When I was a university, I had set a bench press in one room of the apartment I was renting, but when I tried my maximum weight at that time alone, I have collapsed as I couldn't lift it. The bar was approaching near the cervical region, as close as several cm until the neck was going to be choked. I had the experience that, I thought "Wow! I'm going to die!" then I mastered up all my power to put one side of the barbells to the floor, and raise the other side, to survive the pinch. You shouldn't do such a stupid thing without securing safety, alone, so I would like the reader to never imitate this, but at that time I think that more than my usual power was generated. This is a bad example (embarrassing example?), but What kind of condition would you set as "a state of high urgency" for you? I think that it raises the possibility that the work load which will concretize in the self-asked question and secure the "exception of the principle of size" can be used.

(2) Eccentric contraction

The state where the muscles contract while the length of the muscles becomes longer is called eccentric contraction. For example, when jumping off from a high place, if you leave it to the momentum and bend the hip joint and knee joint, you will land with your buttocks. Occasionally it may lead to coccyx fracture and lumbar fracture, so in most cases, brakes are applied by lower limbs when jumping. Also, prevent falling with your face by putting your arms forward when you fall to the ground. Like that, the muscles that work during braking have an eccentric contraction, but at this time it is thought that an exception to the principle of size is occurring.

3) Kiai and Shouting

There is an experimental result that maximal muscular strength increases when you exercise your muscular strength and you emit a kiai or shout. To demonstrate instantaneous muscle strength, it is a short sound such as "Ha" "Uh" "Ah", and the maximum muscle strength tends to increase with the sound that extends the endings such as "Ahh" and "Uuh" for sustaining muscle strength Also, we know that the maximum muscle strength is greater for voiced sound than for unvoiced sound.

The daily practice of exercising muscular strength with loud voice and trying out the length and different kinds of voices to be output according to the muscular strength demonstration time may be able to demonstrate great power as an exception to the principle of size .

4) Hint

There is also a research result that maximal muscular strength increased by suffusing to oneself. Just before trying the weight that you have never experienced yet in weight training, it feels like "Somehow I feel like I can lift, today" or "I feel like I can win the tournament today" at the warming up stage before fighting in the tournament. I think that there are many people that have been achieved. When we have accumulated good preparation and meet that moment, self-suggestion is applied in "natural form", and the image in the brain becomes clearer and it is thought that it brings positive effect to the movement. Natural form, is the point, if you usually raise only 70 km of barbells, and saying "I feel like I can lift 100kg today" is "impossible" in any kind of possibility. Because there is no reason there, it won't go well at the first place. In regular exercises and daily lives, "conscious of what you have done up to now + α", trying from 70 kg to 71.25 km, and then trying 72.5 kilometers " While accumulating the work to do ", let's create a "natural implication → achievement → confidence" loop.

【7-5 Breakthrough the principle of size by mastering up all power】

I had a conversation with a traditional martial arts teacher , "Is bench press necessary or not" as a topic. According to the teacher, "The movement of the bench press and the movement necessary for the thrust are completely different, so the movement of the bench press disturbs the strikes", so it was argued that the disadvantage is great. Certainly, that claim may be so if you look at the mechanism of exercise from the "physical" aspect. We could say that the movement of the punch while moving the entire body forward, and the movement of the bench press where the back side is fixed, is a similar movement but different movement in fact. However, many athletes who are indiscriminately active do thoroughly exercise weight training and muscle training and give out results.

"Is it for making a strong body?" "For not losing from strikes?" "Because everyone is doing?" I have also pursued the reason for incorporating the weight training as the Society of Fighting Medicine, but now I think it may be "to make route using the exception of the principle of size".

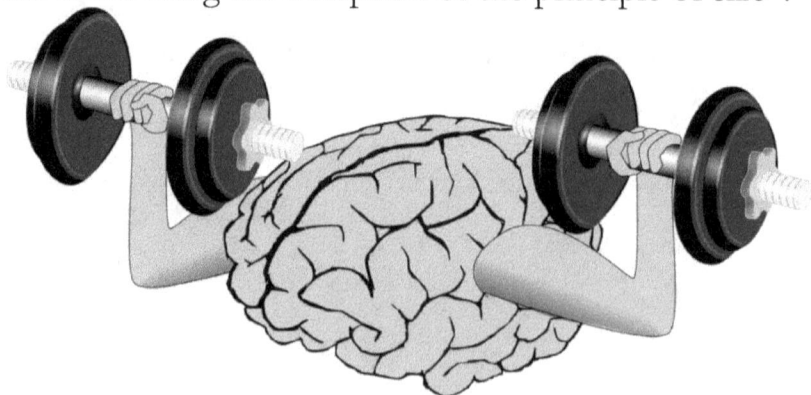

Of course, there is a gap as exercise saying "Make the movements of the bench press directly onto the punches".

Therefore, through the bench press, use the power of the whole body in one stroke, and make it to the brain and body so that suddenly explosive power can be obtained. And then practice punching.

I myself have experience as well, that for some reason I become confident if I can handle high weight weights such as bench press and squats. "No matter how much the opponent beats you, with a single strong punch, can't I turn it over?" A type of confident like that. Even if you cannot turn it over, there is a meaning in the place where you can be confident. Although the mechanism of so-called "self-confidence" has not been completely elucidated, it is hard to think that only confidence follows, without creating much of new circuit in the brain. I think that creating a new circuit is more expanding and strengthening and that having confidence forms a quiet link.

I feel that it is a "convenient?" era that does not require you to experience of "Using all the power you have, to demonstrate the maximum power" everyday, so you also feel the need to make that circuit at the same time. Of course, we do not recommend weight training only. Regardless of what kind of training it is merely "one of the methods" and more effective methods will be born, more and more. There is strength that absolutely cannot be obtained unless you dare tonight against an "opponent who is bigger than you" or "opponent who is several levels stronger". Furthermore, even if it resists the big opponent with full power, even if it is pushed by the opponent at that time, an eccentric contraction occurs, strengthening muscular strength and the neural circuit which can be really used in battle. The important thing in practice is how to lose. It is extremely important for "to lose after being fully pushed out and to lose" to become stronger. If within 2 hours practice the in that 2 hours, I think that leaping hints are hidden in "how to produce such time". Let's proactively establish "the opportunity to mastering up all the power" and go beyond "the principle of size".

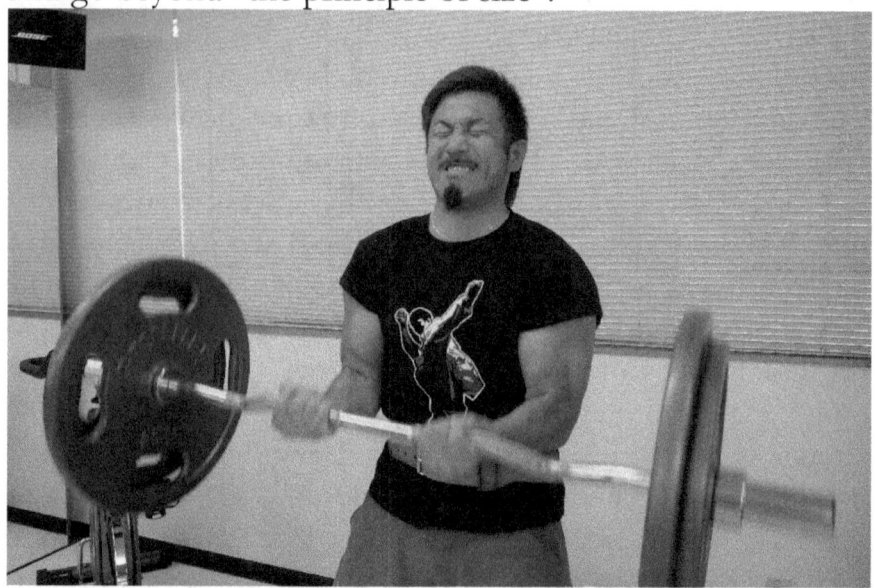

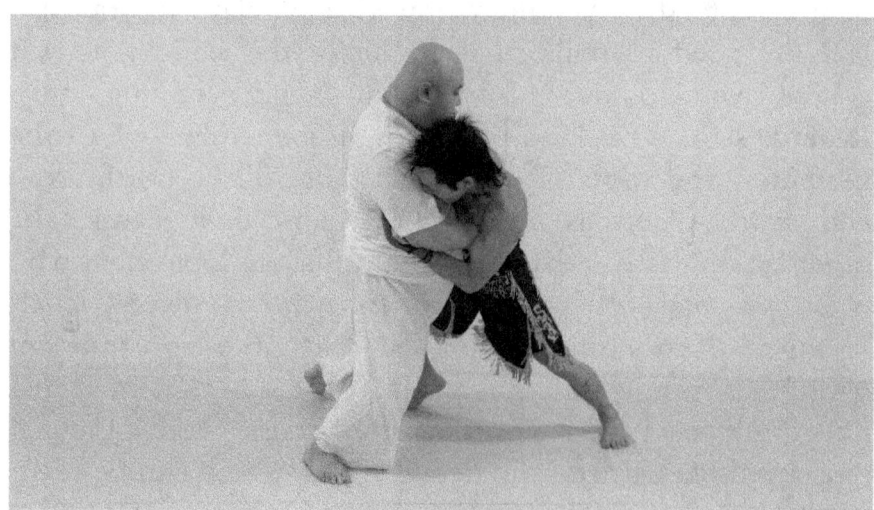

【7-6 Increase frequency of impulses】

I mentioned that it is important to increase the mobilization number of the motor unit in order to maximize the muscle strength, but also the frequency of the impulse to the mobilized motor unit is involved. Impulse is the action potential of an electrical signal traveling through nerve fibers.

Let's experiment here. Hold something like iron arrays, can coffee or PET bottles that do not have a lid open, something that is hard enough and at the size which you are able to hold in your hand. Count down "5, 4, 3, 2, 1" at 1 second intervals, then grasp with your hardest at the timing of "Zero!". Please remember the grip feeling of this moment.

Next, count down "5, 4, 3, 2, 1" at 1 second intervals, then grasp with your hardest at the timing of "Zero!". from there, more grasps with power, 5 times by further counting "Zero! zero! zero! zero!". At this time, do not return the angle of the joints of hand and fingers. Not "Grasp and return", but "Grasp, further, grasp, and further grasp ..." give command from your brain at each timing of "zero!".

What happened to the muscular strength exerted when holding it? zero! I think that you feel that you can grasp more strongly when you issue multiple orders than when it is one time. The more frequently the impulse from the brain is generated, the stronger the muscular strength exercised will be.

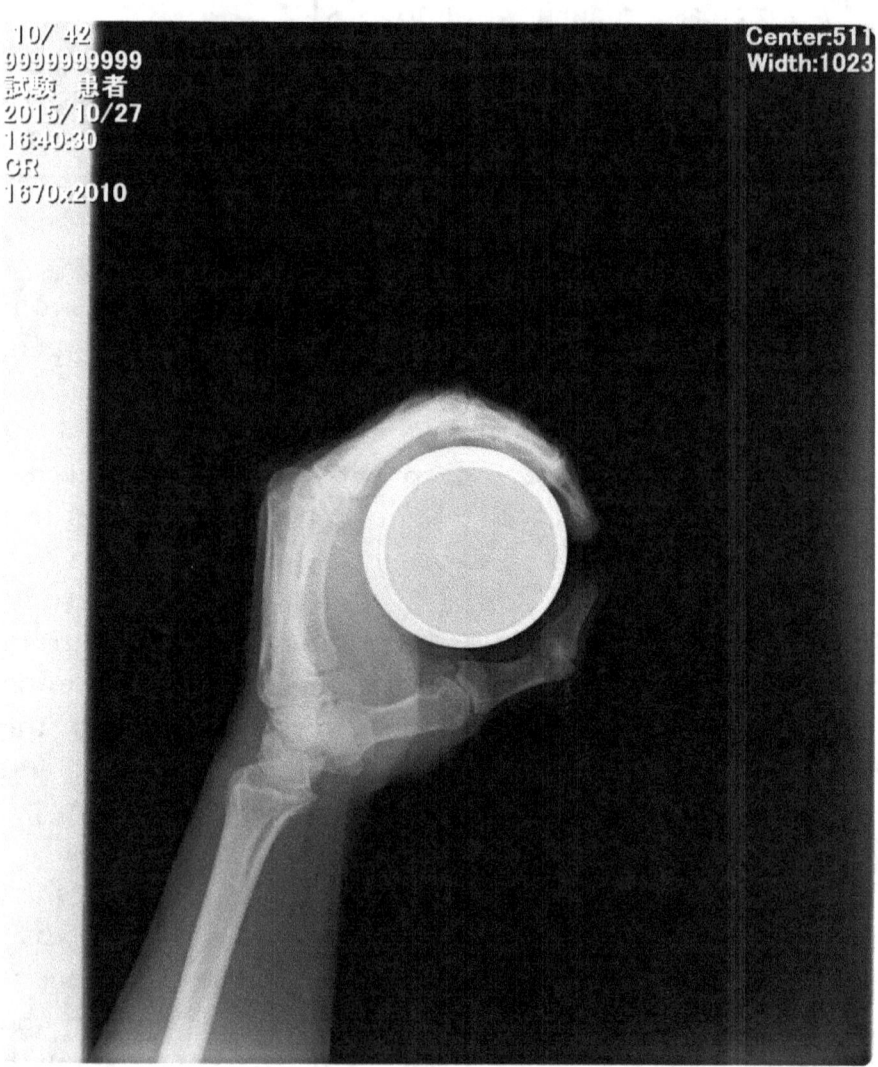

(one zero)

11/ 42
9999999999
試験　患者
2015/10/27
16:40:30
CR
1670x2010

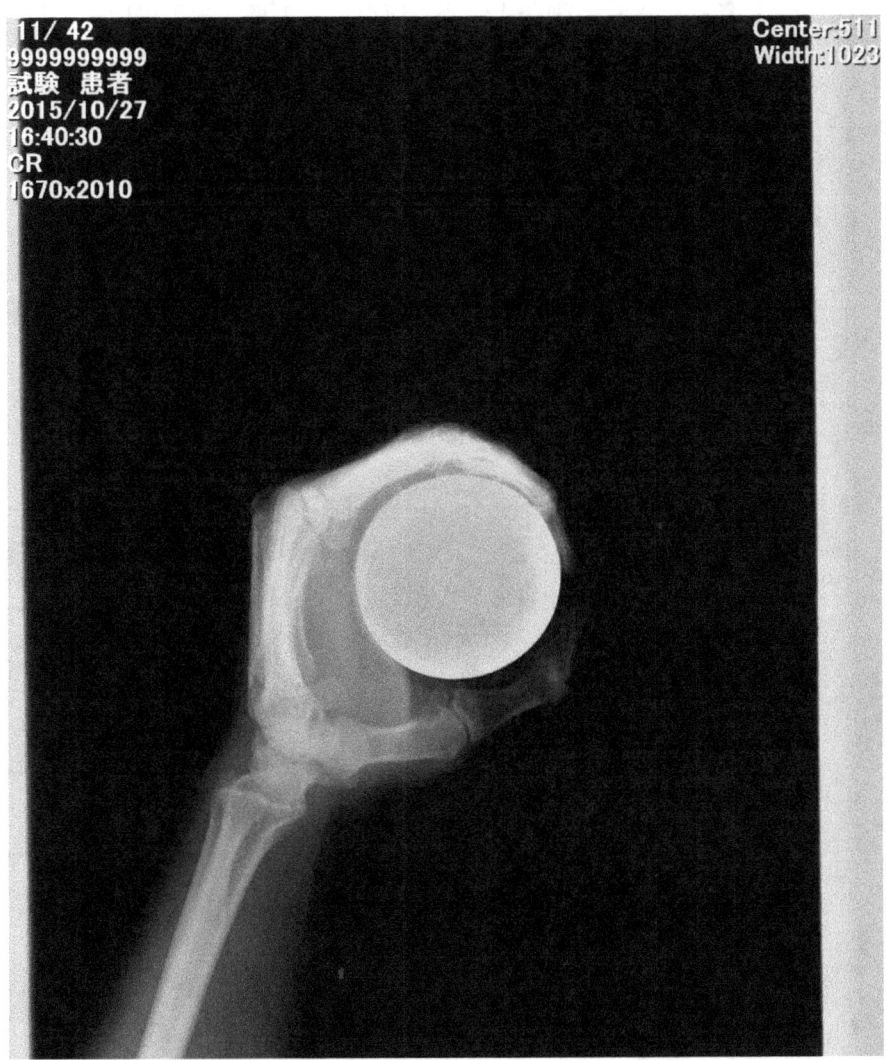

(zero zero zero…..)

【7-7 Frequency of impulse generation and techniques】
This time, let's hit a mitt with one punch.
(A) Pattern that is imagining striking only one punch, and with imaging, working simultaneously to punch once.
(B) In an image of hitting the punch several times, a pattern to hit a punch once

In A, the number of imaging times in the brain is one time, and the output in the muscle is one time.
· In B, the imaging in the brain is performed more than once, the output in the muscle is 1 time.

Compared to A, the frequency of impulses required for punching is higher than that of A, resulting in a strong and fast punch. There is a possibility that many impulses are generated by strongly and frequently creating images of the exercise recalled in the prefrontal cortex of the brain. For the sake of clarity, I explained grips and punches as an example, but please try this practice by "Improving the frequency of impulses" exercise by other techniques and exercise as a base.

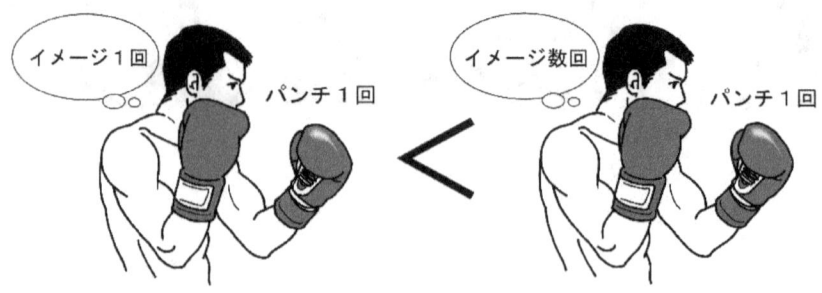

(One image one punch < Several images one punch(

【7-8 One strike one kill and modern masters】

In Karate and Martial Arts, there is a concept of "One strike one kill". With one strike, you knock down your opponent, control your opponent, put him/her in a state which he/she cannot fight anymore. It is a longing for many practitioners. Those whom will continue to practice towards the ideal of one strike one kill. As a lifetime goal, it's very nice and I feel romance in it. And in the scenes of the competition, some fighters accomplish a "one strike one kill". Not under the conditions of "cheating", "opponent not in combat state" and "weaker opponent than me", within the condition of techniques and time, there are rules to comply under the public view, starting with a signal, KO the opponent that comes to defeat you whom is definitely not a weak one, with one strike.

This is an amazing thing!！！Speaking of golf in the first shot hole in one, in baseball in the first hit home run, it may be a further level of miracle skill. It is the contestant who embodies the one strike one kill in the constraints of the competition, I think that he/she is the "modern masters ".

The common feature of the fighters who embodied the one strike one kill at the competition is that they can "chain strikes". And the fighters who are firmly engaged in the practice of hitting repeatedly have accomplished the one strike one kill. Even if it is Mike Tyson of boxing that has realized a shocking one blow KO, even if it is Naseem Hamed, even if it is Francisco Filho of Kyokushin Karate, they can also make fast chain punches and practice that.

At first sight, it seems to be inconsistent, but "to practice chain hitting" is a reason for that, "It is generating impulses in a short time", so the fighters who can chain punch, when impulse at that time is included in one blow, it becomes possible to hit one shot with the frequency of impulse occurrence raised. Sometimes, there are people who practice only single strikes for to strike one strike strongly. They believe that if that blow hits the weak points, then the one strike one kill would be realized. Of course, believing is important. However, in that direction probably only one impulse occurs. (There is no problem if it is a consciousness to increase impulse once). "Modern masters" who embodied "one strike one kill" in competition are not that they practiced only single blows.

One step in walking is part of the whole walking, as an exercise, one strike is a part of a chain punches. Based on the overwhelming basic physical strength and overwhelming momentum, impulses of successive hits can be put in a blow. If the opponent does not collapse with a single shot, it will lead to the next blow without hesitation at the next moment.

Stand up in front of someone who is higher level than you and continue to refine your ability to do something in a highly urgent situation. Set a load a little above the range that you can afford, and mobilize "mastering up all power" to overcome the "principle of size" wall. Such a tremendous detour, is it not the royal road to a one strike one kill?

8 Scapula/Upper limb

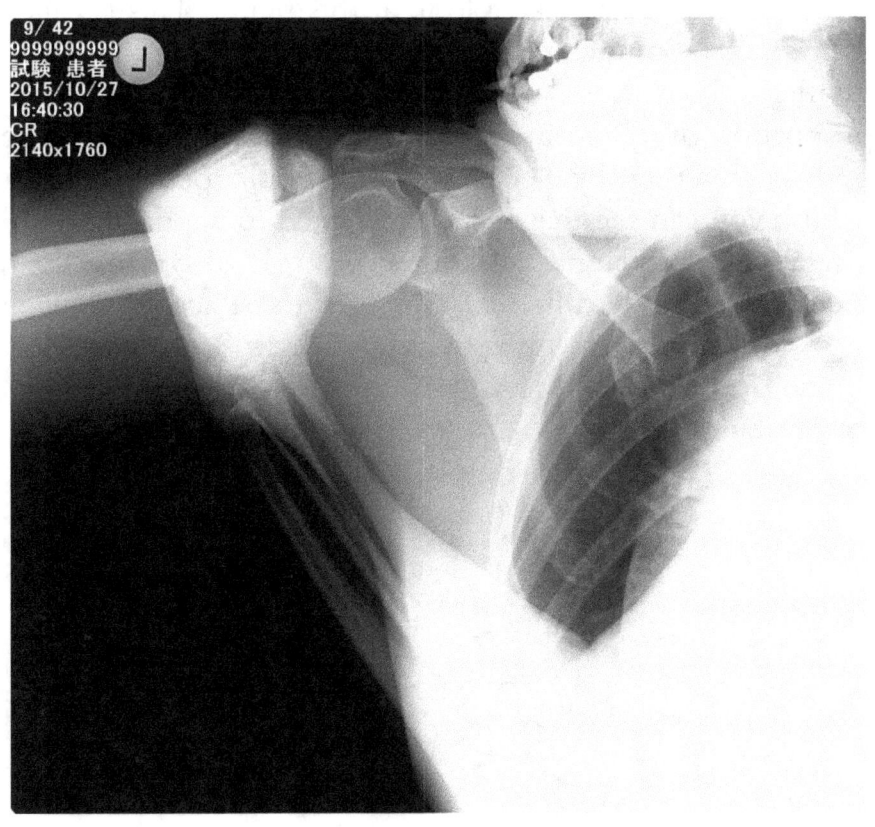

9/ 42
9999999999
試験 患者
2015/10/27
16:40:30
CR
2140x1760

【8-1 Development of Scapula / Upper limb】

First of all, please take a look at this figure. This is called 'Picture of Homunculus' written by Canadian brain surgeon Penfield. It is a diagram that schematically shows the proportion of where in the cerebral cortex the part of the body is governed by electrical stimulation experiments, but I think you can see that the areas related to hands, lips, and tongue are very large. Looking at the role of brain cells in the brain of modern humans, the area to be activated when moving the upper limbs is very wide. So in exercise, moving the hand and its upper limbs leads to mobilizing a lot of brain cells.

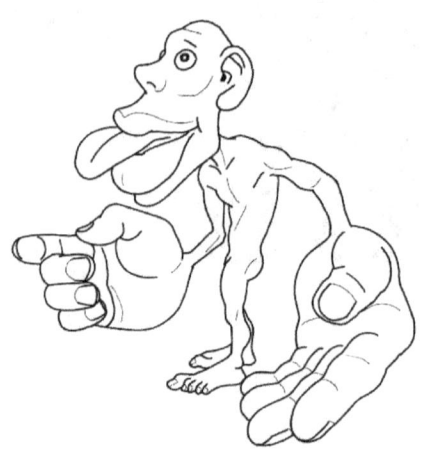

From the sense of modern people, because the lower body is mainly used for movement, it is difficult to recognize that upper limbs are involved in movement (it is also one of the characteristics of human beings), but from the sea to the land upper limbs have played an important role in exercise and mobility in the process of evolution from raised organisms to humankind. Furthermore, it has developed closely with the acts related to "eating" which is the backbone of "survival" such as grasping, tearing, crushing, pushing, and throwing food, that is, the reproductive acts.

Even in exercise of fighting sports and martial arts, how to use the scapula and upper limb affects performance. Let's look at the movement of fighting sports from the viewpoint of how to use the scapula and upper limbs.

【8-2 Punch of Front Hand】

Make a pair with a partner and ask the partner to hold a mitt, and try to punch with the front hand. As I write it in orthodox (left front, right rear), southpaw people please swap the left and right and read.

A) Let's hit the left punch by moving the front arm as main movement from the fighting stance.

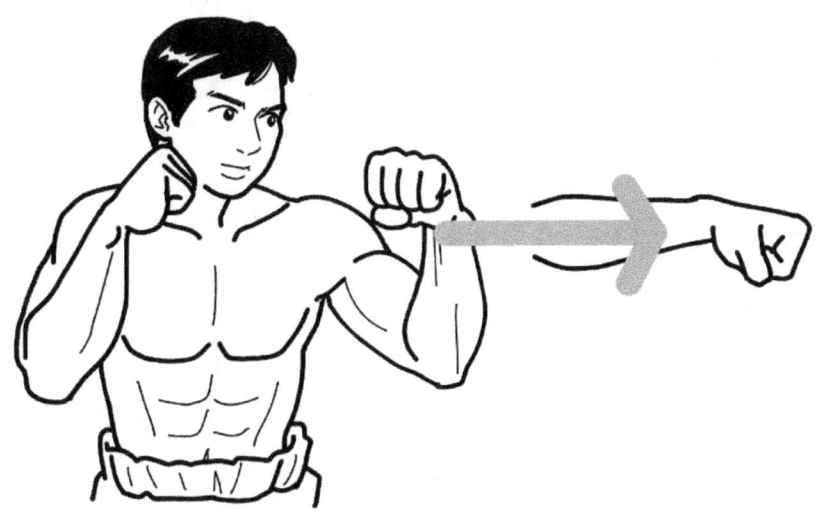

and then,

B) Place the elbow of the right upper limb at a place about 5 cm to 15 cm from the stance, then try the left punch the next moment. At this moment, keep it in front of the scapula, fix the place of the elbow of the back upper limb (right elbow), adjust the rest of the body to that position and please move by putting out the left punch.

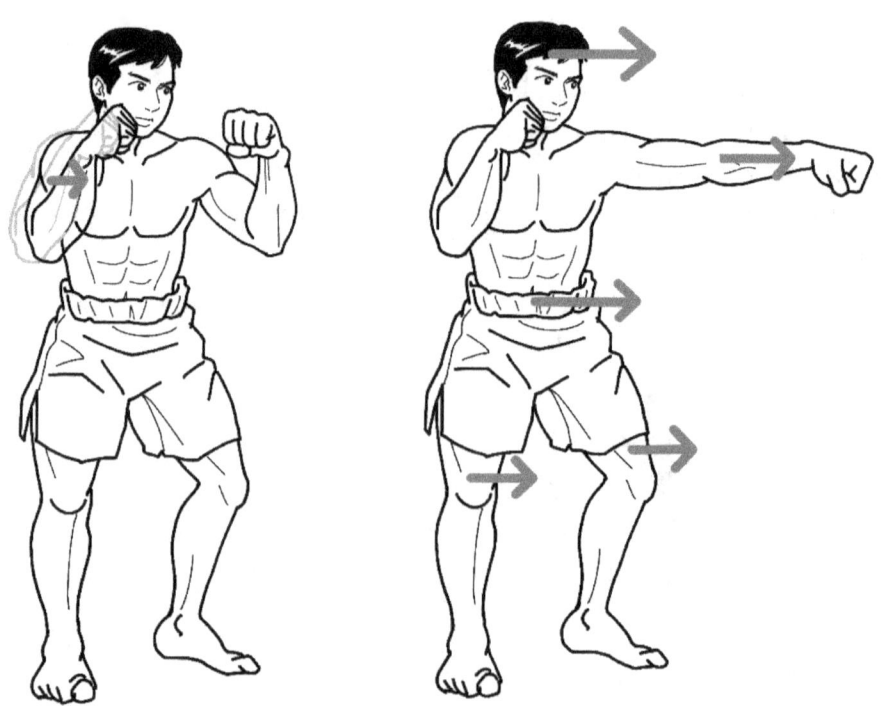

【8-3 Punch of Back Hand】
Next, let's try the back hand punch.

A) In case you hit the right straight so that you put the right fist in front from the fighting stance.

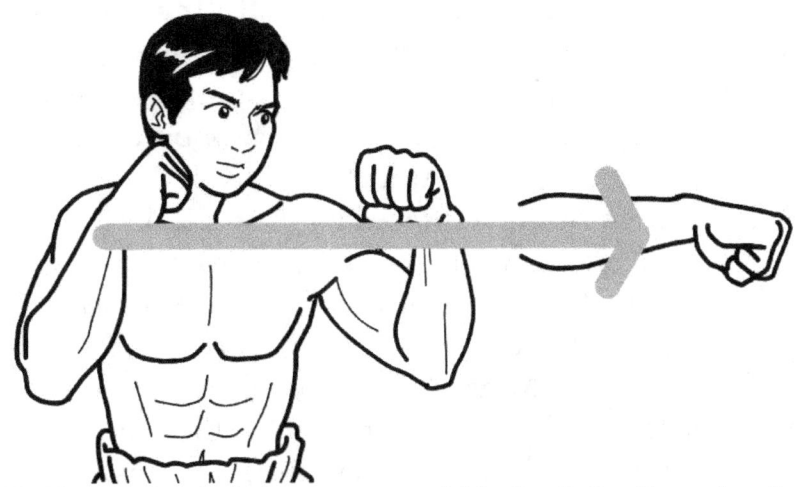

B) From the fighting stance, shift the left elbow by 5 to 15 cm forward with the shoulder blades and strike the right straight punch to fit all the remaining parts to that position

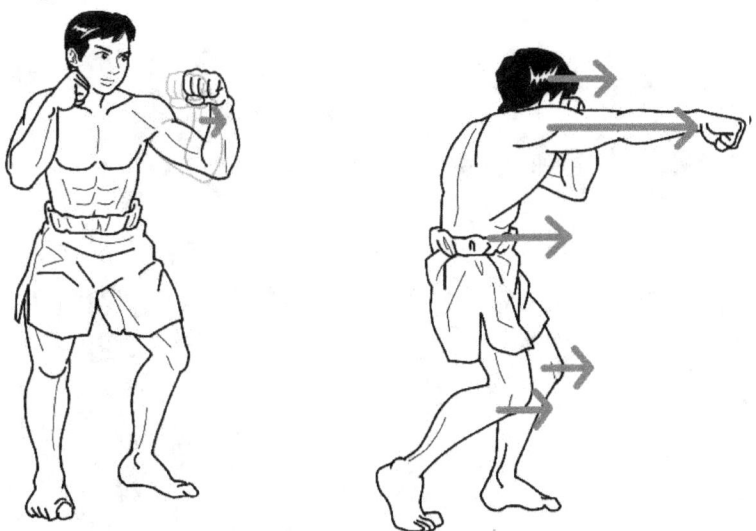

How was speed, power, easiness to generate? In case of A), the brain gives a command to the muscle group for putting the fist forward. So the muscles that participate in

the punch will be the main muscles that give the right fist in front. In case of A), the brain gives a command to the muscle group for putting the fist forward. B) In the case of B), the command comes out from the brain to the upper limb on the opposite side first, then the command is given to each remaining part (trunk pelvis, lower limbs, upper limbs on the punching side). As a result, it is the combination of "movement preceding the opposite scapula" + "movement where the rest goes forward" + "movement of the fist goes forward". "movement of the fist goes forward", the reason I wrote is, "Movement to put the fist forward" and "Move the fist goes forward" are similar in appearance but are different from the exercise . As the skill improves, it changes from the local muscular strength like A to the overall muscular strength with the kinetic chain like B. The image of the exercise recalled in the brain is also larger for B than for A.

(A)

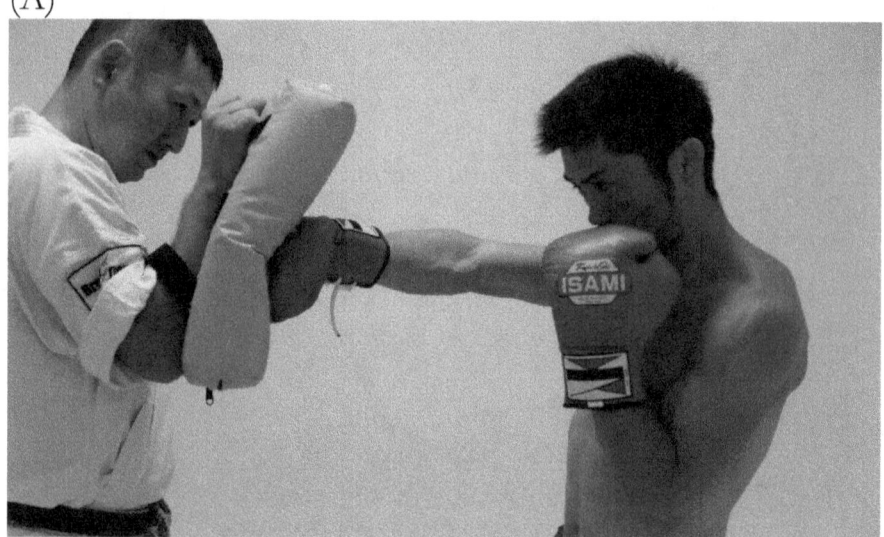

(B)

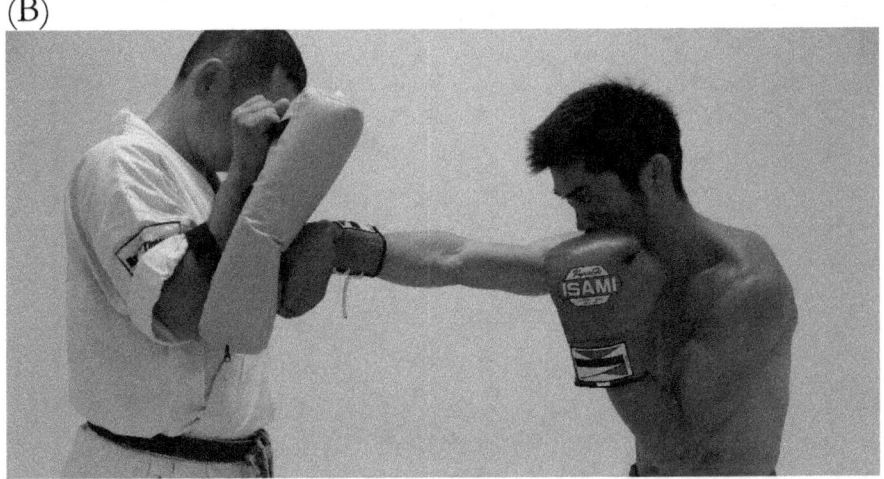

There is a difference between a practitioner who recognizes A's motion as a punch and a practitioner who recognizes the movement of B is a punch and A is a part of the process. Also, B is big as exercise and there are also a lot of muscle groups to participate, so even if the practitioner's punch of doing B does not actually move, a wider range of brain cells participate in the movement of the punch because the image of a large movement is recalled, the muscle group participating in the punch increases.

【8-4 Receive then Return】

Let's try another experiment. Make a pair sitting with your legs crossed opposite from each other and face each other and try punching lightly on the other's chest on the left. Since there is a danger of shaking the heart for children, we ask for only the person who is over 20 years old for the menu. and also the other menus with strike experiment on the chest are applied the same.

A) First, the case you hit a left punch from the fighting pose.

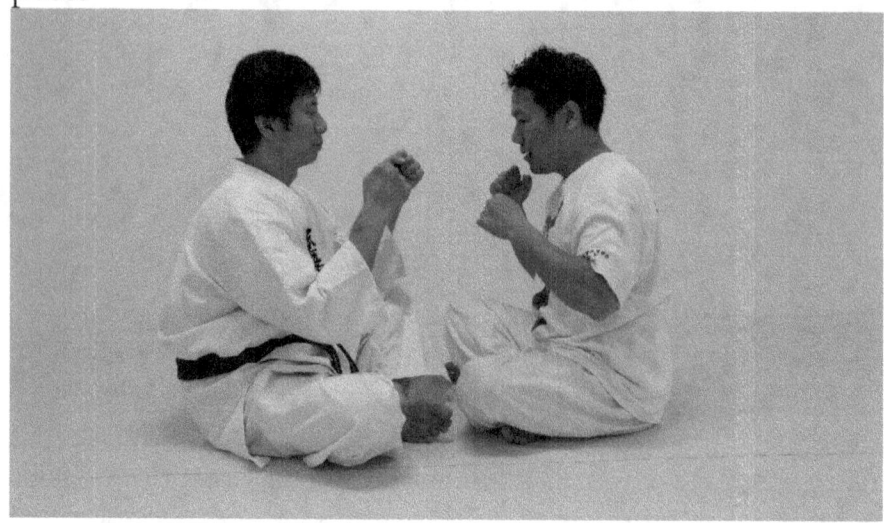

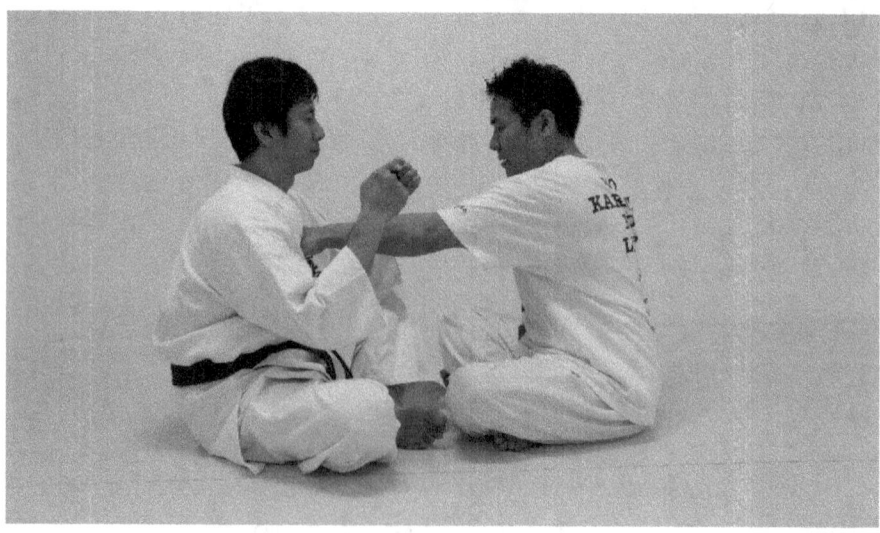

B) Next, the case you hit the left punch with the right upper limb after receiving with outside block or inside block, the basic defense techniques of Karate

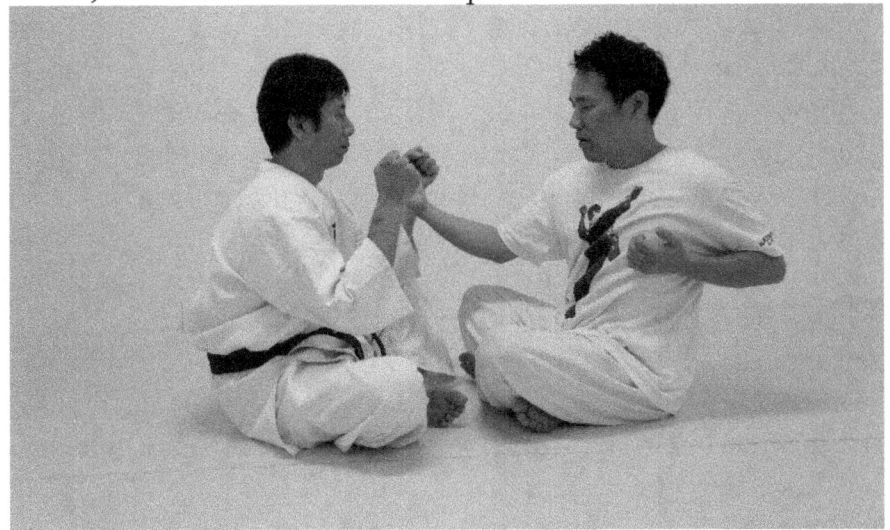

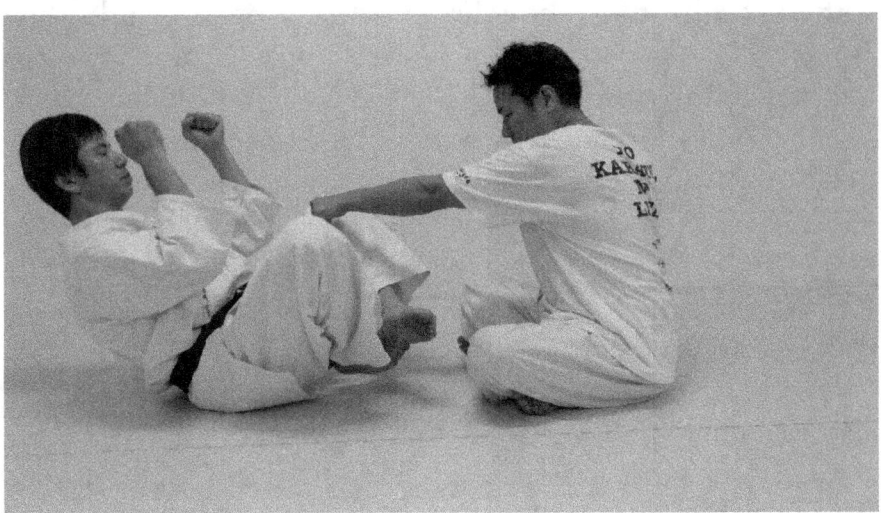

In this experiment, by touching the buttocks to the floor, we are limiting to prevent the forces generated by the lower limbs from being transmitted to the upper body. When introducing the movement of B), the position of the right shoulder blade changes, so I think that you can feel that a left punch matching the position puts out. Many cases of "the movement to advance the shoulder blades on the opposite side" also to the traditionally come down Katas of Karate. The first movements of the katas such as Takyoku and PinAn learned by the Karate schools are also taken from the view of the direction of travel → After setting the direction to go with the right upper limb and shifting the shoulder blades ahead of time → Connect to the desired left downward block. Even from the downward block, and in the process of shifting to the next chase, the direction is determined with the left upper limb received, shifted with the shoulder blades(scapula), and then connected to the lunge punch. In addition, "movement to attach a fist to a body trunk" called a Hikite (pulling hand) also becomes "to move a part other than a fist up to the position of a fist" not only "attract a fist to a body" in the kata. "Before getting on the left, it will work well if you move the right in the first place (and vice versa)", "When moving, you move easily with the scapula ahead, it is easy to move", "Move the body to the position of becoming a Hikite" These messages are hidden inside of it. There are also "Kamae (fighting stance in Japanese)" and "Fighting stance" for fighting sports and martial arts competitions. As the word "Kokoro ga(ka)mae (direct translation is "heart" "Ready". Expression of "condition ready" in Japanese)" is said, the stance itself is already a start of movement.

First-class fighters are skillful in how to use defense and stance too. In fact, the pace is on the opponent side if you ", make move of defense, only when the opponent attacks". "Because the opponent plays Rock, I will play Paper" "Because the opponent plays Scissors, I will play Rock" This is the case starting from your opponent, so it seems to be compatible with the case, in fact the pace is on his/her hand.

Even when your opponent does not attack you, try moving the stance, try to create a state that you don't even make a stance, mix in the defense technique for a instant, change the distance while keeping the safe state with the defensive posture, such a "gimmick from myself" starts the flow. In Muay Thai, making stance by holding firmly with both hands, you may create a state in which it is difficult to get the counter, a situation where the attack of the opponent is easily caught in the stance, and closing the distance and capturing the next moment. It is possible to become a clue to attack by going forward while firmly defending. It is, to utilize the offensive defense, and the active defense. A fighter who goes up in a competition can set up such "change" from himself. While taking action from his/her side, make use of defense techniques and defense state to move the opponent. Am I using the defense techniques and the stance only when my opponent attacks? Or am I actively using the defense techniques and the stance for "the next moment"? The difference of this consciousness is very big difference. Mr. Gichin Funakoshi, the great meritorious person who has developed it to international well known, KARATE written in various languages, has left the word "There is no first strike in Karate".

Interpretation as a word of commandment that "karate is a technique to train the heart and protect yourself, so do not attack from yourself" is commonly said, but when you look back at the transmitted form from the kinematic point of view, I feel that the utility of body control "receive then return" is somehow hidden as another truth.

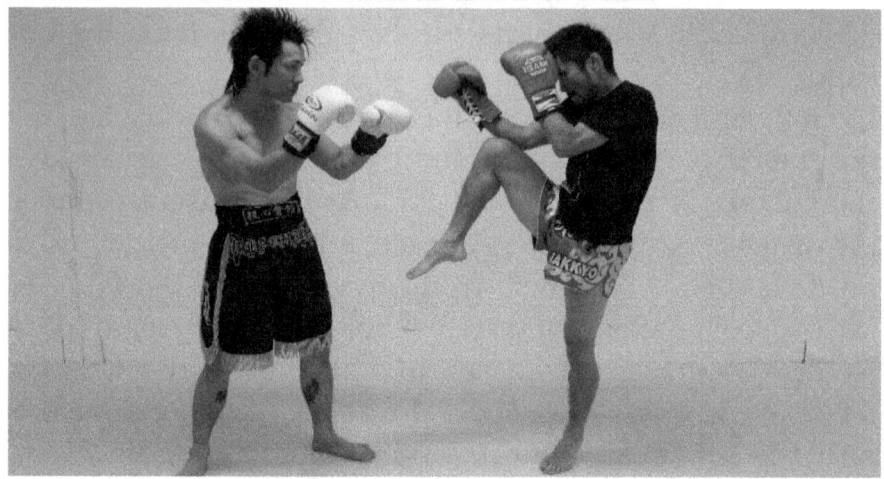

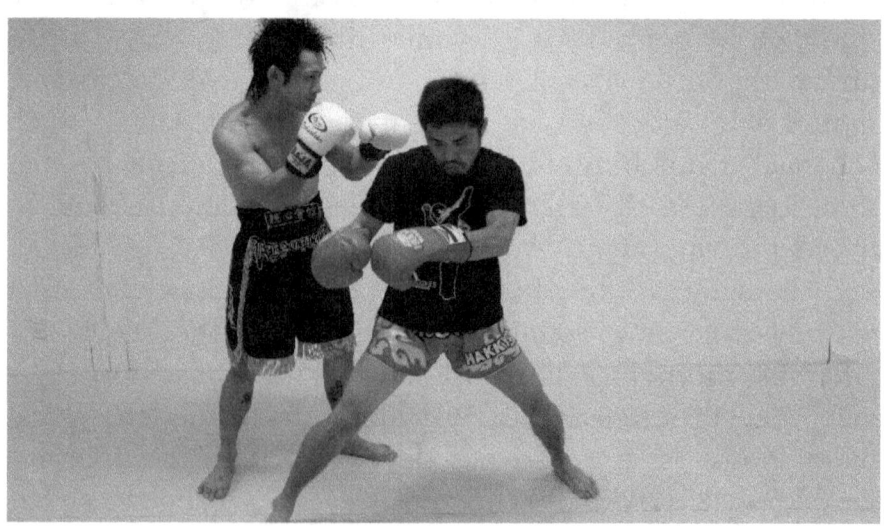

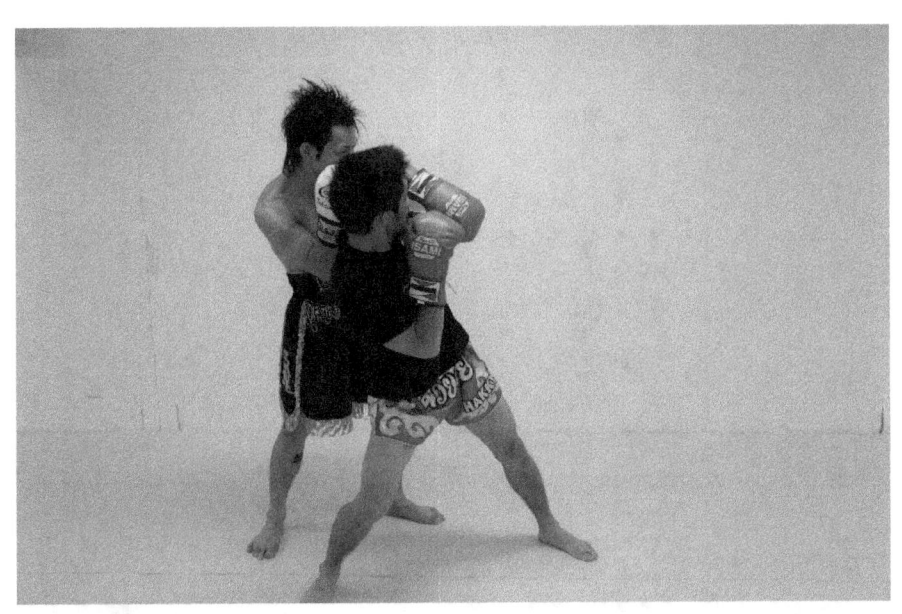

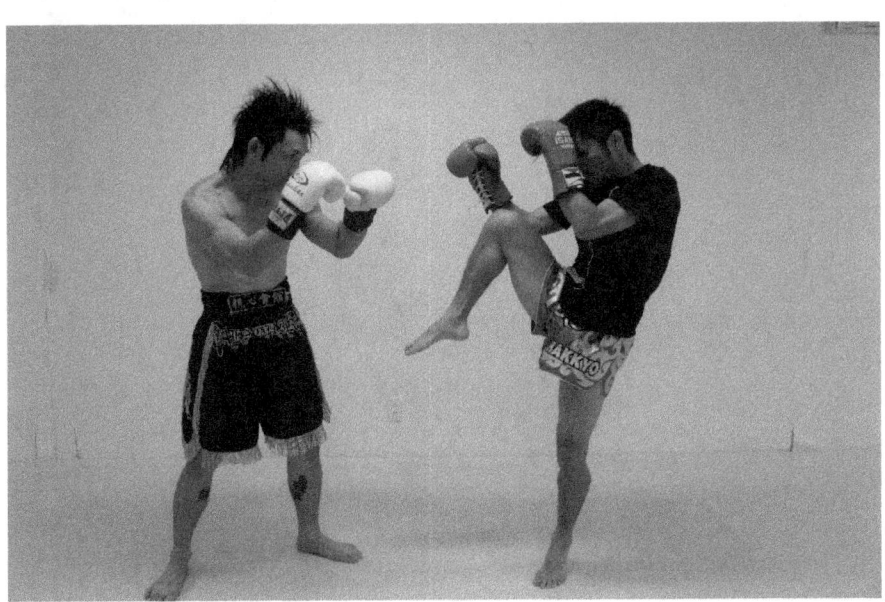

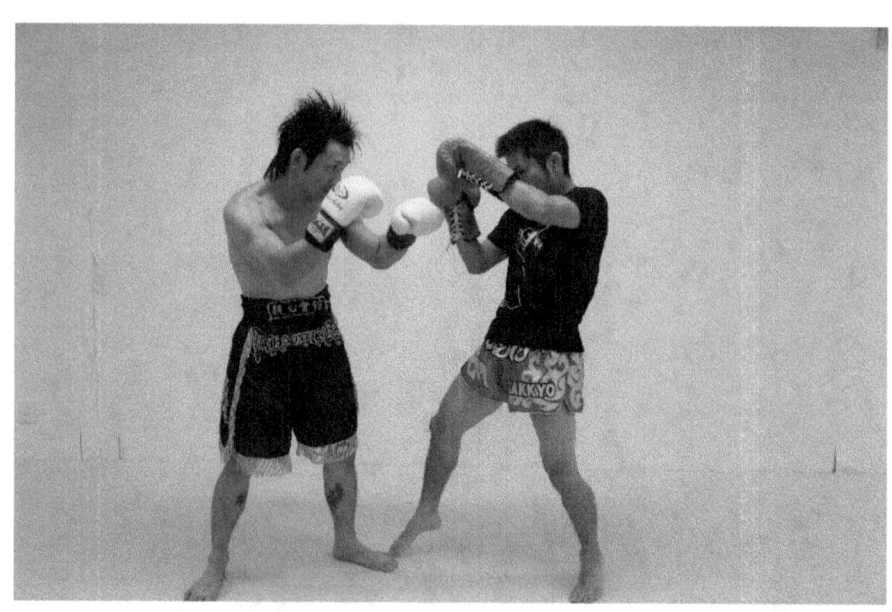

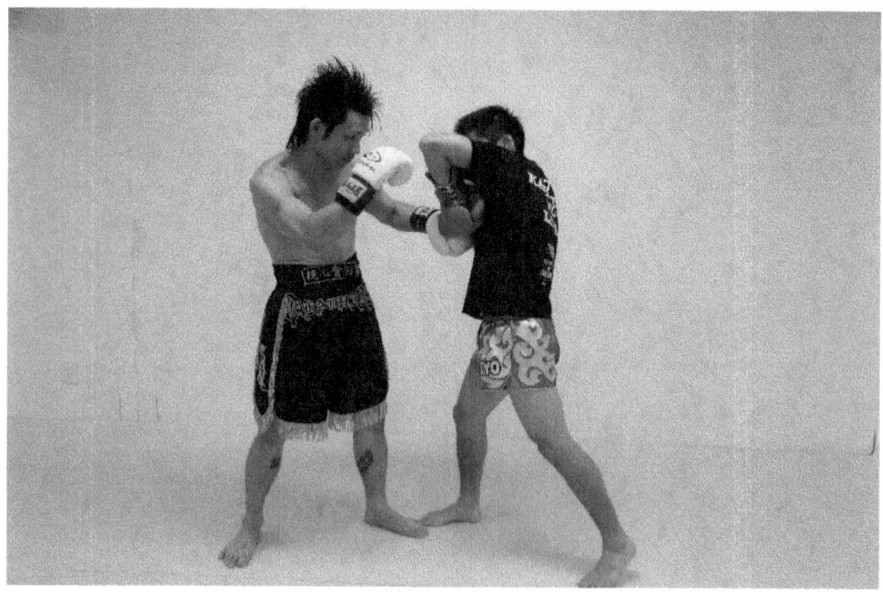

【8-5 Parry and Outside Block】

Parry which is practiced in boxing and kick boxing. It is a
defense method of moving the upper libs from the outside

to the inside relative to the opponent's punch, changing the course of the opponent's punch and stopping the punch. In the case where the opponent strikes the right straight with the orthodox stance, there are many cases that are instructed to guard using the left upper limb, and there are not a few fighters who actually do so. On the other hand, Karate also has outside block as a traditionally come down technique of defense. Applying an external force to the opponent's attack from the outside to the inside, that part is the same, but the outside block has a movement before that. When blocking with the left forearm, first shift the right upper limb towards the opponent. At this time, the right upper limb has already become a barrier to the opponent's punch course, and deviation is caused in the assumed distance for the opponent. At the next moment, while pulling the right upper limb, it defends the opponent's punch with the left forearm. Along with these movements, the left hip joint moves in the extension direction and the right hip joint moves in the bending direction. Outside block of Karate is accompanied by preceding movement of scapula, and using both upper limbs, it is a blocking technique of "whole body exercise" including lower limbs and trunk in type and basic, I teach that discreetly. In the case of outside block, since the right upper limb and lower body of the unaffected side will also be in full-motion exercising full operation, it will be easy to get stretched reflection there, and reaction of gravity and gravity will also be easy to use, so counterattack can be done very quickly.

(Parry)

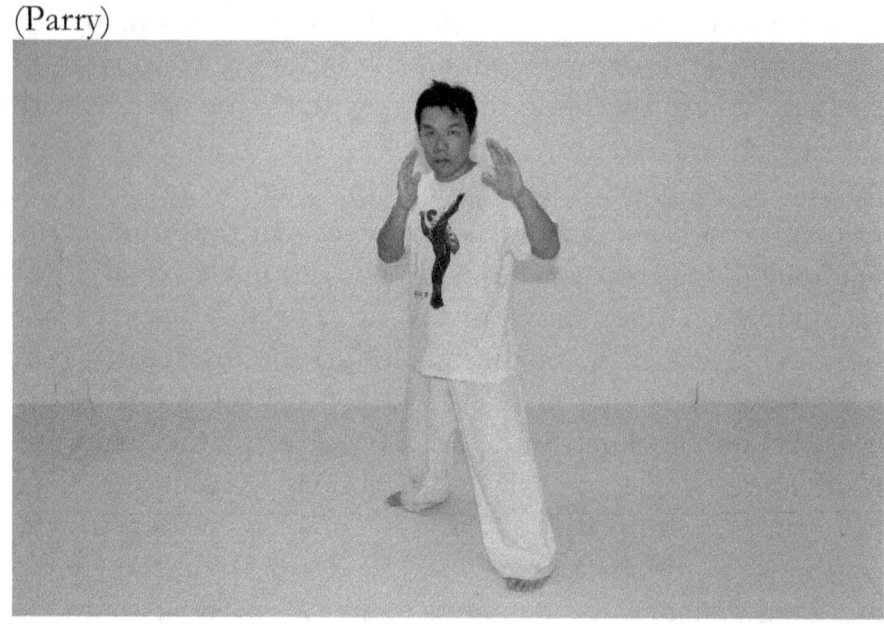

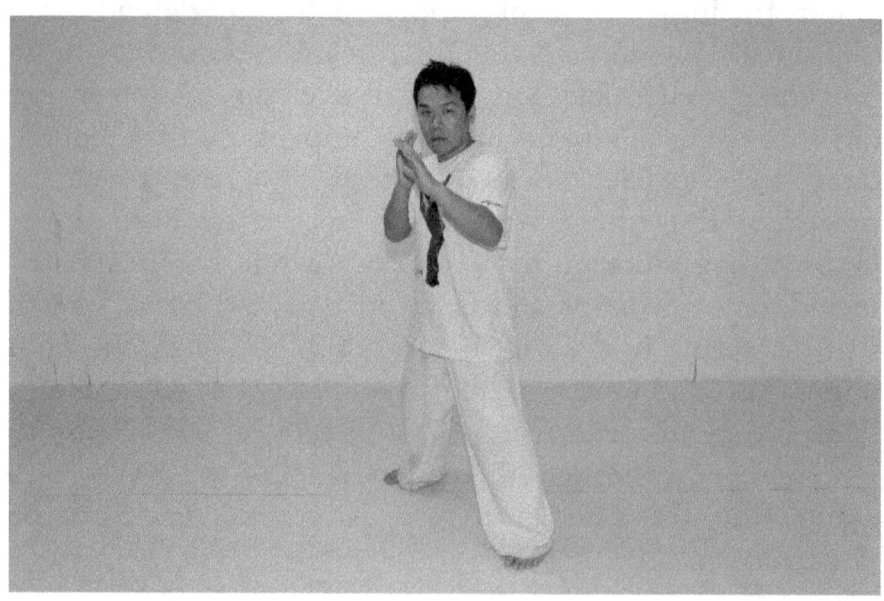

(Sotouke-Outside block)

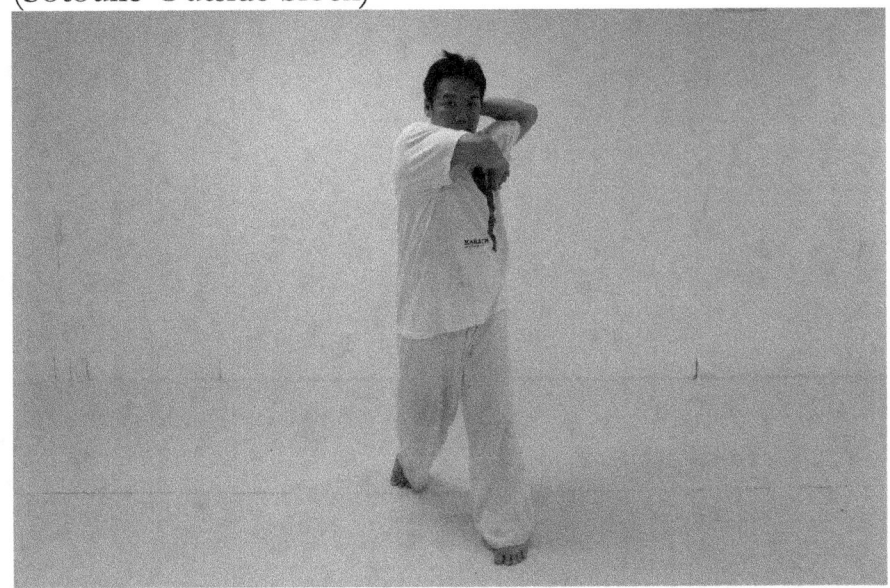

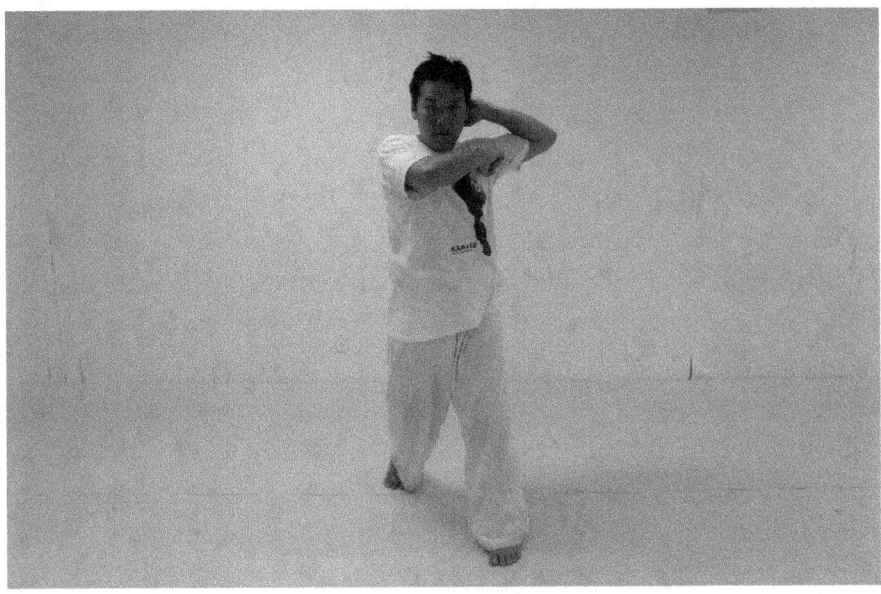

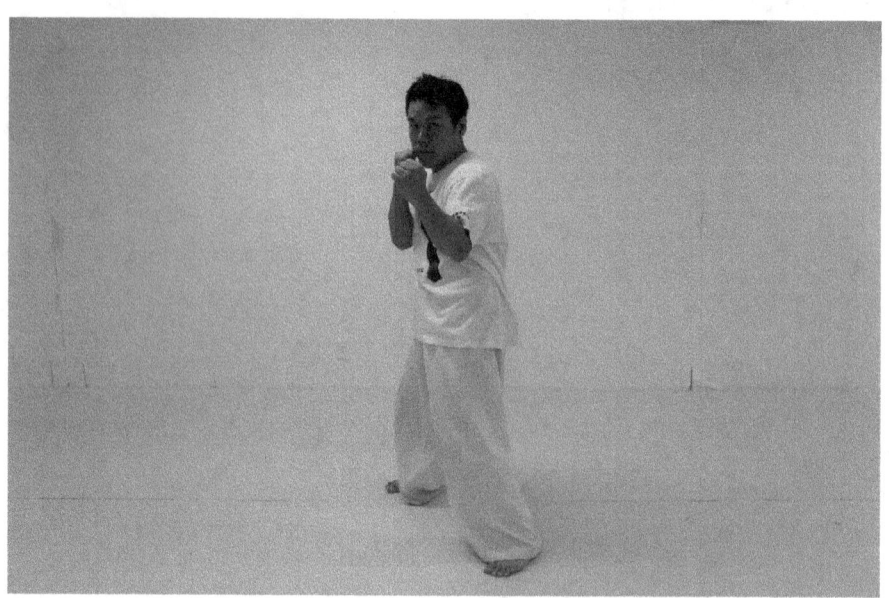

Of course, there are also a lot of fighters practicing it in kick boxing, boxing and mixed martial arts, and there are many karate fighters blocking only with the command of the upper limbs. There seems to be some Karate dojos of the policy that only sparring and mitt practice, without practicing basics and kata at all.

Although I mentioned in the point of visual function, the kata of Karate appears to be "useless" as it's with very big movements. And that is correct in a way. If everyone sees it and understands it, it will reveal what kind of training is being done to the enemies. It is inspired by the "Only those who know, would understand" because it is meant to be made "not to useful at first glance". When the pitcher throws the ball towards the catcher, they say they throw to the back net behind the catcher. If you throw it towards the catcher, the speed will drop and it will be easy to hit. With this same principle, it is effective to create huge neural circuits in the brain - nerve - muscle through large movements on a routine basis. In the load of movement with difficulty, a hidden rule that practices large movements with large images and generates large impulses while concentrating it on small scenes in actual situations. The work of installing to the progressive "competition" while elucidating the essence put in the movement of the traditionally transmitted katas through the battle, and the task of installing it in the movement of the tradition with the traditional katas. The task of finding out common points is very deep and it is a time trip of "visiting old, learn new".

Originally the katas were created by the fighting people. It's not that Katas existed first then there were battles, but there were battles then Katas were created. Locks the secret of the strength cultivated in the life risking battles and the law which reduces the risk of life, into the katas. There is a part which visualizes and conveys some movement with movement as "shape" in the katas. Katas are about how wide the foot is, where the line of sight is, how the direction is, how much is the height of the pelvis, where the position of the fist is, so that everything is fixed with rules, so that in the acquisition process Although it cannot be used freely, there is a possibility that "you can move freely if you keep the points you should protect in inconvenience." It is like, the difference between hit randomly the keyboard of piano without any basic skills, and learned basic finger works, scale, melodies and rhythm and play freely is different like another dimension, so, move freely within the fight is not move however you want, but assembling several basic patterns together, subtract, multiply to select accurately while moving, is the answer. There are several correct answers as to how to notice what you notice there when doing a kata, how to interpret it, and how to feed it back to your strength while doing firmly the contest which is a contemporary battle. Not only do you pass on the form as a traditional art but the development of the katas as an excellent gear living in the competitions is expected more and more from now on.

(Parry)

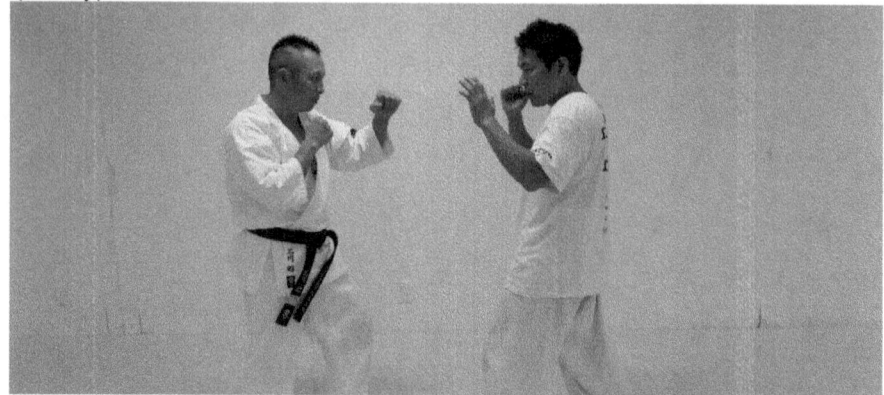

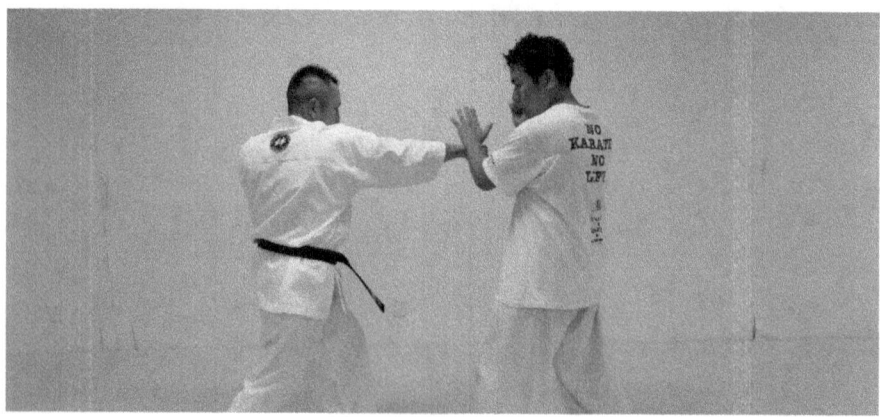

(Sotouke outside block)

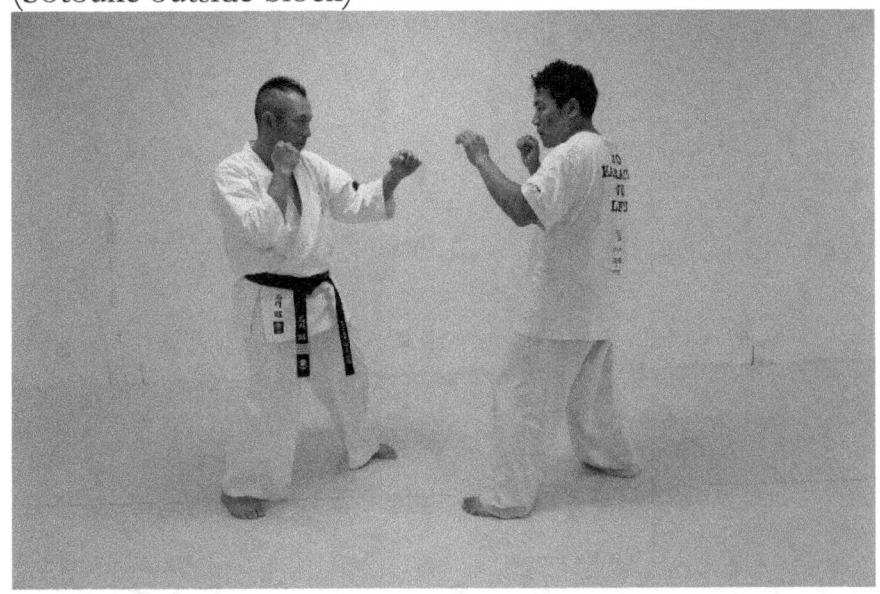

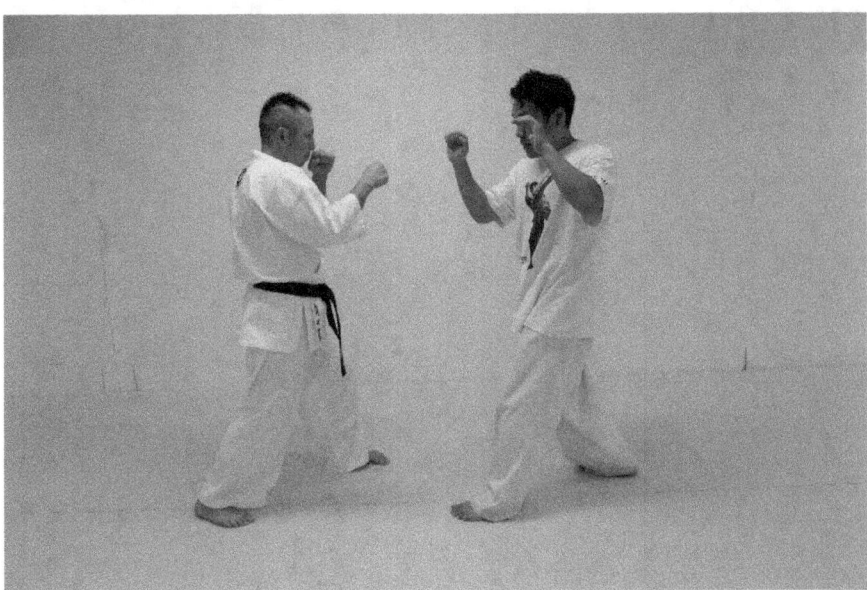

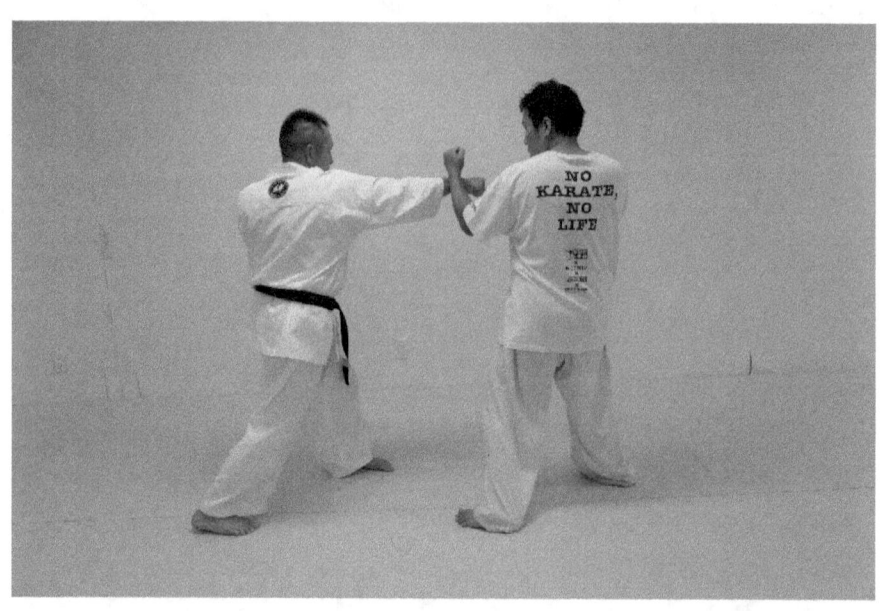

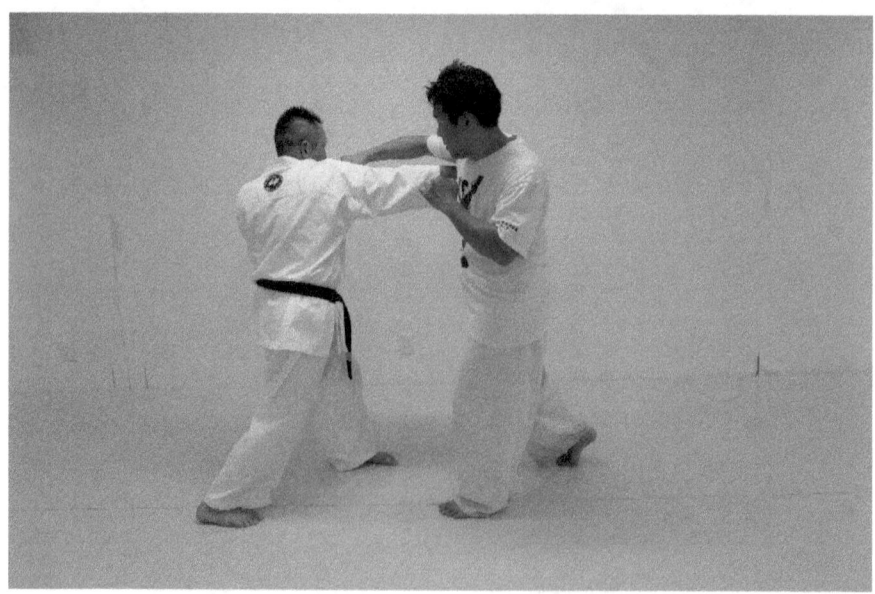

【8-6 How to receive reaction of punch】
   I wanted to know the secret of a strong punch inevitably, so I did an X - ray filming.

1) When you hit without changing the position of scapula

2) When you hit with the scapula doing abduction

A picture taken by irradiating radiation vertically from above. Of course, the subject is myself (lol). Looking at the relation between the humerus and the shoulder blade, which is the bone of the upper arm, I think you can observe 2) the humerus is being received on the joint surface of the shoulder blades on the image. You can see the connection of a bone and a bone sandwiching the cartilages. In comparison with this, 1) is receiving the reaction on the humerus at a place not on the joint surface. Anatomically, it is receiving the reaction of the punch at the site called soft tissue including the ligament, the joint capsule and so on. A fighter with a strong punch firmly receives the reaction with a strong scapular blade and a fighter who damages the shoulder has been received with a weak soft tissue for every punch. A fighter with 1) form hits the unnecessary load on ligaments and so on as he/she hits more and more.

In the Karate's kata, put a hand of the fist on the ribs and side flanks. Even in boxing and kick boxing, comprehensive, and even Karate competitions, I can keep my fist away from my trunk, "why do I have to explicitly include the movement of sticking the fist or forearm to the trunk?" For many years I had been wondering.

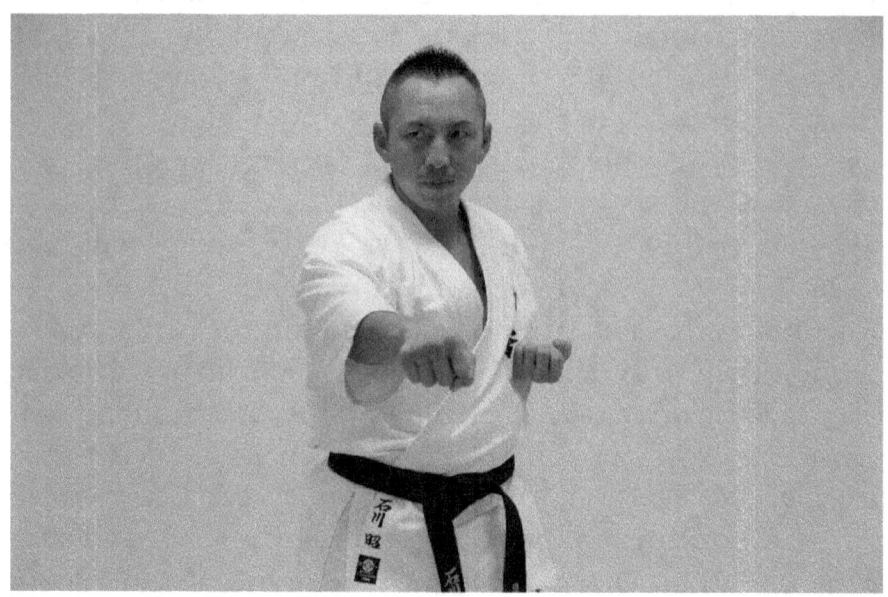

While clarifying and researching from the viewpoint of fighting medicine, a possibility popped out. It is about, when you put out a punch, even just one moment, integrate the movement of pulling the upper limbs to the trunk (the movement to move the scapula towards inner rotation direction), shoulder blades become easier to abduct, it becomes being able to receive the reaction with a bone and a bone. I wonder the reason why the fist in the kata contact with the trunk, and the reason why the thrust is rolled out, so that the upper limbs and trunk cause friction, was suggesting the positional relationship between the scapula and the upper limbs?

Type A

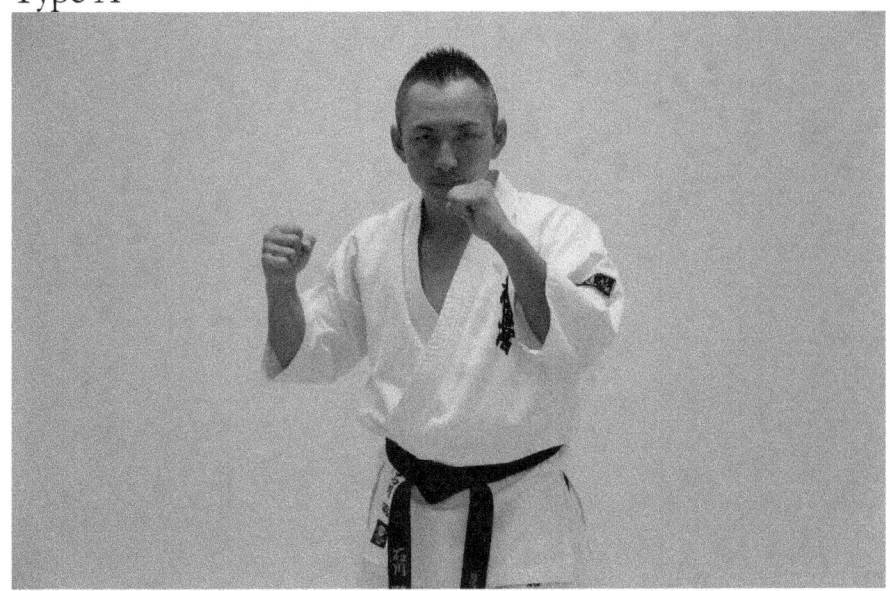

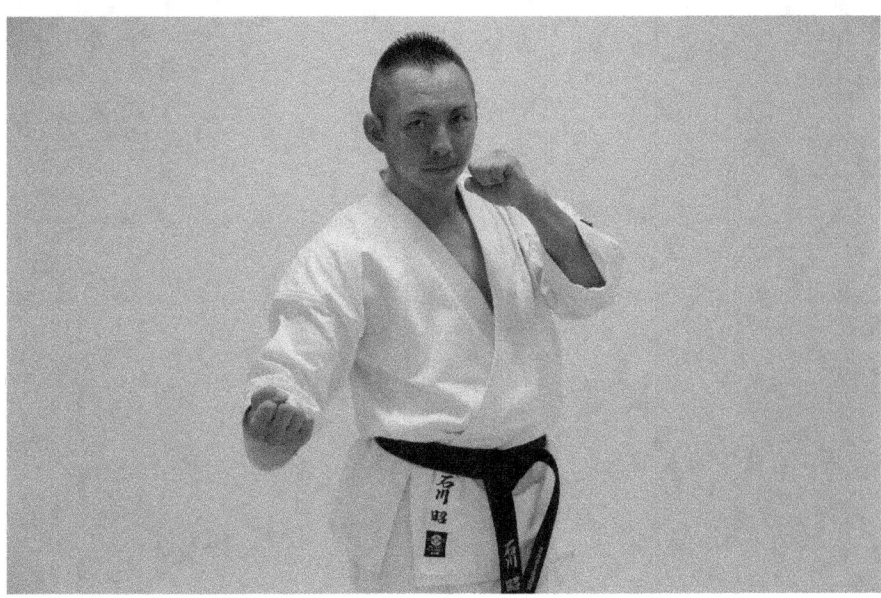

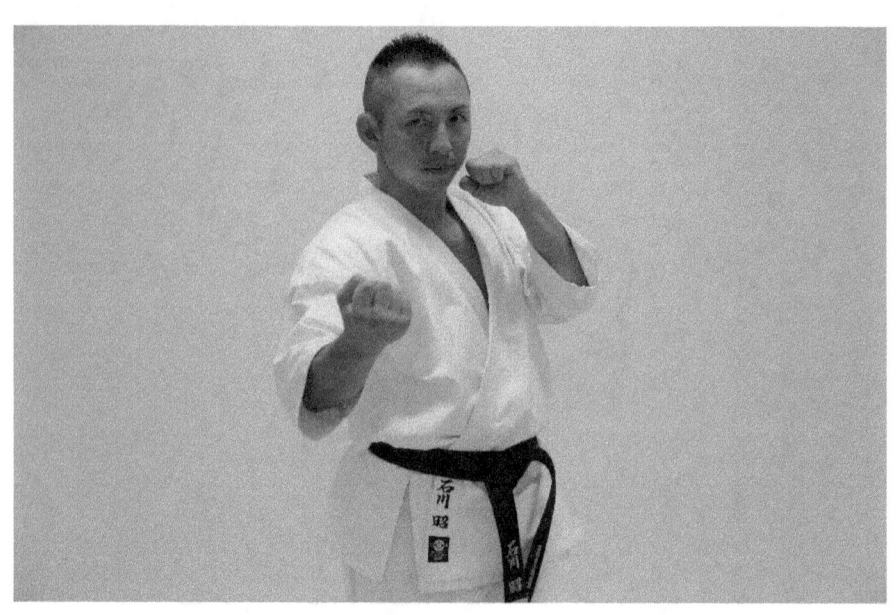

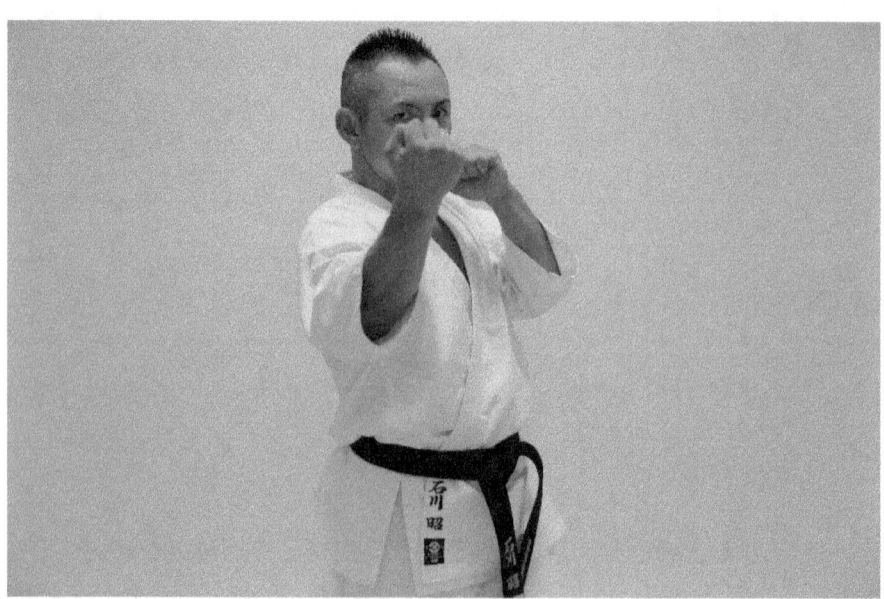

Type B

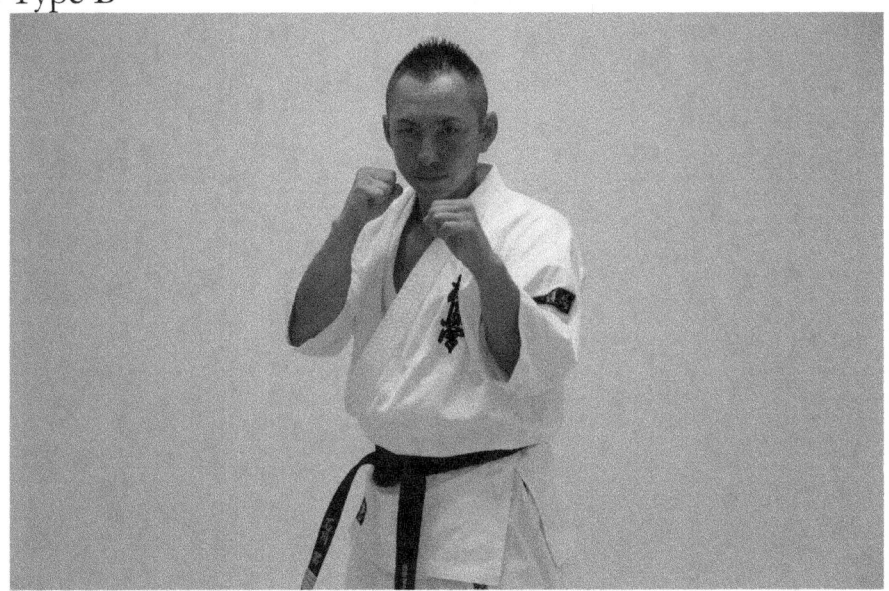

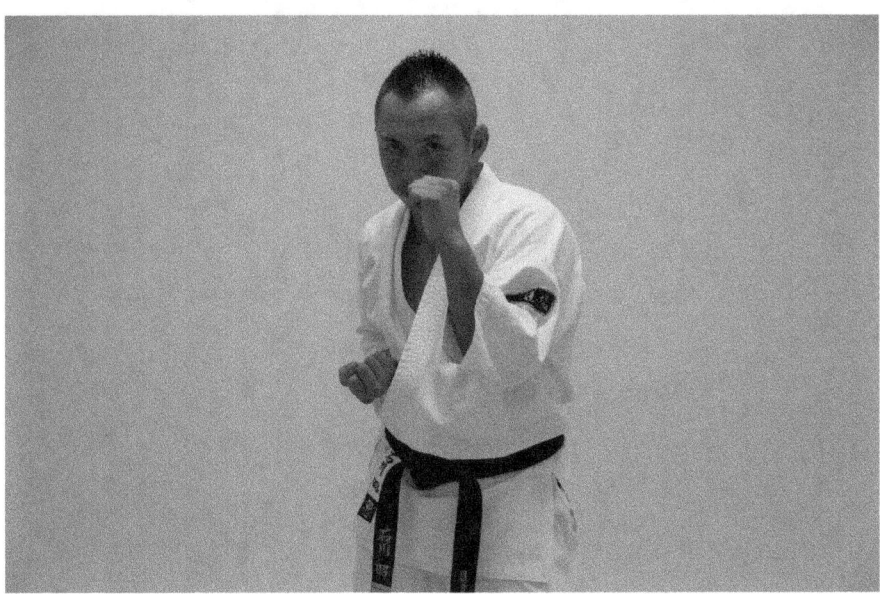

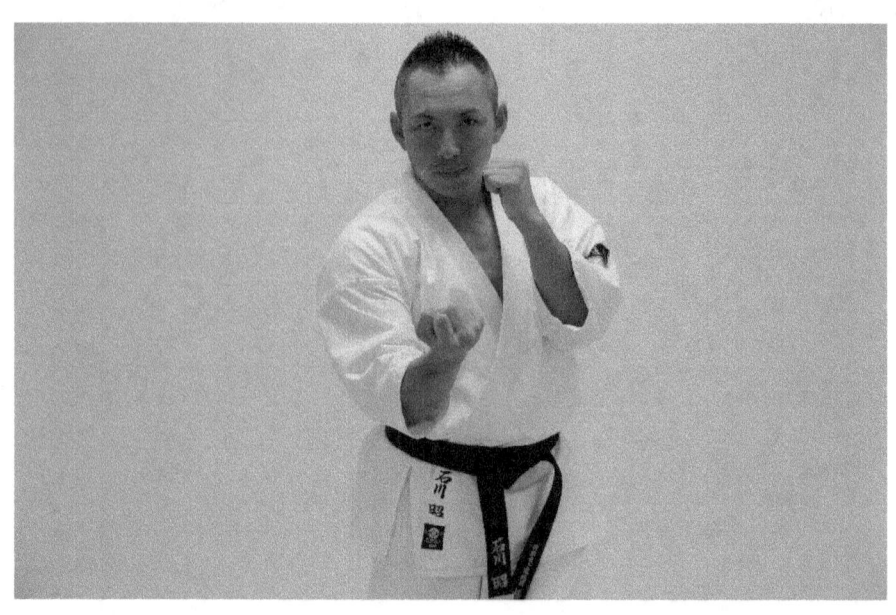

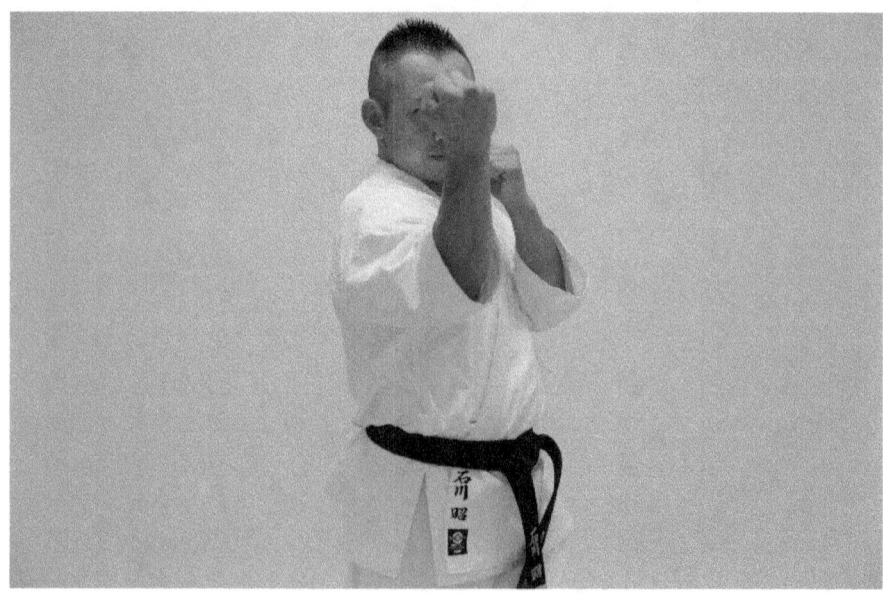

When the scapula securely receives the upper limbs, the muscular strength becomes very large. If you lie on your back and extend both upper limbs without rolling the scapula and you extend the upper limbs with abduction of the scapula, the latter is large enough to support a person's weight. In addition, it is a work that is good at handstand, handstand walking is also a work of making muscular strength around the scapula and maneuverable magnitude of human's shoulder blades.

If you seek to improve performance in fighting sports / martial arts, risk of injury or failure may be reduced. The opposite is also true. "Pursuit of techniques" and "risk avoidance" will start towards compatibility when pursuing the direction of "where and how to receive reactions".

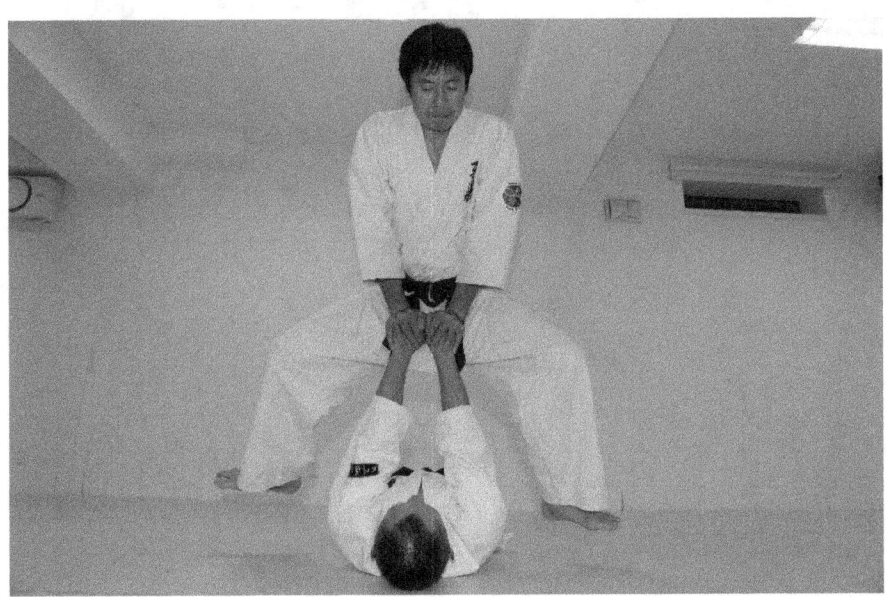

(abduct scapula to support partners)

【8-7 Kick】

How do the scapula and upper limbs work in kicking movement? Let's look at the movements of the scapula and upper limbs in the right middle roundhouse kick (middle kick) with orthodox stance. From the fighting stance,

A) The case of both of the scapulas are fixed and the right middle roundhouse kick is kicked.

B) Firstly, place with the left scapula forward, next moment, put the right scapula also forward, then right middle roundhouse kick.

A-1

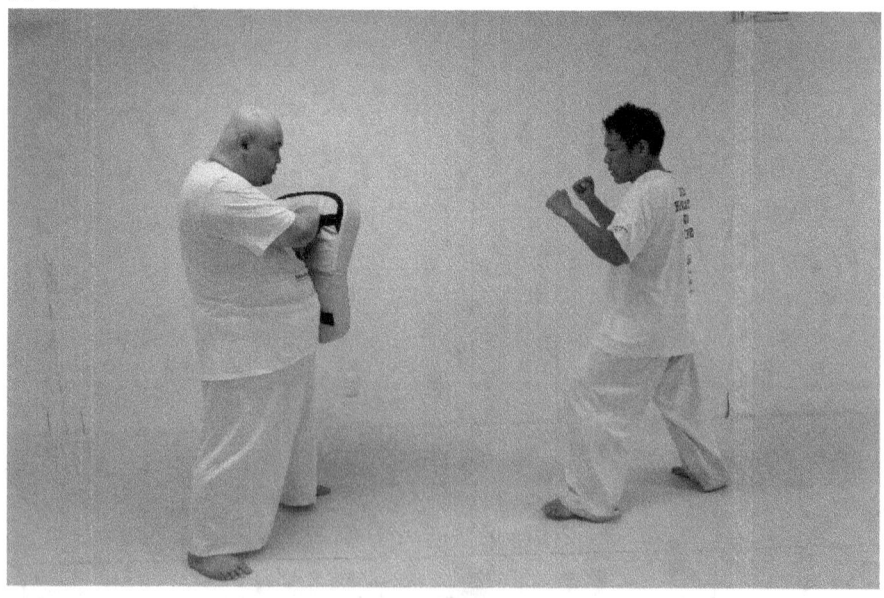

A-2

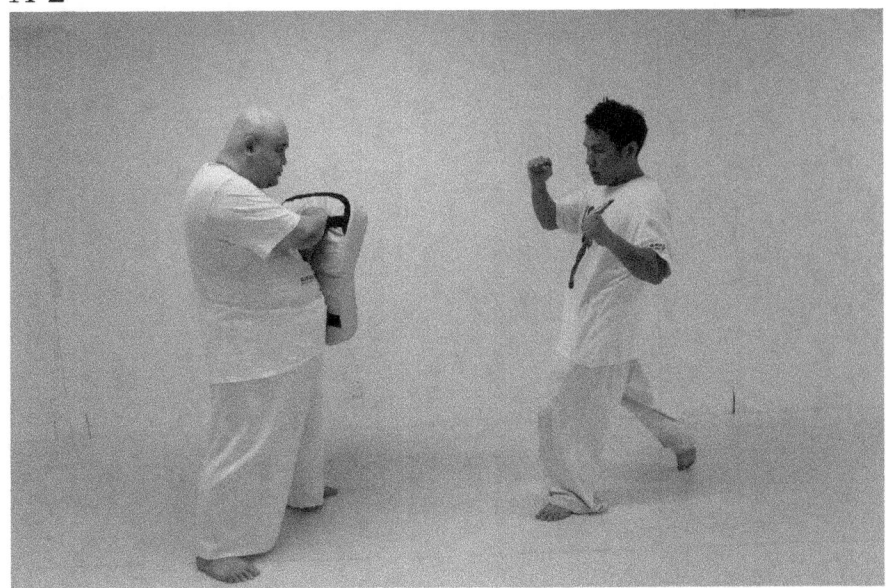

A-3

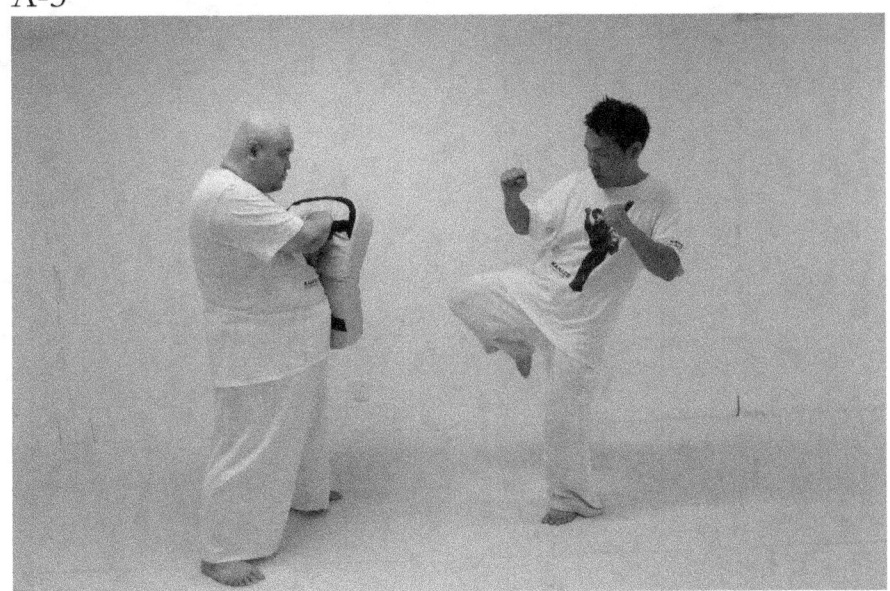

A-4

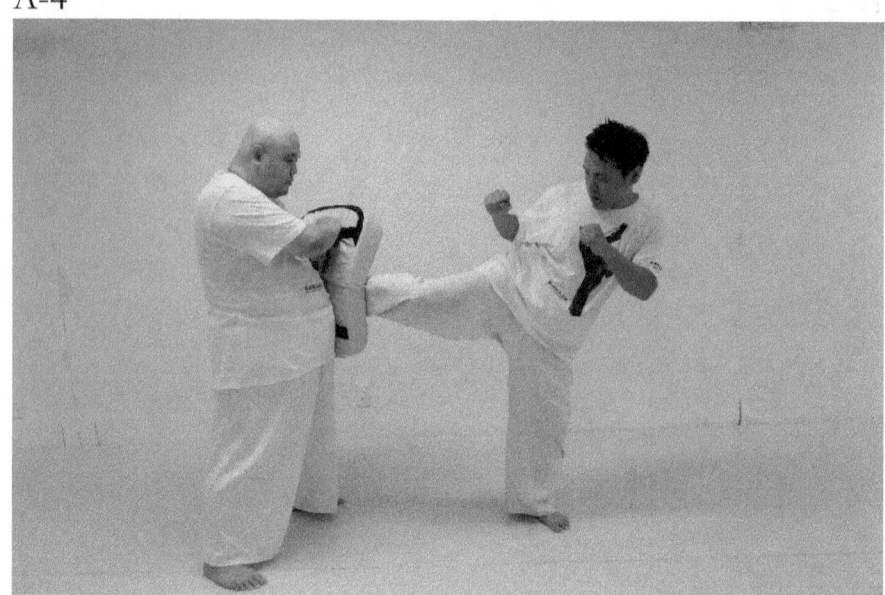

B-1

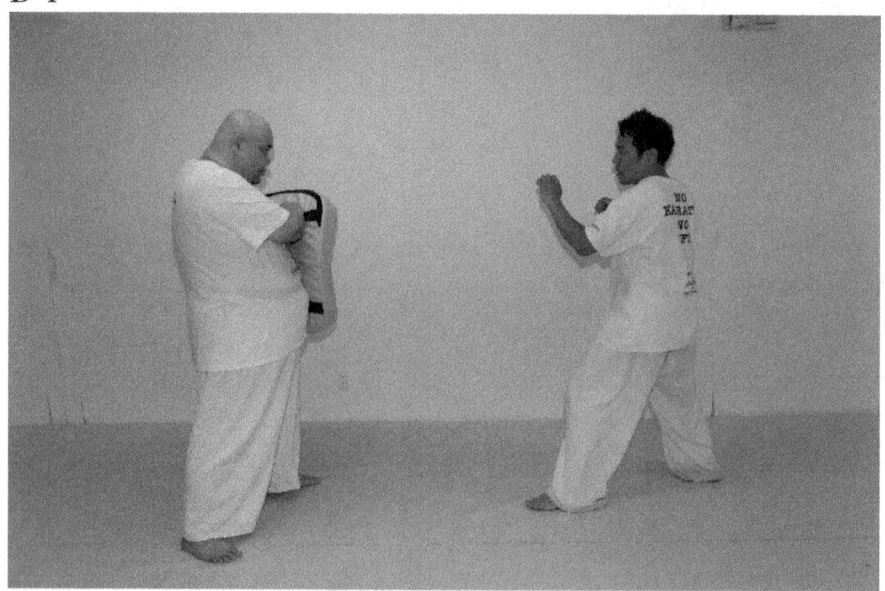

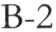
B-2

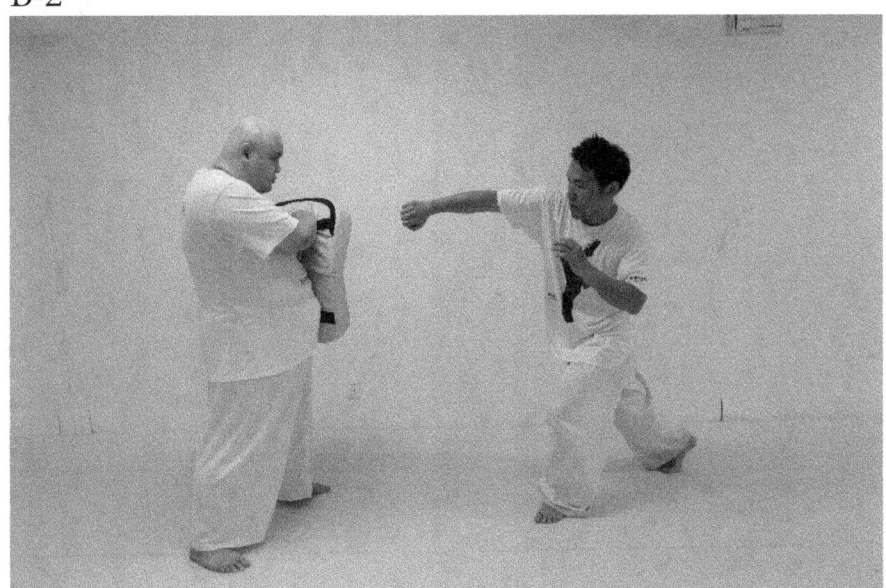

B-3

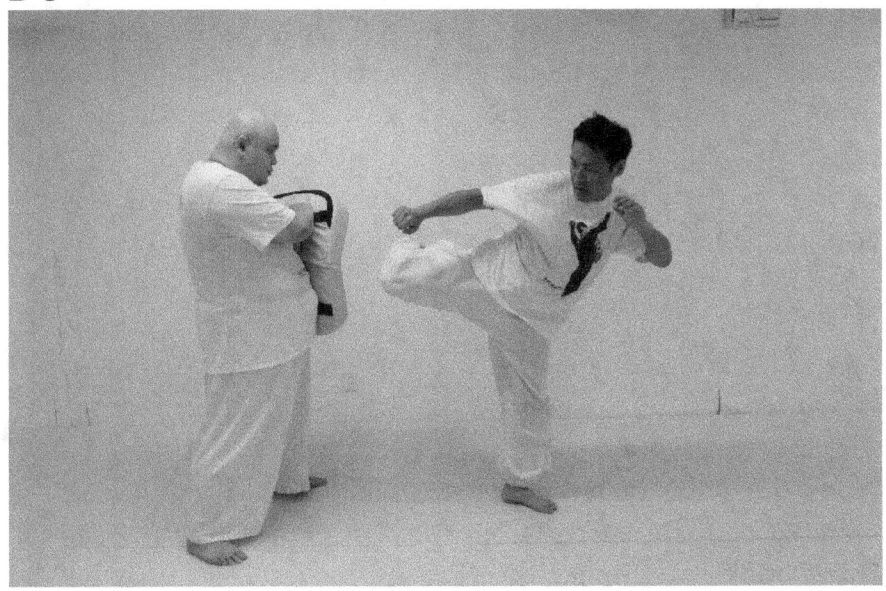

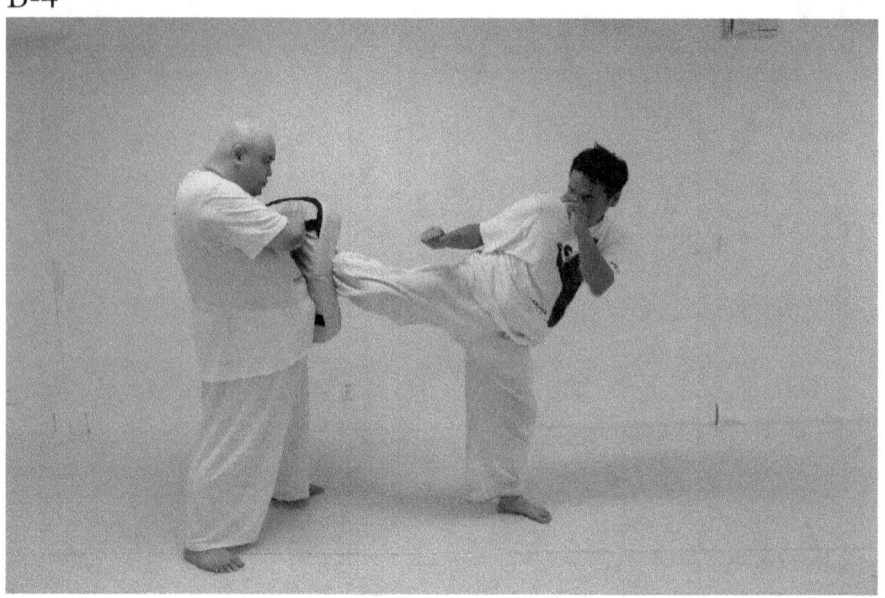

When you kick in style B), the left and right upper limbs extend the muscles necessary for kicking at the next moment, making it easier to realize more speedy and powerful kicking. The same is true for kicking and guarding. Instead of guarding with the arm alone, if you connect the kicking while shifting the position of the scapula forward, a movement of the body that kicks naturally tend to occur is generated. As kicking practice comes in, consciousness tends to go to the lower limbs, but if you review the way you use the upper limbs and the scapula, that alone may increase your power and speed. Analyzing the movements of players who are good at kicking, they move the upper limbs, especially the scapula, sufficiently to connect the flowing kick. When moving the upper limbs left, right, and moving the upper limb in advance as image of the kicking trajectory (if you trace the kicking course to draw with the upper limbs), it will produce impulses to the muscle groups needed for kicking Recalling the image of movement, it will be possible to connect to kicking. Imagining several times to kick once, that attracts the change for the power and speed occur, like from imagining one kick to kick once, to 3 times of imagination of "left → right → kick", and moreover, generating the images 5 times like "eye → cervical spine → left → right → kick" every time you move one part.

【8-8 Evolution and Development】
Primates mainly living on trees, such as gibbons and chimpanzees, will move to swing in the air like "overhead ladder" using the upper limbs rather than the lower limbs to the ability to grip the branches strongly. They are moving with the upper limbs. The anatomical feature of the primate living on these trees is that the spine is close to standing upright to the ground. It is said that the relative muscle mass of the muscle group that moves the scapula of human is more numbered than the type of primate that lives on trees, and is more than four primed locomotive primates.

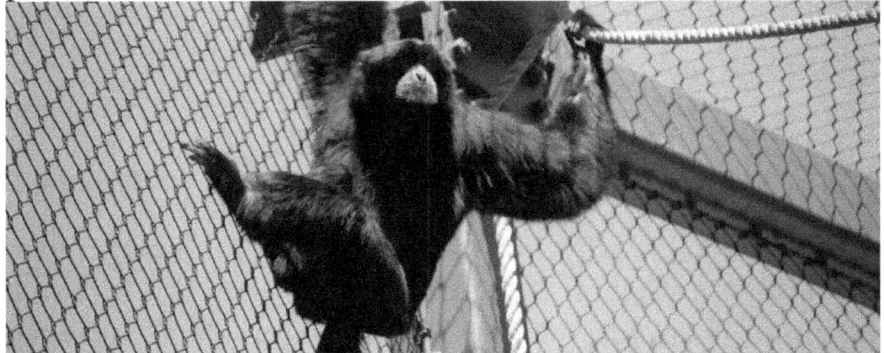

"The muscles associated with our scapula are strong!" This is wasting if you do not use it! Behind the scenes where human beings are able to move with biped walking, as a preliminary step, freedom and muscular strength of the upper limbs including the shoulder blades and the uprightness of the trunk and pelvis are acquired. After that, it is said to have acquired biped walking in the center of the lower limbs. As a remnant, when you walk, when you run, you swing your arms. It is a proof that when it is "On your mark, get set, go!", "Get set" in a footrace on a sports day, the shoulder blades and upper limbs are leading the movement of the shoulder blades and upper limbs to move efficiently as exercising by bringing the arm forward before the shoulder blades forward.

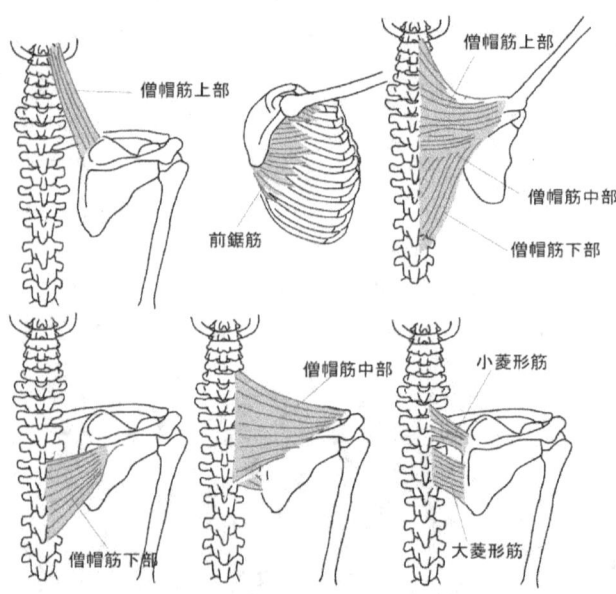

Also, when a baby becomes able to "sit down", then nextly 4-leg walking is completed as "crawl", after the period of "grasping standing", "grasping walking" and then "biped walking" become possible, with the developmental process, the scapula and upper limbs take the steps of "supporting weight" → "lifting up and pulling up" → "supporting with upper limbs" → "become free". Thus, the upper limbs and the scapula have also played an important role in human evolution and development.

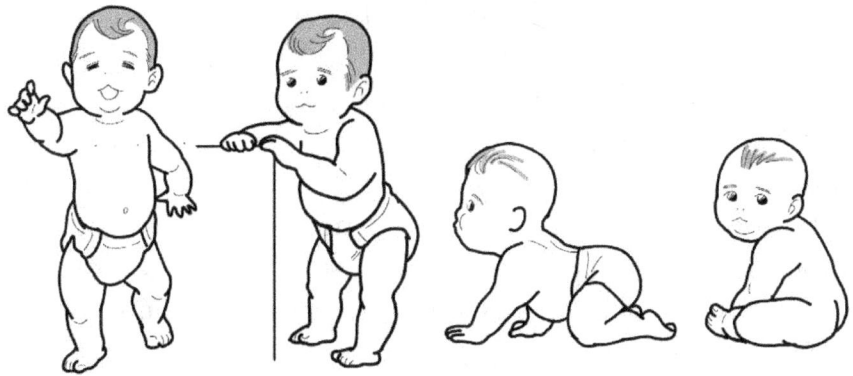

During exercise, the command "move" from the motor cortex of the brain comes out and the time to move is faster than the lower limbs, because the upper limbs are shorter than the lower limbs. As can be seen from the picture of Homunculus mentioned above, when looking at the amount of nerve cells in the brain, the number of nerve cells related to the upper extremities, especially hands is very large. The more you use your hands and fingers, the closer the fingertip nerve cells and brain work, the more brain nerve cells will work. Moving the hands, the upper limbs, that makes the brain gets further activated, making it easier for the target movement to be realized. When the movement is about to stop during a match, it tends to consciously "try not to stop the foot", but if you firmly move the scapula and the upper limb, the lower limb becomes easy to move. It makes weight transfer easier. The condition that the scapula do not move so much because of the strain in the tension, because it can become a factor that hinders the movement of body weight of the whole body, is "dangerous". "If you think that you are not moving during a game, try moving the upper limbs and scapulas anyway" is one of the official formulas that can be used.

Even in boxing and kick boxing that wearing gloves, if you only use rock and paper in the glove, that is a very wasteful story. It is because the exercise is restricted by the glove. How much hands and fingers can move within the constraint of gloves? As you pursue, the movement will definitely change. First-class players are not bound on freedom by gloves, but are freely handling them as effective weapons in battle. Even in judo, jiu-jitsu and mixed martial arts, you can move your scapulas to create a kinetic chain, find a better way to grip, find a way to grasp, make use of stretch reflexes of your fingers, fit joint angles, and more. If you pursue the movements of the scapula and upper limbs, I think that you will find more hints for further leap.

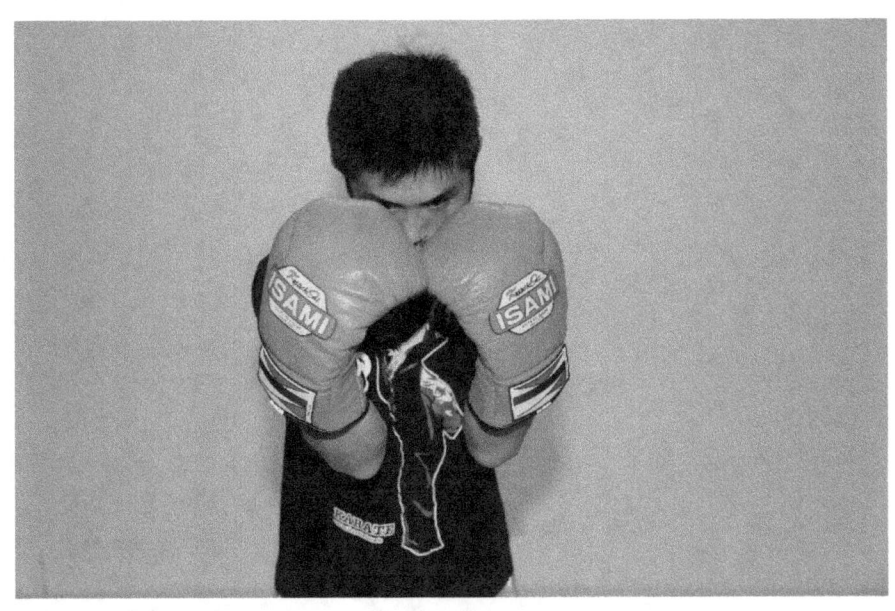

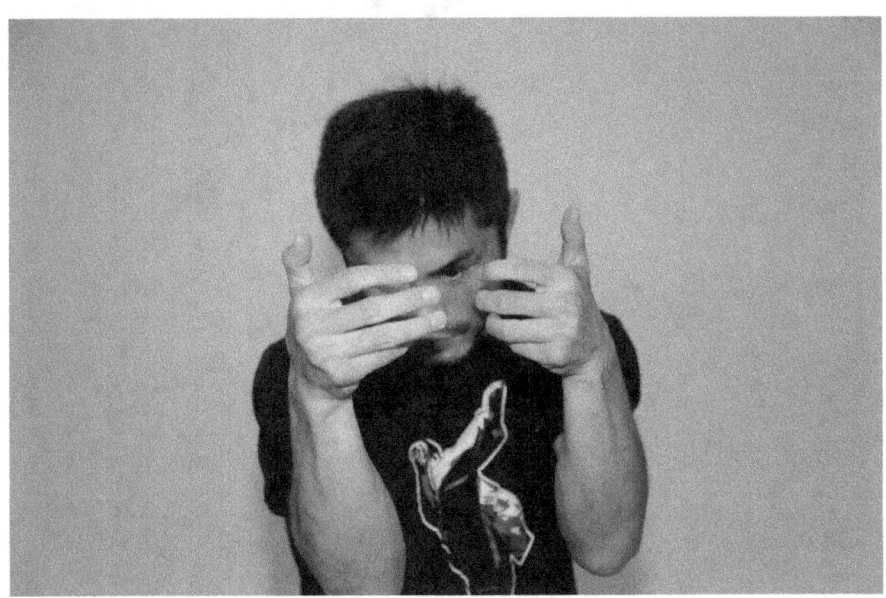

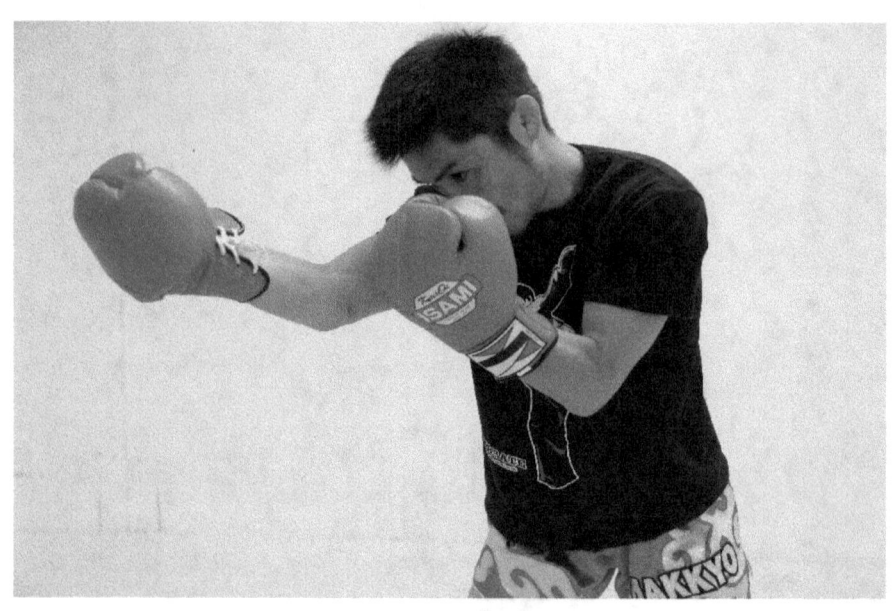

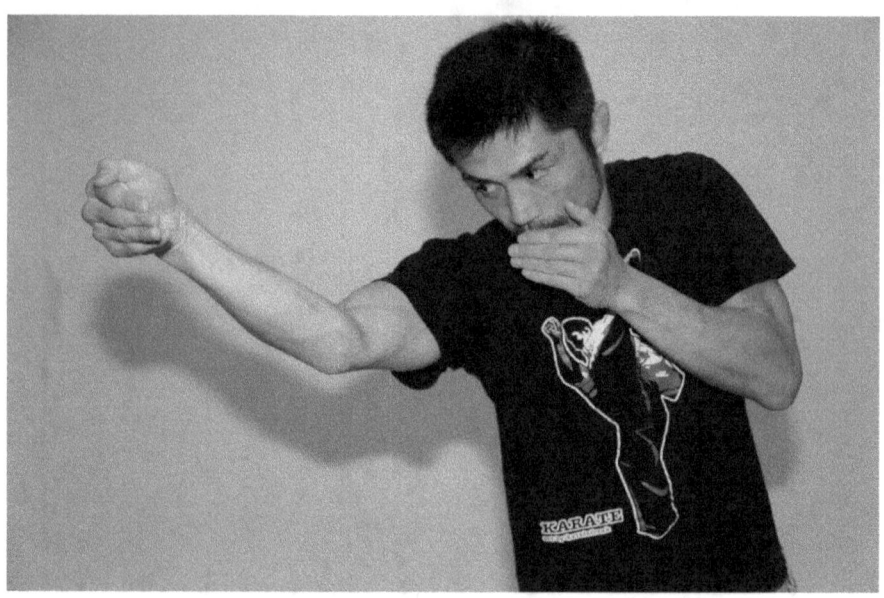

9 Base Of Support & Movement

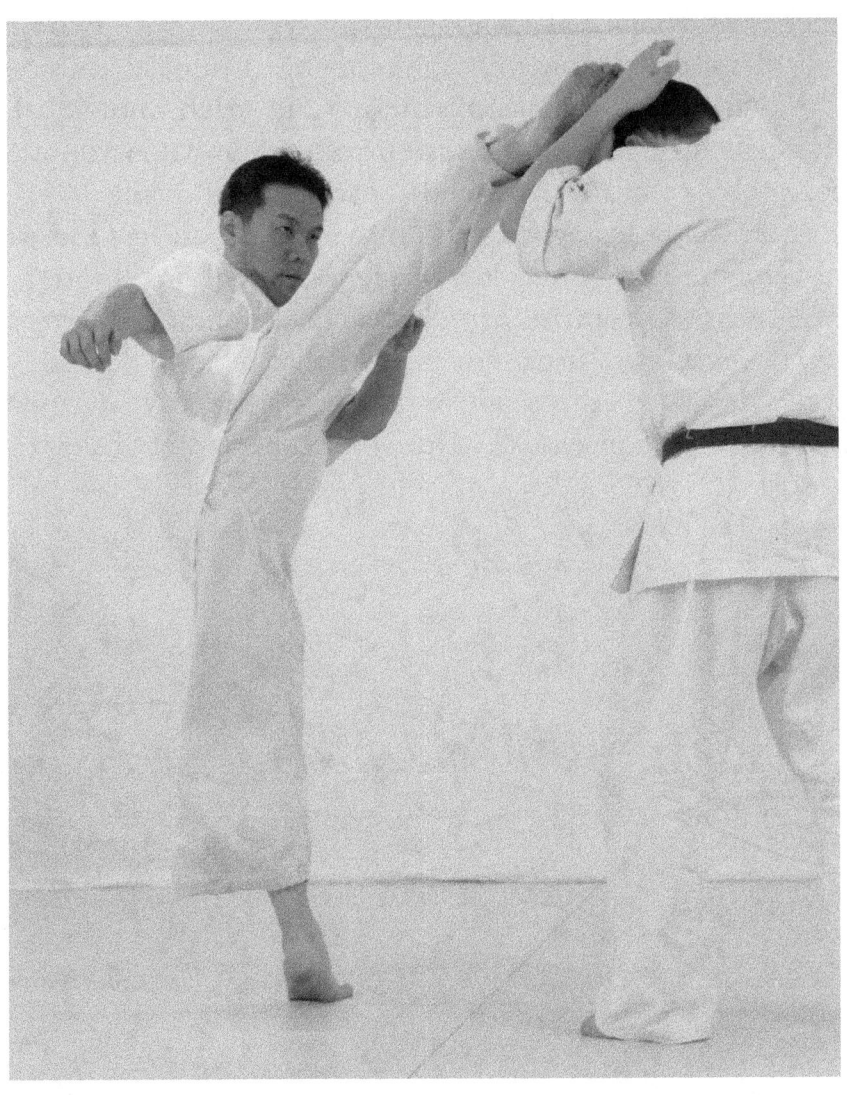

【9-1 What is moving?】

What is the meaning of "moving"? Is to put out many punches and kicks? Tackle aggressively? Using footwork? Controlling the opponent with grappling? I think that there is "moving" in each competition and each individual. "Move" is diverse, each one is correct. Even when you are sleeping, your heart, eyes, and muscles are moving, so it's also one of the categories of "moving". So, what kind of "movement" is required in the scenes of fighting sports / martial arts? Of course it will change depending on rules and conditions, so it cannot be said that what is definitely good. However, there is "a concept that may change movement if conscious". One of them is the base of support.

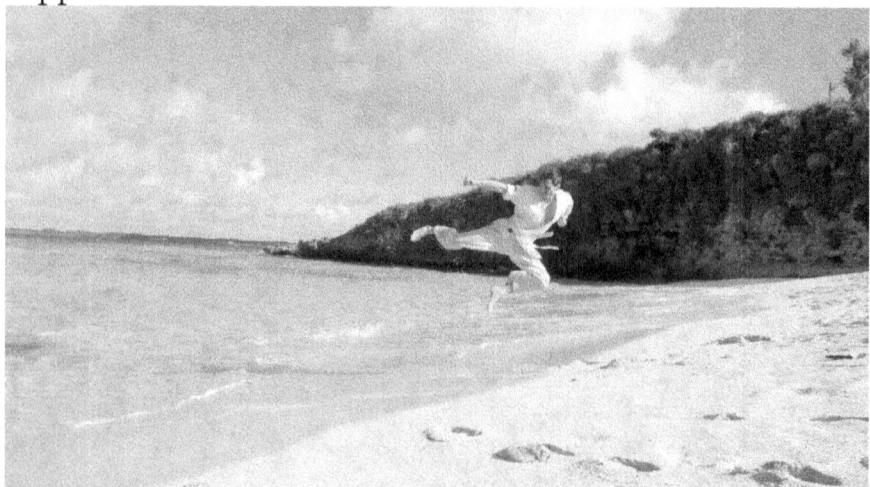

【9-2 What is Base of support?】

Base of support is a term used in rehabilitation medicine, kinematics, etc. It is a range that surrounds the surface that is in contact with the floor, and may be easy to understand if you think of it as the area of the surface that supports the body. When standing with two legs, the range that connects the outside including both feet soles is the base of surface. When standing on one foot, the ground touching area of the sole of the foot becomes the supporting base plane. When standing with two legs and one cane, the range formed by the outside of both feet and the cane is the base of support. If you sit on the floor grasping your knees, the area that connects the outside of the buttocks and the bottom of the sole, if you lie on the floor with face up, if the range that connects the outside of the ground touching area on the back side, stand with 4 legs, And the area connecting the outside of the ground plane of both lower limbs, are the base of support.

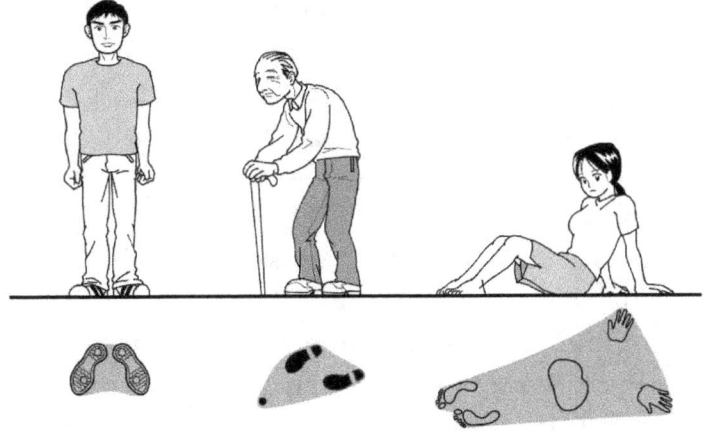

The wider the base of support, the more stable it becomes. Rather the moment when planting yourself than the moment you are running, even more when sitting, become smaller risk to lose balance and fall. Conversely, "being able to move stably even with a small supporting base surface" means, matching high level as exercise, and high exercise capacity.

When a football player shoots, when grasping the ground with a shaft foot, the base of support is a part of the contact area of the shaft foot. When a figure skate athlete is turning at high speed with one foot, the base of support is only a small point. "It is not possible to walk without the use of a cane" and "you can walk without using a cane" is clearly the state that the latter is "movable", the direction "move steadily while reducing the base of support" direction will lead to better performance.

From the viewpoint of base of support, movements such as walking and running are performed most of the time with one foot ground. When the walking person stops, both feet are installed, the base of support becomes large, and when you sit there, the base of support gets even bigger, and when it is lying it gets even bigger.

When observing the movements of top fighters well, there are few scenes that they are always standing with both feet during the match. Always at least one of the feet is away from the ground, and the base of support changes instantaneously. Also, looking at strong fighters such as mixed martial arts, jiu-jitsu and judo, they are not stopped. Even at grappling, they continue to move while changing the ground plane frequently. When you recapture the event of "moving" in the scene of fighting sports and martial arts as "to keep changing the base of support", you can see whether it is moving or not.

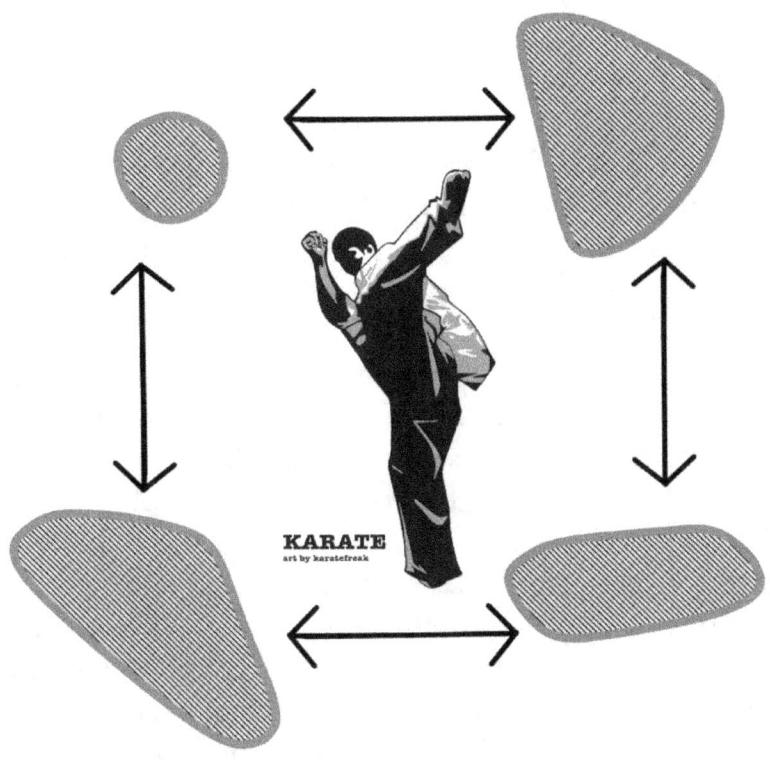

(First-class fighter changes)

【9-3 The number of strikes/trial and error】
We will introduce cases where movement is improved by changing the base of support. In boxing and karate, the offensive point is often added to the judgment when KO cannot win the game. Is it evaluated by judgment which one actively attacked? In that case, it becomes an important factor whether or not to get the number of strikes. When I was a competitor, in order to practice to get the number of

steps, I planted both feet and repeated punches with heavy iron arrays on both hands and repeated training to increase the numbers. As a result, the number of strikes when there was a stamina came out. However, it did not change very much when entering an extra round, extra-extra-round.

Techniques for changing the base of support will become very effective in order to be able to get the number of steps and become a fighter who can be hit repeatedly. Let's move from the orthodox stance to the ground, alternately touch the ground with the back foot and the front foot. Then, can you tell that when the right fist displaces the forefoot away from the ground, and the left fist displaces slightly forward when the back foot is separated from the ground? Just by changing the base of support back and forth, the position of the fist changes from the original place.

The fighters who can hit repeatedly, this method is applied to their punches. When you try to move the fist by stepping on both feet, the muscles to move the fist exhausted, but stopping on both feet, standing on one foot, one foot moves the fist from its original position. It uses the displacement as it is and leads to the number of steps. This movement is common to the positional relationship between the base of support and the upper limb, which is seen when dashing on the spot, and it is easy to move without difficulty.

The exercise menu I used to do was to plant the feet and put out the hands. In the process, it was fine if I could realize myself for an unreasonable movement and be able to improve it, but the time I found how to hit a stroke accompanying the change of the base of support was much later, at the time when I watched a video of a genius boxer. With that boxer, Manny Pacquiao. Brilliant achievements of the champion of the major world title in 6 divisions as well as he is a hero of the world that Asia gave birth to a Philippine parliamentarian member, as an actor, and as an active fighter. His shadow boxing training was always in a move, including the lower limbs, the whole body was moving, stopping the feet and putting out only the fists didn't exist.

When finding a secret part of the super high-level number of strikes to the flowing shadow boxing image in which the rotation speed of the punch and the change of the base of support matches spectacularly, the number of steps is controlled by the change of the base of support, I found what I could do and I was impressed.

As a result, it's not wrong to say that I was doing "wrong training" or "useless training", but learning the right training from the beginning, and hypothesising to try and do, are not the same. Without the accumulation of wrong training, there is no discovery or impression there, and it is said that the nerve cells in the brain will be activated at the moment when the exclamation mark turns on like "!!!". In the first place, both the human body and the brain change more and more. So, the necessary training will change as well. As with role playing games such as Dragon Quest and Final Fantasy, choices, priorities, necessary times, paths of getting stronger. I think that "trial and error" is the essence of becoming strong. Sometimes it is necessary to avoid "mistakes" and "waste" as much as possible, sometimes it is necessary to seek efficiency, but also when we need to jump into the ocean of "mistakes" "waste" and seek out better movements out of them is necessary sometimes. There is not only one way to climb a mountain to get stronger. Individuality comes out in the way of climbing. The important thing is a cycle of trial →

verification → improvement → trial. I think that it is important to listen to your body.

However, severe injuries and unrecoverable accidents, irreversible damage such as eyes and brain, which threaten the athletes' life and instructor life, should be avoided as much as possible. Light injuries are also "signs that must change something," and it is sad that they cannot do the "trial and error" themselves.

Pushing arms

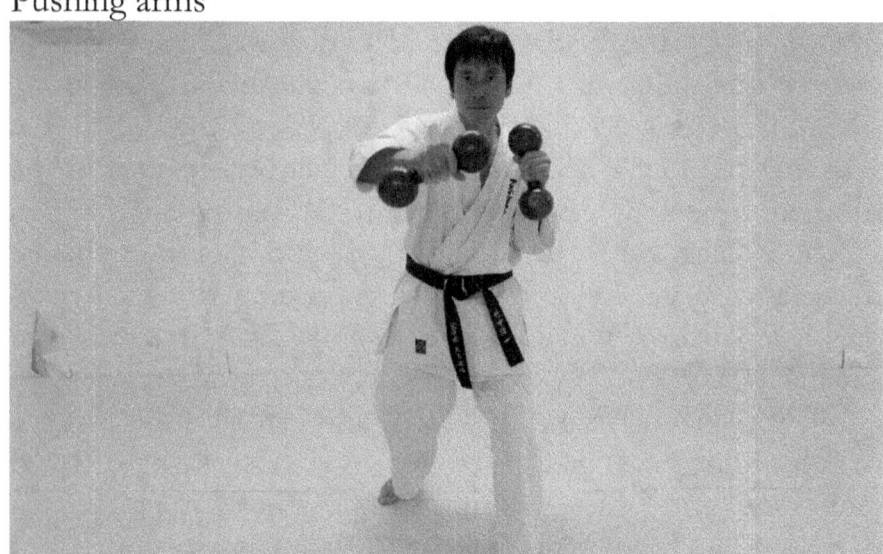

Changing base of support

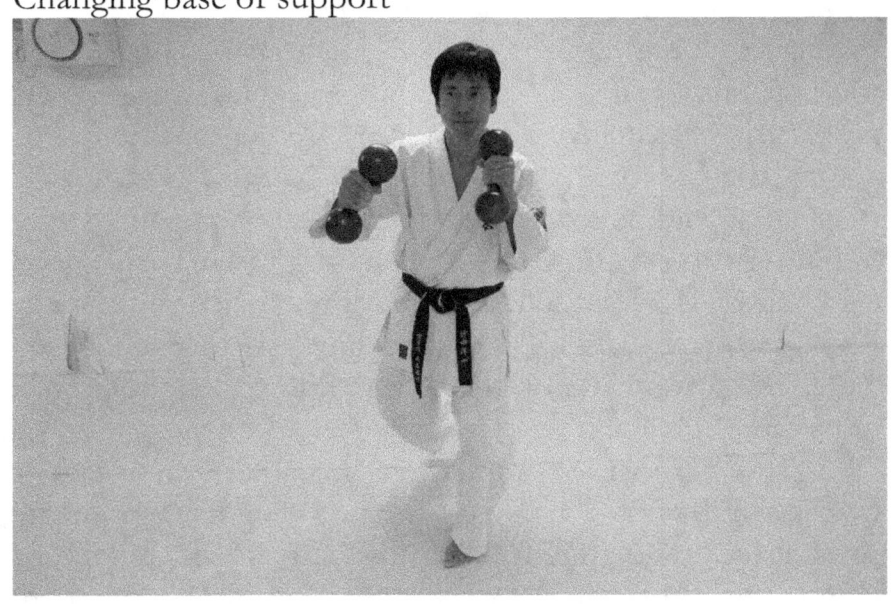

ways

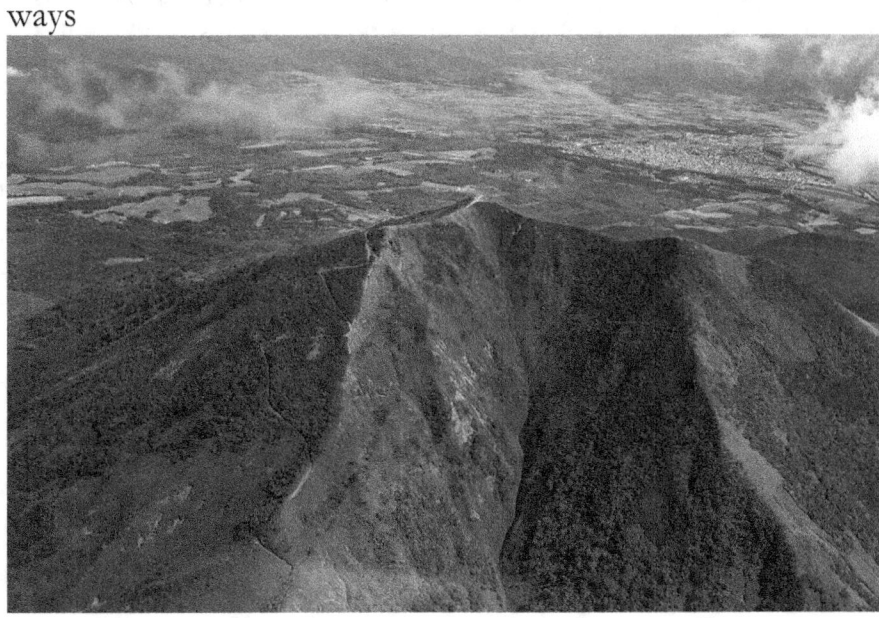

【9-4 Test to know your own movement】

Analysis of the movement of the fighters who said, "I'm good at mitts and sandbags, but I cannot move as I expected, in matches or sparring", "When the habit of putting the base with the supporting base on both feet is attached" could be seen many times. Even taking a position with footwork in football, the person himself has noticed the habit of striking the feet on both feet when putting out a skill, hitting, poking, kicking, tackling, and throwing from there. Because it is not there, the flow of motion once stops there.

For the purpose of improving this, there is one foot sparring in the practice menu for controlling the supporting base surface. We conduct sparring with a high degree of safety like light touch, with only one foot grounded. "Either right, left, please ground only one foot, OK, simultaneous grounding of both feet prohibited" will be performed. If you set this condition and test it, you will feel difficulty in movement if you are in the habit of "There is no skill if the base of support does not become both feet at once". By doing the appropriate skill of the technique at that time, by optimizing the base of support of the step, "ability to move even on the small base of support", "defense capability using control of the base of support" "escape of damage when you receive it hints on how to use various bodies such as "How to use" will be obtained.

Single leg kickboxing sparring

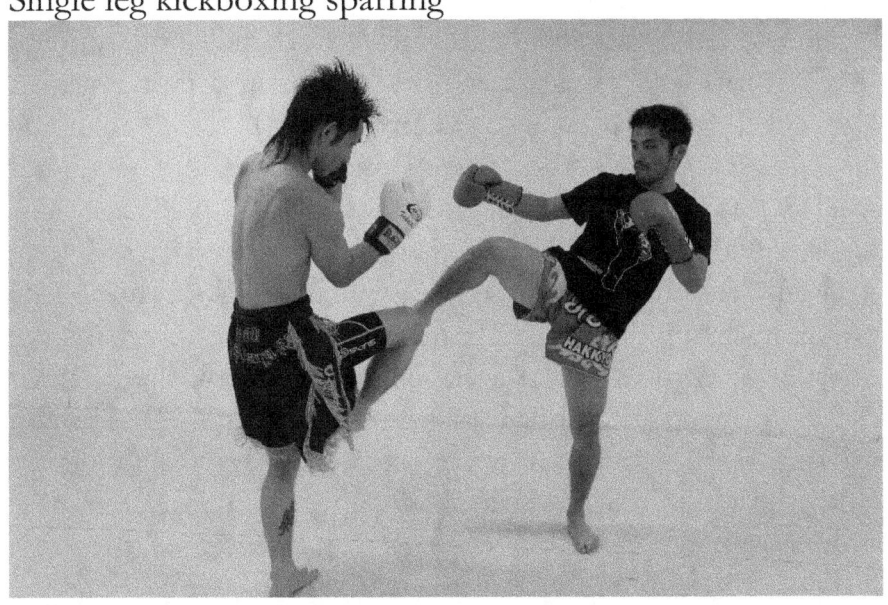

Single leg karate sparring

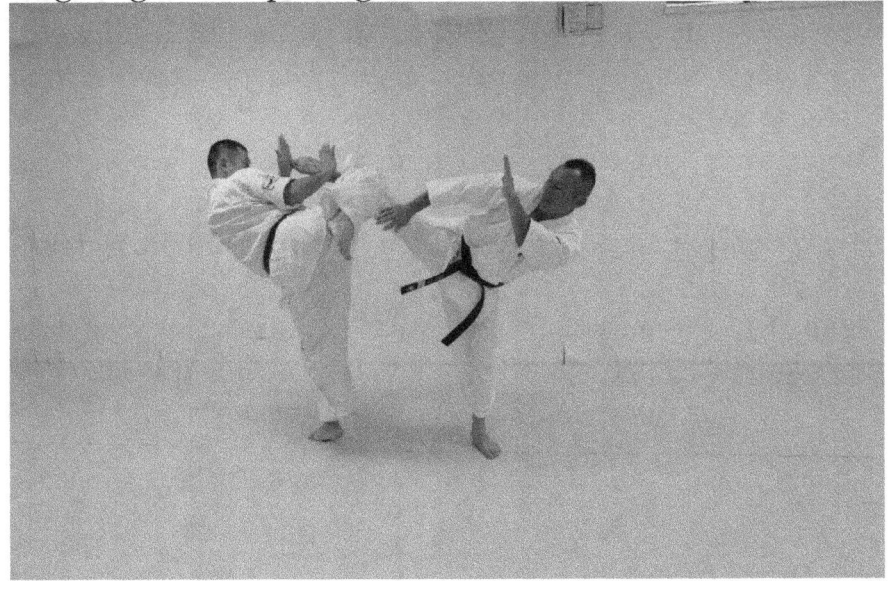

In the dojo and gym, you may be instructed to "stably balance on the feet and stably with both feet and put out skills from there". Of course, that is an important practice. However, to further aim from there, I think that the direction to control the base of support leads to a higher level of movement. In the first place, human walking walks while breaking the balance. When moving forward, one foot comes out in front. Its feet touch the floor, apply the brake, and function as shaft feet. In the next moment, the other foot comes forward, so walking is established, and if you do not put the other foot forward, you will fall. Human walking is the most energy efficient in animals living on land, the ability to travel long distances is hardly fatigued, even compared to other animals. The secret of the high walking ability is the technique of "walking while breaking the balance". So, "Keeping a stable balance with both feet and putting out skills" "While breaking the balance, I value where to put the next step, putting out the skills and stabilizing" is a big difference even they look the same at first glance.

People who can move with one foot on the ground can move with no problem even if both feet are grounded, and if external force is applied to the opponent, movements such as one foot → both feet, or widening the foot width, hands if it is a grappling, " You can stabilize it by using the technique of widening the base of support in a moment ".

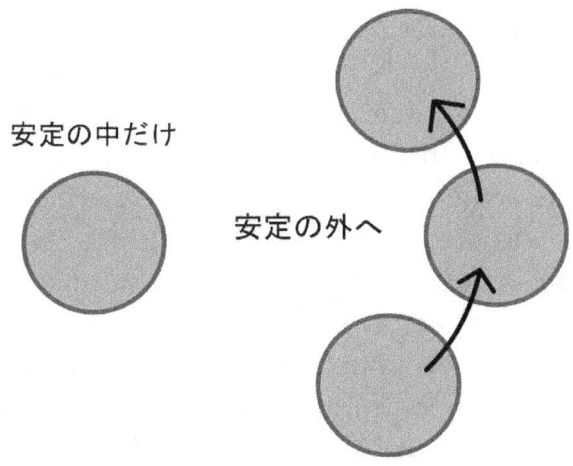

安定の中だけ

安定の外へ

【9-5 Mankind's "moving" fate】

The Japanese characters "動(move)" is a combination of "重力(gravity)-consists from 2 character combined". It will be "移動" only after 移(shifting) 重力(gravity), and "運動 (exercise)" to 運(carry) 重力(gravity) well. It is "活動 (activity)" that utilizes gravity.

If the supporting base surface is the base of support, it connects that, keep changing the base of support = keep moving. The history of mankind is also the history of movement. The ancestry of human beings born on the African continent is supposed to have traveled to the southern tip of South America, which is 50,000 km away. Humanity do not move to one place to install but has moved to search for a better environment. In premodern times and modern times, we have developed transportation network and expanded the range of movement to the sea, the sky, and the outer space as well as land movement.

Why have human beings expanded the scope of their activities to that extent? One of the reasons is the characteristics of the brain. The brain has developed with new stimuli. When you move, the environment changes, everything you see, listen, what you touch, what you feel, what you feel, the space of your life, the image that comes from it ... everything is a new stimulus. Even though the baby cannot do so much, it opens a big eyes for new information and open minded to sensory inputs. It is never closed. By growing up and becoming able to ride a tricycle, when you learned the pleasure of moving by moving by yourself, you can move far away with your own will on a bicycle, you can feel it enter "freedom" together with information input. Conversely, it is said that solitary confinement in prison is the most painful because new information is blocked at all. The brain cannot bear no stimulation. Therefore, it will create a hallucination and a vision and help the brain.

"Move" → "A new stimulus is input" → "An image advanced by memory is created" → "Further moving and heading for a new stimulus"

In such a loop, the brain and the body mutually act while growing. Those who conspicuously and closing more than people who are progressing more steadily with open minds and who are moving and creating environments shine sparklingly, maybe that is appealing to themselves also make mankind fateful "to move" Fighting sports and martial arts competitions are the battle of "whether you can move or not". At the same time, it is also a battle of "to let the opponent cannot move" KO settlement is the best example of it, and suppression of judo is "the side unable to move, loses". To be thrown by the opponent is that you cannot make gravity on your side, it will damage yourself, and the joint lock gets you at the moment when you stop moving. (We can say that there is nothing to be locked if you continue to move.) "I do not move" has a right meaning, but if "I cannot move", then I cannot win. The fighting sports and martial arts competitions have aspects that manifest themselves in the interpersonal 'movement' which is the characteristic of mankind.

When I was a high school student, Master Katsuou Yamamoto, the founder of combat karate Yoshukai Karate which I was a member. He instructed me, "People who line up at the first of the lines of alignment, people who go to take the mitt fastest, people who intend to draw water into the bucket for the first time at the time of cleaning will be stronger". At that time, it was young so I arbitrary interpreted it as "to win the first place is important", but as I get older, not only in fighting sports and martial arts, but also in various scenes and phases, realize the importance of "move" everyday. And I think that it would be nice if I could become a person who could move, through "moving my body". Since the movement of fighting sports / martial arts is fluid, it is not easy to objectively evaluate it, but I'm pleased if I could help you visualizing and imaging even in practice scenes with the introduction of "new ruler" called the base of support.

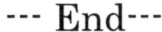

--- End---

Recommendation

UFC fighter, Kiichi Kunimoto

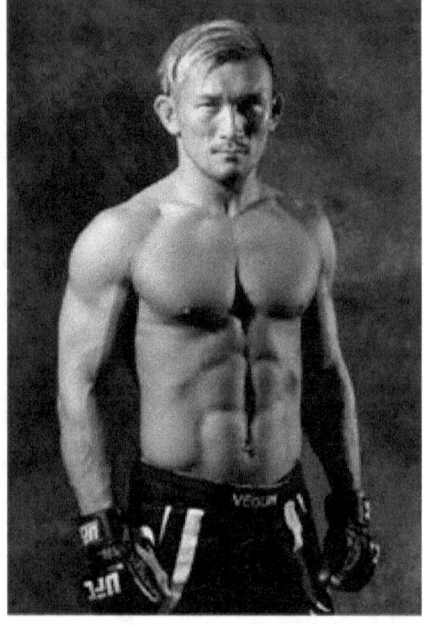

The time I first met Dr. Futaesaku was not much later than I became a professional fighter. I placed my base in Tokyo, and learnt a lot of how to use the body and brain, as well as techniques and the image trainings. Every single time I had an inspiration and could meet a new myself. We made our goals. Me as "Fighting in the best qualified arena called UFC", Dr.F as "Spread the Fighting Medicine to the world wide" Had been cooperating each other and working hard on each side throughly. and with a luck, my debut came true in January 2014. 3 wins straight. I have since been feeling my improvement. If you have a will of wanting to be stronger even a tiny bit more than now, I strongly, fully recommend this

100 men fights achiever, Karate legend Kancho Ademir Da Costa

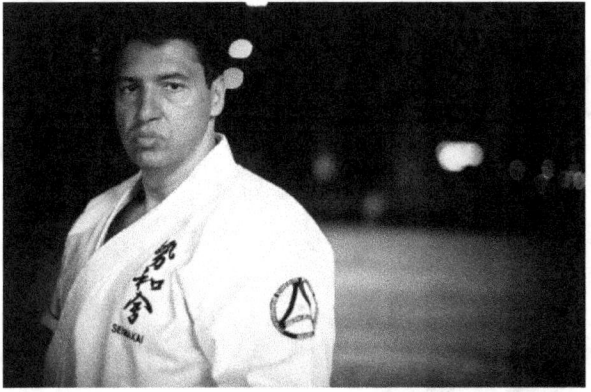

I congratulate Dr. F for his incredible work for the health of the practitioners of the martial arts. His scientific research about the best way to prevent injuries in hard training - which the athletes are submitted - and the correct way to practice some techniques, will help both professional fighters as the beginners, to have health and quality of live. I suffered many injuries caused by the hard trainings without any scientific orientation. Now, with the research of Dr.F, the new generation of practitioners of martial arts will have a correct orientation to practice the martial arts with a healthy way. My sincere thanks for this as important work for the martial art and budo. Osu!

Kyokushin WKB CEO, Kancho Pedro Roiz

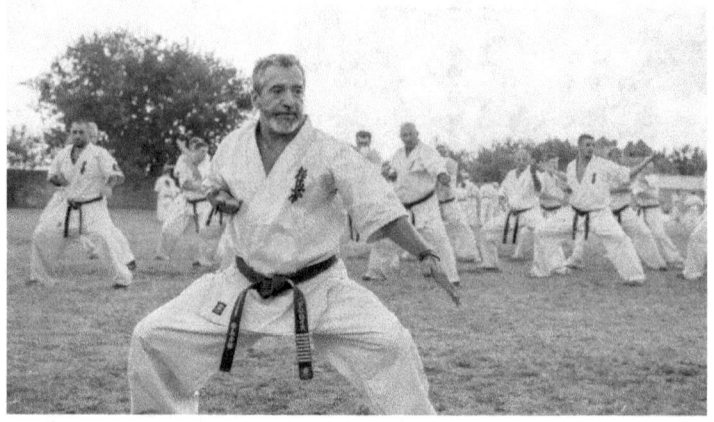

This book has been well received within the martial arts community and I especially cannot recommend this amazingly well researched and well written book enough. Fightology is possibly the best scientifically written martial arts book to be published. Reading this book will open new doors to the execution of techniques and will give a better understanding of our Martial Arts. Through its pages we will get a better work foundation to achieve greater results in our athletes and, furthermore, a better understanding of how the internal energy works. This exquisite book is the result of years of exhaustive work, carried out by the preparation and the scientific rigor of a doctor, combined with the first-hand experiences of a martial artist. Dr.F is a lover of these arts, and his insatiable hunger for researching allowed him to contact some of the most reputed teachers, with whom he has worked extensively in the study of body motion. He is not just a scientist with sufficient basic knowledge of anatomy, physiology... to carry out this deepening task. He is also "one of us", able to address this study from our perspective, from the knowledge of a martial artist. And this is what makes the analysis much more adjusted to our demand. From these lines and from the great affection I have for him, I would like to express my appreciation and admiration for this great work, wishing Dr.F all the success he deserves, and hoping that he always keeps that clean gesture on his face.

MMA legend &
Arm wrestling World Champ
Gary Goodridge

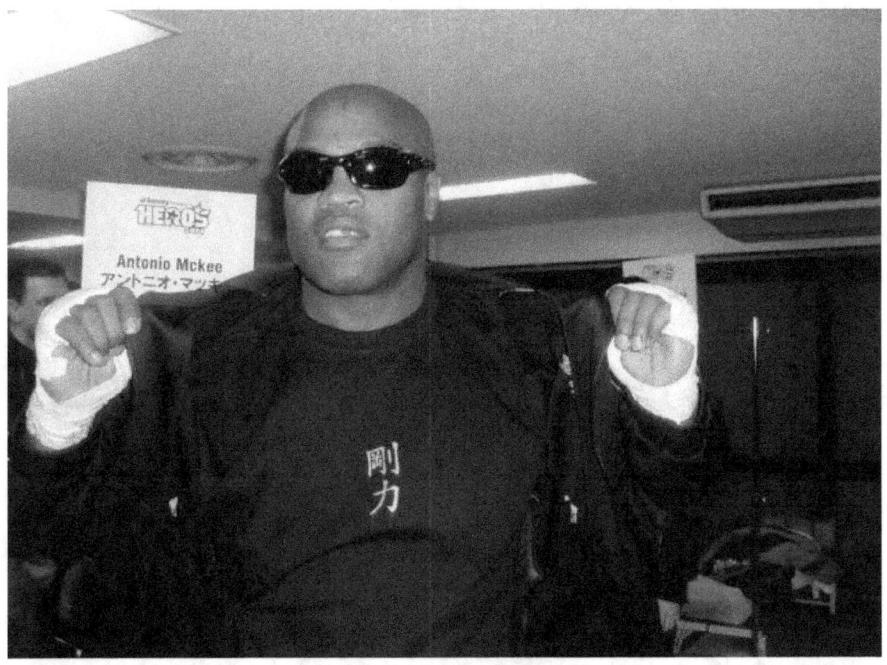

Dr.F was my team doctor as I was a professional fighter for a few years. Worked my corner on several different occasions. I am sure he will be more then competent to do any job as helping out in MMA or any fighting organizations.

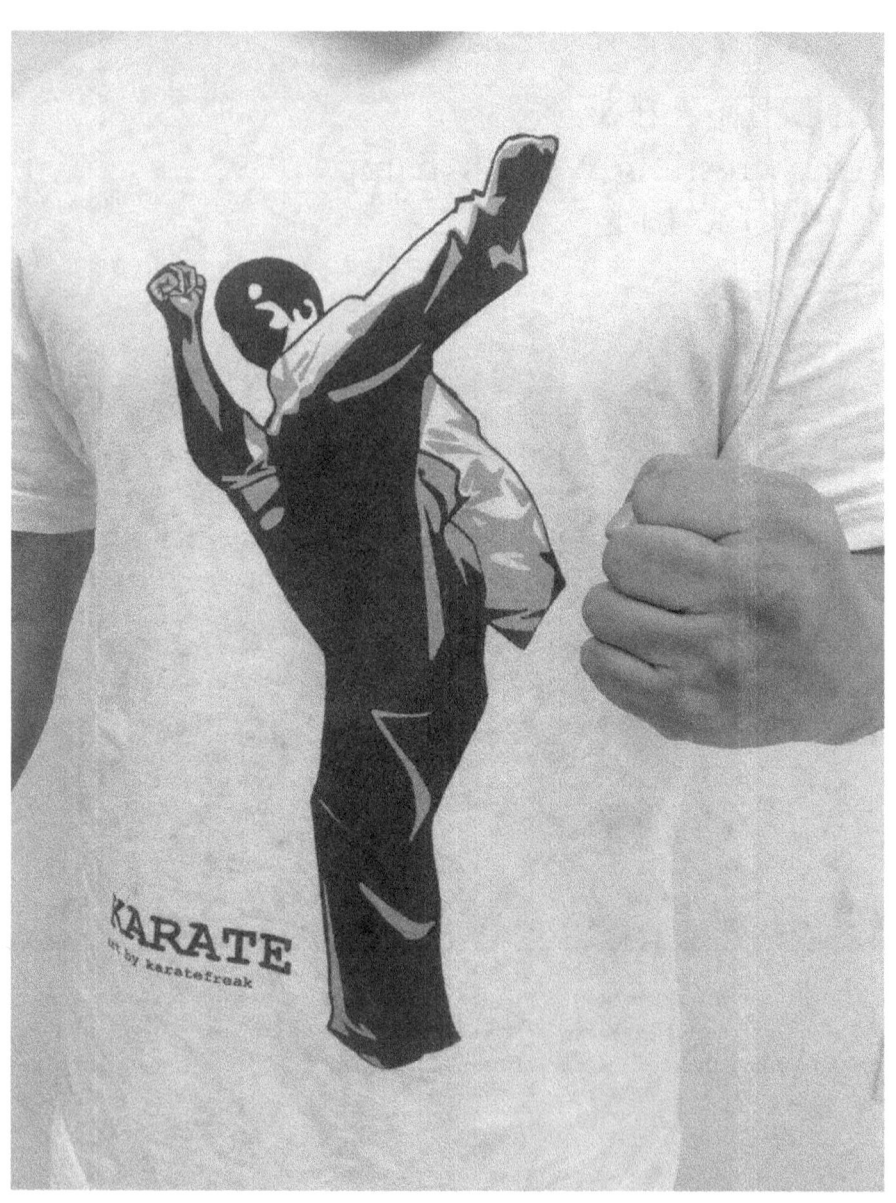

Takuya Futaesaku (a.k.a "Dr.F")

is a Sports Medicine Doctor from Japan famous for his work in supporting many professional fighting sports athletes from Karate, Muay Thai / Kickboxing, and MMA. Dr.F developed a strong interest in the martial arts since he was a child. He initially began training in full-contact Karate and became a Karate instructor during his high school years. While studying at Kochi Medical School (Kochi University), his enthusiasm for fighting sports led him to apply his medical knowledge (such as anatomy, kinetics, kinesiology, etc.), using the term - "Fightology" to encompass his medical research on Fighting sports. His medical science approach in fighting sports is a very new and exciting concept, with his work attracting attention from martial arts enthusiasts around the world. His "Fightology" seminars, which have been held in Australia, Spain, Chile, Costa Rica, Hong Kong, and Paris have been very popular and in turn recognizing Dr. F as a true innovator in fighting sports. Aside from his "Fightology" seminars, Dr.F is also a famous contributor for various Japanese sport magazines such as Ironman magazine, Full Contact Karate, Coaching Clinic and more recently Fight and Life magazine. He is also the author of "Fighting Sports for Juniors", "Medical Science Of Fighting Sports" "Self improving Training learning from Top Fighters" and the DVD producer of "The Anatomy of Knockout Vol1&2", and "The Kinematics of Fighting Sports Vol.1 to 7" - all of his works are ranked 5 stars on Amazon Japan. Today, Dr.F continues to develop "Fightology" with medical knowledge, research, and passion. He is looking forward to raising the level for combat sports enthusiasts all around the world. He is also recognized as music tour doctor, Supporting Prince family, George Clinton &P-funk, Tower Of Power, Candy Dulfer, John Blackwell and more top artists. His book about Prince, Words Of Prince" got no.1 best seller in soul music, amazon USA.

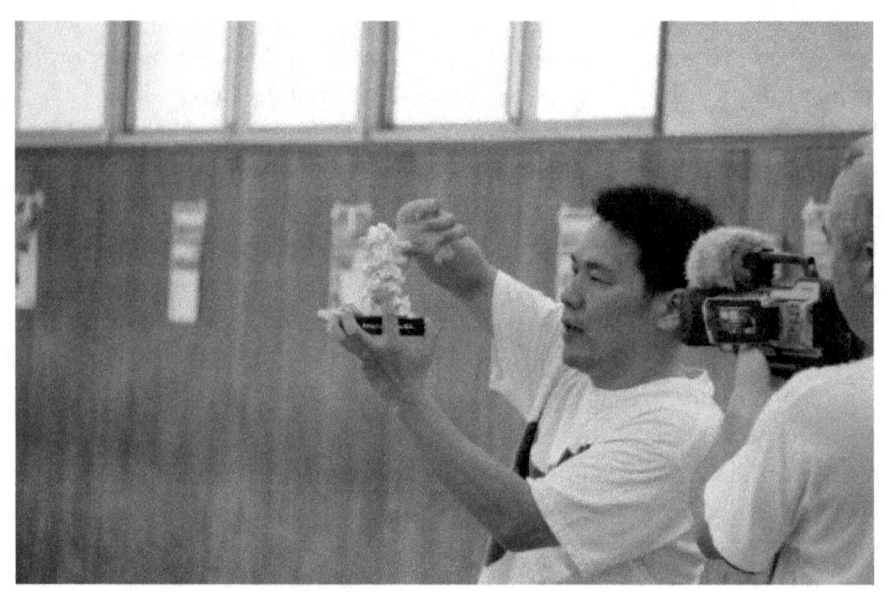

＜Contact & Booking＞

No Karate No Life official page
https://www.facebook.com/nokaratenolife

Facebook
https://www.facebook.com/takuya.futaesaku

Instagram
https://www.instagram.com/takuyafutaesaku/

ありがとうございました。
Thank you very much

押忍
Dr. F

June 7 2018